Augmentative and Alternative Communication
in Acute and Critical Care Settings

Augmentative and Alternative Communication
in Acute and Critical Care Settings

Richard R. Hurtig
Debora A. Downey

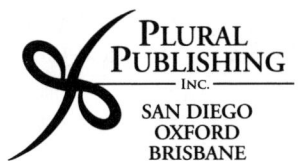

SAN DIEGO
OXFORD
BRISBANE

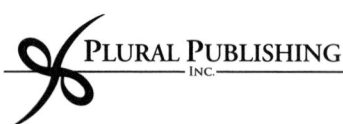

5521 Ruffin Road
San Diego, CA 92123

e-mail: info@pluralpublishing.com
Web site: http://www.pluralpublishing.com

49 Bath Street
Abingdon, Oxfordshire OX14 1EA
United Kingdom

Copyright © by Plural Publishing, Inc. 2009

Typeset in 10½/11 Garamond by Flanagan's Publishing Services, Inc.
Printed in the United States of America by McNaughton and Gunn, Inc

All rights, including that of translation, reserved. No part of this publication may be reproduced, stored in a retrieval system, or transmitted in any form or by any means, electronic, mechanical, recording, or otherwise, including photocopying, recording, taping, Web distribution, or information storage and retrieval systems without the prior written consent of the publisher.

For permission to use material from this text, contact us by
Telephone: (866) 758-7251
Fax: (888) 758-7255
e-mail: permissions@pluralpublishing.com

Every attempt has been made to contact the copyright holders for material originally printed in another source. If any have been inadvertently overlooked, the publishers will gladly make the necessary arrangements at the first opportunity.

Library of Congress Cataloging-in-Publication Data:

Hurtig, Richard.
  Augmentative and alternative communication in acute and critical care settings / Richard Hurtig and Debora Downey.
       p. ; cm.
  Includes bibliographical references and index.
  ISBN-13: 978-1-59756-079-5 (alk. paper)
  ISBN-10: 1-59756-079-0 (alk. paper)
  1. University of Iowa. Hospitals and Clinics. 2. People with disabilities—Means of communication. 3. Communication devices for people with disabilities. 4. Critical care medicine. I. Downey, Debora. II. Title.
  [DNLM: 1. University of Iowa. Hospitals and Clinics. 2. Communication Aids for Disabled. 3. Communication Barriers. 4. Critical Care—methods. 5. Intensive Care Units. WL 340.2 H967a 2008]
  RC423.H863 2008
  616.85'503—dc22
                                                                                    2008035843

Contents

Preface ix
Acknowledgments xiv

1 History of AAC 1
   Defining AAC 2
   A Brief History of AAC 3
   How Technology Has Impacted AAC 6
   Etiologies That May Benefit from AAC 11
   ASHA's Stand on AAC 12

2 Challenges 15
   Access Challenges 16
   Opportunity Challenges 17

3 The Impact of Assistive Technology (AT) in Acute Care Settings 21
   Review of AAC in Acute Care Settings 25

4 Assessment Protocol 29
   Videos for This Chapter 35

5 Switches as the First Step to Establishing Communication 37
   Nurse Call Systems: Alternatives and Modifications 42
   Standard Switches 47
   Advanced Technology Switches 49
   Iowa Smart Switch 57

6 Iowa AAC Templates 59
   One Button Template 60
   Two-Three Button Templates 61
   Grid-Pattern Button Templates 62
   Simple Buttons with Links Template 62
   The Iowa Template 66
      Top Level Menu Page 66
      Feelings Pop-Up Page 68
      Pain Pop-Up Page 69
      Entertainment Pop-Up Page 69

v

	Chat Menu Page	71
	Medical Questions Pop-Up	71
	Jokes Pop-Up	72
	Room-Control ECU Pop-Up	72
	Bed Control Pop-Up	74
	TV Control Pop-Up	74
	Help Pop-Up	75
	Personal Pop-Up	77
	Novel Message Generation	79
	Rate Enhancement Strategies	81
	Videos Associated with This Chapter	88
7	**Mounting and Access Issues**	**89**
	Device Mounting Solutions	90
	Hand-Held Implementations	91
	Bed Tray Implementations	91
	Bed Rail Implementations	96
	IV Pole Implementations	98
	Switch Adaptation and Mounting Solutions	102
	Adapting Switches	103
	Mounting Strategies	103
	Videos Associated with This Chapter	124
8	**Pain Management**	**125**
9	**Environmental Control Units (ECUs)**	**127**
10	**Bad News—Communication Issues**	**133**
11	**Cases**	**141**
	A. Solving the Language Barrier	141
	B. Maintaining a Personal Voice—Adding Humor	147
	C. Don't Assume Full Understanding	151
	D. Don't Assume Too Little Understanding/Be Prepared for Surprises	153
	E. Voicing Anger Case	154
	F. Codependency	157
	G. Failure All Around	159
	H. Against-All-Odds: Success	161
12	**Setting Up and Funding an AAC/Assistive Technology Service**	**163**
	Current State of Affairs	163
	Organization of an AT Service	164
	Staffing	166

	Equipment	169
	Training	170
	Assessing Staff Needs	170
	In Service Training	174
	Online Tutorials	175
	Competency Assessment	176
	Funding Issues	179
13	**Useful Products and Links**	**181**
	The MacGyver Kit: Essential Tools and Materials	181
	AAC Manufacturer Links	182
	AAC Resource Links	182

Appendix A. Assessment Scenarios   *183*
Appendix B. Major AAC Manufacturers   *193*
Appendix C. AAC/AT Resources   *195*
References   *197*
Index   *203*

Preface

The connection between an understanding of the mechanisms underlying human communication and advances in electronic speech generation and microcomputers offers us the possibility of enhancing acutely ill patients' ability to communicate and control their environment. This book is the product of a collaboration of a psycholinguist with a tendency to be a tech-nerd and a speech-language pathologist with many years of experience working with children with developmental disabilities. The development of our program for implementing alternative and augmentative communication (AAC) in intensive care settings is the result of an evolutionary process. The principles underlying our approach emerged from the convergence of our individual learning trajectories. This book provides both the technical details related to our implementation of AAC in the intensive care units at the University of Iowa Hospitals and Clinics (UIHC) as well as the particular principles and strategies that we have found might enhance the communicative abilities of critically ill and often intubated patients. We feel that we learned a great deal from each case and to that end we include an account of a number of individual cases that we feel illustrate some key issues that can determine the differences between success and failure.

Psycholinguists are trained to design and execute experiments that often include presentation of speech materials and recording behavioral responses with an assortment of switches. As such, they have familiarity with the software and hardware issues that are entailed in AAC systems designs. Many years ago, a colleague inquired whether somewhere in Hurtig's little black bag of switch technologies, he could find something for a young child with severe limitations due to cerebral palsy. The request was not to figure out how to connect this child to a traditional AAC system but rather to see if he could give the child control of an electronic toy. From his perspective, the task was fairly trivial and involved simply taking a large microswitch and using it to close the circuit from the batteries to the toy's motor. Today, numerous commercial products are available to give children with limited motor skills the ability to control toys and other electronic devices in their environment. The child and her parents were delighted, and more importantly, the child had the ability to demonstrate intentionality and the potential to use some form of AAC system. This case illustrates the important connection between the ability to control one's physical environment and one's ability to participate in effective communication.

Without language, we are limited in how we function in our environment. Language enables us to extend our reach and ability to meet our physical and psychological needs. Even though I am healthy, my height may preclude me from reaching and obtaining objects I desire that are placed on upper shelves. In the most narrow context, my linguistic abilities enable me to seek the assistance of others; in a broader context, language allows me to collaborate with others to develop a tool that would allow me to independently get the objects that my physical limitations would otherwise preclude. Children learn that they can get what they want equally well by moving their limbs or by moving their articulators to produce an abstract code for speech, signing, or writing. It all becomes so automatic that we are rarely, if ever, conscious of the interplay of what we do directly and what we accomplish through the use of language. Even our use of language is tied to context, such that the message is not necessarily coded entirely in the string of speech sounds or signs we produce. We see this interplay in a mother's ability to respond to her infant's cry, not because the child has differentiated a "hungry" cry from a "pick-me-up" cry, but because of an understanding of the temporal context in which a cry occurs. At perhaps the other extreme of the lifespan, one can get one's spouse to bring a desired object without using the object's name or a specific referent marker by saying "get be the thingamabob from the whatyamacallit." Again, it is the reading of the context not the parsing of the linguistic string that leads to the effective communication. Similarly, we encounter lots of cases where an individual might say "your tone of voice told the whole story" or "your face betrayed your true meaning." What is important to take away from such observations is that, when we are confronted with the loss of our primary communication channel and we seek a substitute, we often forget that our other channels of communication might have remained intact. In this technological era, we sometimes mistakenly believe that the device or prosthesis replaces the entire communicative ensemble rather than just a single component. If your facial muscles are intact, why give up the easily produced "furrowed brow" that can quickly and effectively communicate your state of mind. It is remarkable how many individuals who are introduced to alternative and augmentative communication systems focus on laboriously producing an utterance to describe their reaction rather than utilizing the simpler and often unambiguous facial gesture. A hallmark of our approach to implementing AAC is that we try to always remember this dynamic interaction of the diverse behaviors that make up human communication. Regardless of whether we select a high- or a low-tech AAC system, a major part of an effective solution is getting users to recognize the need to combine the technology we offer them with whatever residual components of natural communication are still under their control.

Imagine that tomorrow morning, when you awaken, you are not in your bed at home but rather in an unfamiliar setting surrounded by people and sounds that are totally alien to you. What makes things worse is that you have no idea of how you got there and you quickly realize that (1) you can't move your arms and legs, (2) you can't talk because there is an endotracheal tube in your mouth, and, (3) there appear to be catheters and lines penetrating your entire body.

- How do you find out what happened and more importantly what will happen to you?
- How do you let people know you want to participate in decisions about your medical care?
- How do you assert yourself so that the medical staff and family and

friends know what your wishes are with regard to your care and treatment options?
- If you had the foresight to have left an advanced medical directive or living will, how do you let people know that you have prepared such a document and that it outlines the procedures you approve of and those you wish to decline?

One problem with advanced medical directives is that we often write them when we are in good health and have defined "quality of life" from an able-bodied perspective. That perspective makes some interventions like ventilatory support and tube feeding unacceptable and justifies "do-not-resuscitate" orders. But things may look very different from the perspective of the hospital bed or wheelchair. Having changed one's perspective and as a consequence one's wishes, how do we communicate what we want done here and now in the intensive care unit?

AAC was developed to allow individuals with either developmental or acquired communication disabilities to effectively communicate in a variety of settings. Over the history of AAC, resistance to alternatives to natural speech often has kept individuals from being afforded the benefits of AAC systems. This can be seen in the reluctance of parents to have their children use low-tech language boards or any system that would not lead to the use of natural speech. Likewise, individuals with acquired communication disorders have been reluctant to accept having to give up use of their natural voice. In both cases, it is the belief that AAC can only yield a limited form of communication with a broken form of language. Some of this reluctance to accept AAC systems, low- or high-tech, can be attributed to the belief that communicative autonomy cannot be achieved with any system that does not allow novel utterance construction. Parents of children with developmental disorders as well as adults with acquired disorders worry not only about the limitation on expression, but also about the stigma that using an AAC system may impose. These are legitimate concerns but ones that can be addressed by system design, appropriate training, and counseling.

The process of doing an evaluation for AAC candidacy and the construction of a system for a particular individual is seen as a complex process requiring both considerable expertise and time. As such, it is not one which is undertaken unless there is both a reasonable expectation that the individual would benefit from having an AAC system and that the time and resources are available to undertake the effort of designing and implementing the system. Individuals with short life expectancies or individuals whose communication disabilities are seen as temporary are not often considered candidates for AAC. But the need for these individuals to communicate is no less than that of any other nonspeaking person. Because of the longstanding belief that significant time and effort are needed to successfully implement an AAC system, working with such patients has not been seen as an effective use of resources. The successful use of AAC by many nonspeaking individuals with degenerative diseases like amyotrophic lateral sclerosis (ALS) has in part called into question many of these longstanding beliefs about AAC.

Critically ill patients tend to experience a range of unfamiliar and often upsetting communication problems caused by potential cognitive, sensory, or language barriers that distance them from their family and caregivers. Many of these "voiceless" patients often reported having experienced feelings of anxiety, insecurity, and panic during their stint on mechanical ventilation (Bergbom-Engberg, 1993). The nursing literature notes the use of non-vocal behaviors (i.e., mouthing words, gestures, and head nods) as primary modes of communication used by critical care patients. Inconsistency in the choice of communication mode as well as a great deal of variability in nurses' and family members' abilities to lip read or interpret gestures can create confusion and frustration for critically ill patients, families, and caregivers during what may be viewed as the most critical period of the patient's life. Given the medical and psychological state of such patients as well as the transitory nature of their limited communication, addressing their communication issues has not been a high priority of most hospital based speech-language pathologists (SLPs). However, the patients, family members, nurses, and others involved in the care of such patients must cope with the less than optimal communication that is a consequence of intubation and ventilatory support. Although complications with and limitations of communication in the critically ill had long been ignored, they are emerging as a treatment priority for critical care units (Menzel, 1994). The physical limitations of patients in critical care units often leave them unable to express themselves in any consistent manner and as a consequence they cannot participate effectively in their care, medical decision making, and in critically important emotional and social interactions.

The Joint Commission of Accreditation of Healthcare Organizations (JC) now mandates that all hospitals identify the communication status of each of their patients at admission (JC requirement [IM.6.2], 2005). AAC systems can provide a means by which individuals can alert healthcare staff of their physical and emotional needs (e.g., pain, positioning, or respiratory care) with the added positive outcome of a reduced need for restraints and sedation. Thus, the use of AAC can empower patients with no functional speech and/or minimal control of motor function to become active participants in their medical care. By enhancing communication and independence in critical care units, AAC should reduce the anxiety patients often experience. Thus, the time for introducing AAC systems in acute cure settings is now.

This book characterizes the issues and problems associated with the implementation of AAC in acute care settings. The presentation is based on data from over 200 cases in which some form of AAC was implemented at The University of Iowa Hospitals and Clinics (UIHC). We also include some case presentations to illustrate some of the issues that we have encountered and the implementation strategies that we have developed.

An extensive historical perspective of AAC can be found in Zangari, Lloyd, and Vicker's excellent paper (1994) and in Beukelman and Mirenda's text (2005). An important part of the recent history of AAC is the expansion of the etiologies of individuals that may benefit from AAC. As both assistive technologies have evolved and our awareness of the populations that can benefit from their implementation has grown, the place of AAC in the SLP's scope practice has become more explicitly defined. Both the American Speech-Language-Hearing Association (ASHA) and the Council for Clinical

Certification (CFCC) have identified AAC among the knowledge and skills requirements (KASA) for clinical certification in speech-language pathology.

To assist the reader in implementing AAC in acute care settings, we provide a large number of illustrations of both hardware and content solutions that have emerged from our experience. The companion DVD provides full color versions of all of the illustrations in the text as well as a number of video clips that illustrate a number of beside assessment strategies and AAC implementations. We had the good fortune to be able to shoot many of the bedside images and the videos in the UIHC Clinical Nursing Education simulator facility. Because of patient confidentiality and privacy issues, we have opted to mostly use healthy volunteers for most of the illustrations and video clips. We do want to thank one patient for granting us permission to use a few images of him in this text. The companion DVD also provides many examples of communication board layouts that can be implemented with a range of AAC systems.

Acknowledgments

We would like to acknowledge the help and support of Ginette Boudreau, Mark Miksch, LouAnn Montgomery, Karen Stenger, Michelle Wagner from the UIHC Department of Nursing; Jessica Daniels, Jenna Kessel, Julie Ostrem, Theresa Prisco, Arik Wald, David Wood, and Lauren Danna Zubow from The University of Iowa, Department of Communication Sciences and Disorders; Dick Huber from the UIHC Center for Disabilities and Development; Abby Arens, Meagan Cole, Brian Crabill, and Shelby Kobes for serving as demonstration patients in our video clips; Steven Kono for letting use images of him using our adapted switches; and all the physicians, nurses, physical therapists, occupational therapists, respiratory therapists, and rehab engineers who staff the UIHC inpatient units.

1 History of AAC

Our ability to communicate is unique and powerful. Imagine if you had something to say but no way to say it. How would you feel? How would you react when your actions or attempts to communicate were misinterpreted? Now, imagine that your inability to communicate limits your ability to effectively convey vital information regarding your overall health which may include end-of-life care. Imagine not being able to tell your family how much you care for them during critical periods in your life. Your feelings might be those of frustration, anxiety, and fear. These feelings could result in a sense of hopelessness which, in the extreme, can lead to depression. Although you might think that such an experience is unlikely to happen to you, the fact is that it could; especially, if you are one of the tens of thousands of Americans who undergo surgical interventions that can result in temporary postsurgical intubation. The inability to speak during temporary intubation due to ventilator therapy is reported as an unforgettable experience marked with feelings of anxiety and fear leaving the patient with a sense of panic (Nelson et al., 2004). These feelings tend to linger with patients far beyond their physical illness (Jones et al., 2001).

This inability to communicate, whether temporary or permanent, must be addressed. The research is clear; nonoral patients admitted to intensive care units report the inability to communicate as being one of the most frustrating and stress-provoking experiences; (Costello, 2000; Dowden, Honsinger, & Beukelman, 1986; Fitch, 1987; Fried-Oken, Howard, & Stewart, 1991; Gries, 1988; Hafsteindottir, 1995; Hudelson, 1977; Jablonski, 1994; Menzel, 1994; Stovsky, Rudy, & Dragonette, 1988; Villaire, 1995). The prevalence of individuals with severe communication impairments varies greatly depending on the country, age group, and types of disability surveyed (Beukelman & Mirenda, 1998). According to the American Speech-Language and Hearing Association (ASHA, 2004), there are more than 2 million people in the United States who are unable to speak or use handwriting as an effective and efficient means of communication. Beukelman and Mirenda (2005) suggest that 1.3% of all individuals or 3.5 million Americans present with communication impairments significant enough to preclude the use of natural speech to allow for functional communication in a range of contexts with a variety of communication partners. Matas, Mathy-Laikko, Beukelman, and Legreseley (1985) reported that 0.3% to 1.0% of this population are school-age children. A National Health Interview Survey in 1992 of elderly adults indicated that 0.6% to 1% of individuals age

65 or older used some form of assistive technology for communication (Blackstone, 1989). Most estimates of prevalence are based on data concerning individuals for whom communication disabilities are more permanent. There are no definitive incidence data for individuals for whom communication impairment is temporary. Typically, we think of this population as being comprised of postsurgical patients who require some form of ventilatory support. Most of these patients receive care in an intensive care unit. Approximately, 6.7 million patients are treated in ICU settings and 36% often experience some form of ventilator therapy (Angus, 2004). Angus reported that 56% of these patients in ICU who received ventilator therapy were males. The average age of these patients was 65.5 years, with an age range of 19 to 100. The most common etiologies that Angus (2004) reported included:

- Acute myocardial infarction
- Cerebrovascular accidents
- Pneumonia
- Acute respiratory distress syndrome
- Medical conditions acquired as a result of trauma
- HIV/AIDS and related conditions
- Metastatic cancer

Our experience in pediatric intensive care units (PICU) also has included children with a wide range of etiologies including developmental disabilities that can compromise the respiratory system and/or require surgeries that may necessitate postoperative intubation. Many adult and pediatric patients in the UIHC Burn Unit have also required ventilator therapy.

These demographic data suggest that there are a large number of patients who as a consequence of being on ventilators are unable to use normal modes of communication. The need to manage this population of temporarily and permanently impaired communicators falls to the subspecialty of Augmentative/Alternative Communication (AAC).

Defining AAC

Work on Augmentative/Alternative Communication involves the study and, when necessary, compensation of temporary or permanent restrictions of speech-language production and/or comprehension, including spoken as well as written modes of communication (ASHA, 2004, p. 1). The term *augmentative communication* refers to the use of aids or techniques that augment or supplement existing vocal or verbal communication skills. *Alternative communication* involves the use of communication methods or strategies in place of natural vocal or verbal abilities (Reichle, York, & Sigafoos, 1991). According to ASHA, AAC should be thought of as a system composed of four key elements: symbols, aids, strategies, and techniques (ASHA, 2004). *Symbols* represent objects, actions, and relationships that can vary in terms of their "guess ability" or transparency of meaning (ASHA, 2004; Beukelman & Mirenda, 2005; Glennen & DeCoste, 1997; Reichle, York, & Sigafoos, 1991). They can include spoken, signed, or written words, as well as gestures and graphic symbols. The term *aids* refers to devices used to convey or receive messages. These can range from low-tech communication boards to high-tech speech-generating devices. The term *techniques* refers to the range of modalities used to transmit the message from picture exchange to written and spoken language. Lastly, the term *strategies* refers to the manner in which symbols are used to afford quick and effective communication (ASHA, 2004). Recently, the term AAC has been linked with the term Assistive Technology (AT), which has been described as the use of aided tools to improve skills, abilities, lifestyle, and independence for individuals with disabilities (Beukelman, Garrett, & Yorkston, 2007; Glennen & De Coste, 1997, Higdon, & Higdon, 2004; Light, 1988). The range of assistive technology tools includes sensory aids, such as hearing aids and glasses, physical aids such as pointers and grips, as well as signage (Braille) and voice output devices for the visually impaired.

A Brief History of AAC

The term Augmentative/Alternative Communication (AAC) is one that has been in the professional speech-language pathology mainstream since the early 1980s (ASHA, 1981; Glennen & Decoste, 1997; Lloyd, 1985). Prior to the 1980s, the term "nonoral" was widely used (ASHA, 1981, Munson, Nordquist, & Thuma-Rew, 1987). AAC, as we know it, began in the 1950s with many clinicians using a form of AAC to enhance the communication skills of individuals whose oral and laryngeal structures were not intact or who were "nonoral" (Brown, 1954; Coleman, Cook, & Meyers, 1980; Musselwhite & St. Louis, 1982; Owens & House, 1984; Shane & Bashir, 1980; Silverman, 1980; Zangarie, Lloyd, & Vicker, 1994). These clinicians often offered the use of electrolarynges, and/or paper and pencil options for laryngectomy or glossectomy patients to enhance their communication (Glennen & Decoste, 1997). The genesis of AAC research began in the early 1960s. This may have been due to an important shift in thinking to include individuals with limited or sparse verbal abilities. Pioneers in the field began to implement the use of communication boards with cognitively impaired and/or physically impaired individuals (Coleman, Cook, & Meyers, 1980; Musselwhite & St. Louis, 1982; Owens & House, 1984; Shane & Bashir, 1980; Silverman, 1980; Zangari, Lloyd, & Vicker 1994). For example, in the early 1960s, the Non-Oral Communication Systems Project began at University Hospital School at the University of Iowa Hospital's and Clinics (UIHC). The University Hospital School was a residential facility for children with a range of developmental disabilities. Often these children were nonverbal but eager to communicate. The multidisciplinary staff of speech-language pathologists, occupational therapists, physical therapists, and classroom teachers began to try novel approaches with these children and immediately recognized the need to advance knowledge through research. This gave birth to the Non-Oral Communication Systems Project, conducted over a 10-year period from 1964 to 1973 (Munson, Nordquist, & Thuma-Rew, 1987). This was the first study of its kind to track the use of AAC in individuals with impaired neuromotor systems. In the original project paper by Kladde (1974), nine factors were identified as guidelines for determining candidacy for participation in the nonoral project. They included:

1. A comparison of present functional communication abilities to potential expression via a nonoral mode;
2. Overall prognosis for oral improvement;
3. Motor status;
4. Intellectual status;
5. Intrinsic motivation;
6. Attitudes toward communication;
7. The amount and type of professional assistance available;

8. The extent of staff interest and cooperation;
9. Parental interest and cooperation.

Although the general philosophy of intervention may have changed, Kladde's nine criteria continue to be part of the foundation for AAC assessment. Beukelman and Mirenda (2005) recommend the need for clinicians to gain some sense of the individual's linguistic, operational, social, and strategic competencies when assessing an individual's ability to use an AAC system in an efficient and effective manner. Thus, today's list does not look much different from that of the original nonoral project.

During the 1970s, advocacy for social change resulted in more inclusion of individuals with any type of disability in both educational and vocational settings. Speech-language pathologists began to serve individuals who previously were not in the general mainstream. The advent of Public Law 94-142 and the Rehabilitation Act of 1973 gave rise to the public's awareness of individuals with significant communication impairment. This revolutionized the need to accommodate such individuals, provided them with AAC systems, and allowed AAC candidates to be mainstreamed into classrooms across the country. The need to consider AAC systems for individuals with limited communication, but not necessarily nonoral individuals, grew significantly. However, candidacy was often withheld until the individual "failed" traditional speech and language therapy services (Shane & Bashir, 1980). The belief that the use of any form of AAC would stifle an individual's ability to learn or to be interested in learning to communicate orally remained high. The field continued to be more interested in the form of communication instead of the function of communication. Silverman's (1980) research was pivotal in changing the belief that the use of AAC would impede subsequent speech development.

Another important shift in AAC service delivery involved the emergence of interdisciplinary teams. Speech-language pathologists, occupational therapists, rehabilitation engineers, linguists, deaf educators, and physical therapists began to work together and hone their expertise in this area. The greater involvement of speech pathologists led to AAC being viewed as an area of expertise within the field of speech-language pathology. In recognition of this, ASHA formed an Ad Hoc Committee on the Communication Processes of Non-speaking Persons in late 1970s.

The 1980s saw continued growth and interest in this aspect of the scope of practice in speech-language pathology. ASHA released its position statement on non-speech communication which affirmed the need for speech-language pathologists to demonstrate working knowledge of and training in topic areas related to communication development of persons for whom speech may not be the primary mode of communication (ASHA, 1981). The emergence of systematic research and the need for its dissemination resulted in the formation of the International Society of Augmentative/Alternative Communication (ISAAC) and its subsequent support for the first quarterly AAC journal, the *Journal of Augmentative/Alternative Communication*, in 1985. To date, the *Journal of Augmentative/Alternative Communication* continues to be recognized as a major source of information in the field. The scope of practice in the AAC specialty also continued to evolve as evidence showed that there was no individual too physically challenged that could not benefit from some form of AAC intervention. Similarly, clinicians also questioned the need for the previously suggested higher level cognitive prerequisites (Kangas & Lloyd, 1988; Reichle & Karlan, 1985, 1987, 1988; Romski & Sevcik, 1988).

By the 1990s, the service delivery model for AAC had moved to a zero exclusion model. An important affirmation of the broader need for AAC services occurred in 1992 with the Communication Bill of Rights promulgated by the National Joint Committee for the Communication Needs of Persons with Severe Disabilities (Table 1-1). The Communication Bill of Rights outlined the needs of individuals with severe communication impairments and their rights to have access to AAC systems.

Table 1-1. Communication Bill of Rights

All persons, regardless of the extent or severity of their disabilities have a basic right to affect, through communication, the conditions of their own existence. Beyond this general right a number of specific communication rights should be ensured in all daily interactions and interventions involving persons who have severe disabilities. These basic communication rights are as follows.

1. The right to request desired objects, actions, events, and persons, and to express personal preferences, or feelings.
2. The right to be offered choices and alternatives.
3. The right to reject or refuse undesired objects, events, or actions, including the right to decline or request all proffered choices.
4. The right to request, and be given, attention from and interaction with another person.
5. The right to request feed microphone back or information about a state, an object, a person, or an event of interest.
6. The right to active treatment and intervention efforts to enable people with severe disabilities to communicate messages in whatever modes and as effectively and efficiently as their specific abilities will allow.
7. The right to have communicative acts acknowledged and responded to even when the intent of these acts cannot be fulfilled by the responder.
8. The right to have access at all times to any needed augmentative and alternative communication devices and other assistive devices, and to have those devices in good working order.
9. The right to environmental contexts, interactions, and opportunities that expect and encourage persons with disabilities to participate as full communicative partners with other people, including peers.
10. The right to be informed about people, things, and events in one's immediate environments.
11. The right to be communicated with in a manner that recognizes and acknowledges the inherent dignity of the person being addressed, including the right to be part of communication exchanges about individuals that are conducted in his or her presence.
12. The right to be communicated with in ways that are meaningful, understandable, and culturally and linguistically appropriate.

Source: The National Joint Committee for the Communication Needs of Persons with Severe Disabilities (1992). Guidelines for meeting the communication needs of persons with severe disabilities. *ASHA, 34*(Suppl. 71),1–8. Reprinted with permission.

Through the last decade of the 20th century, AAC service delivery continued to expand. Ratcliff and Beukelman (1995) reported roughly 49% of all speech-language pathologists' caseloads included implementation of some form of AAC. They reported that this increase was occurring across numerous clinical settings. Given the rise in the percentage of caseloads requiring the use of AAC, the field began to examine the need for more extensive preprofessional preparation. Ratcliff and Beukelman (1995) surveyed 204 university programs offering graduate training in Communication Disorders. Of the 119 university programs across the nation that responded, 68% indicated that they offered at least one course specific to AAC. At the turn of the 21st century, 76 universities offered courses in AAC, and the nature of research changed from anecdotal accounts to more evidence-based outcomes studies (Higdon & Higdon, 2004). Today, we are witnessing a second generation of AAC research and clinical practice. Current practice dispels several common myths associated with the implementation of AAC (Romski & Sevcik, 2005). Furthermore, technologic advances have enhanced our ability to implement AAC strategies across the life span and for individuals with etiologies who were previously not served. Table 1-2 reframes some of the common myths about implementing AAC from the perspective of applications of AAC strategies in acute care settings with children and adults.

How Technology Has Impacted AAC

The development of computer technology has certainly impacted all of our lives on a daily basis. Some of this technology is so common that it may be hard to recall a time when we did not have it. Ask any child to recall a time when items such as personal computers, tablet PCs, PDAs, cell phones, and text pagers were not a part of their lives or their parents' lives, and they might respond with something similar to "they have always been around, right?" Many of these technologic developments have impacted our ability to implement more high-tech AAC systems (i.e. voice output communication devices [VOCAs] or speech-generating devices [SGDs]).

When we cross an additional generational line and ask grandparents if they use Bluetooth technology, we find that they are often bewildered by the question. They might think we were asking about a new dental technique. This generational difference reflects the fact that the technology explosion in educational and vocational settings has only impacted the mainstream population in the last decade. But how have these advances in technology impacted the field of AAC?

The two developments that have played the most critical role in setting the course for the development of today's assistive technology for communication purposes include the development of speech synthesis algorithms and the increased power, speed, and memory of microprocessors. Effective speech synthesis, which could be accomplished in real time, allowed communication devices to generate a far greater range of utterances than the early devices which used recorded real speech and required considerable memory on the device. Perhaps the most dramatic development in computing involved the miniaturization of circuits that moved computers from big racks to the desktop and finally into a circuit board smaller than a child's hand.

Table 1–2. AAC Myths

Myths	Realities
AAC should only be considered if all other options have been tried and they have failed	AAC should be used whenever needed to supplement or replace an individuals existing method of communication.
Use of AAC will preclude speech development.	Research shows that AAC interventions can support improvement in overall speech skills
Candidates need to demonstrate a set of minimal skills in order to benefit from an AAC device.	There are no cognitive or linguistic prerequisites for candidacy.
Only for individuals with intact cognition can use and benefit from high tech microprocessor based speech-generating devices.	Advances in technology and the use of computers with individuals with a much wider range of cognitive abilities, makes use of speech-generating devices with lower functioning individuals possible
Determining AAC candidacy requires a long and time consuming assessment so use with short-term patients is not feasible.	Given the range of devices and device access methods even patients with locked-in-syndrome can quickly be started using an AAC system
Learning to communicate with an AAC system requires a considerable amount of time, so it can't occur during short-term hospitalizations.	AAC systems can be introduced to patients at the bedside and they can become functional communicators with only brief instruction.
Adults with acquired loss of speech will reject symbol-based systems.	We live in a world of symbols and icons, so where use of symbols facilitates navigation through an AAC system, symbols are seen as natural and are accepted
Individuals with acquired losses will reject AAC systems with preset message templates	When AAC users see that most natural exchanges are often fairly scripted, they come to understand that any form of communication rate enhancement makes their interactions more pragmatically natural.

With the rapid expansion of the use of personal computers, market force pressures continue to lead to more portable or smaller microprocessor-based technologies. For AAC applications, these developments ensured that devices could be portable and move from home to school or work and back without requiring a moving van. This has also meant that AAC systems could be deployed in hospital bedside settings without interfering with the needs of providing medical.

The use of microprocessors became more commonplace in the AAC voice output devices in the 1980s (Romski & Sevcik, 2005). Up until that time, communication systems were large, cumbersome, and required a considerable amount of inventiveness in assembling diverse components. In 1964, the occupational therapy department at the Children's Center Crotched Mountain Foundation (Greenfield, New Hampshire) began to explore the use of early electronic AAC systems (Miller & Carpenter, 1964). They built several electronic AAC systems. The first capitalized on the use of head control as a means of access. The staff used a secondhand hydraulic dental chair base to raise and lower an easel which supported an electronic typewriter. The typewriter was hinged to an easel to provide variability in the position of the keyboard so that it could be accessed with a head stick.

In a second case, the staff built a circular clock face swept by an arrow that could be controlled by an individual pressing a foot switch. Each position on the clock face contained a message. In this case, the child was instructed to press the foot switch when the arrow was pointing to his or her desired message. These two early electronic devices are offered to demonstrate how significant the changes in electronic AAC devices have been.

AAC devices changed through the ensuing decades. We have come from a time when "portable" communication aids weighed roughly 17 pounds to today's devices that can weigh as little as 1.3 pounds. The size of the devices has changed as well. It was clear to clinicians and to the engineers who were designing communication devices that portability was an essential design feature. There were a number of early attempts to produce a hand-held device prior to the emergence of the PC (e.g., Brooch, Auto-Com, Cannon Communicator, Elkomi 2, Express, HandiVoice, and the Form-A-Phrase; see Zangari, Lloyd, & Vicker, 1994). Perhaps one of the most recent developments which has had a significant impact on AAC has been the development of liquid crystal displays(LCD) and touch screens used in computers, cell phones and PDAs today. The lightweight LCD allowed AAC devices to move from fixed keyboard designs to dynamic display designs.

Today's devices offer a variety of options and features that allow for a broadening of the use of AAC to individuals with a wide range of etiologies that are known to limit the use of unaided communication. Today's AAC manufacturers have created devices that allow for a variety of access options, vocabulary/message options, and, of course, greater portability. Many of these advances in AAC technology have made it possible to consider implementing AAC in acute care settings with an ease and functionality not previously possible.

The portability that is provided by the these newer devices has allowed us to mount them on IV poles with extremely adjustable mounts at the bedside, something unheard of 10 to 20 years ago and definitely not an option 30+ years ago. In the 1990s, the first commercially available communication devices intended for use with the acute care population experiencing temporary or permanent vocal impairment became available (e.g., Vocal Assistant; Zangari, Lloyd, & Vicker, 1994). Although limited in functionality, the use of these devices marked a realization of the need to meet the communication challenges of the acute care population. There are now a number of devices varying from low to high tech that can be used in acute care settings. Each new generation of AAC devices has offered some new or improved functionality that both enhanced communication options and widened the range of individuals who could use an AAC system. Tables 1–3A through 1–3D present information on the functionality for some exemplars of lower to higher tech AAC systems.

Table 1–3A. Low-Tech Devices

SGD Manufacturer	Single Messages	2–4 Messages	8–10 Messages	Digitized Voice	Synthesized Voice	Scanning Options
Go-Talk *Adaptivation*			X	X		
Chipper *Adaptivation*	X			X		
Partner One *AMDI*	X			X		
Partner Two *AMDI*		X		X		
Partner Four *AMDI*		X		X		
Tech 8 *AMDI*			X	X		X
BIGMack *Mayer-Johnson*	X			X		
One Step *Mayer-Johnson*	X			X		

Table 1–3B. Mid-Tech Devices

SGD Manufacturer	Paper Overlay	Dynamic Display	Digitized Voice	Synthesized Voice	Scanning Options	ECU
L*E*O *Assistive Technology*	X		X		X	X
Tech 32 *AMDI*	X		X		X	
M3 *DynaVox*		X	X		X	X
SpringBoard Plus/ SpringBoard Lite *Prentke Romich Company*		X	X		X	X
Message Mate *Words+*	X		X		X	

Table 1–3C. High-Tech Devices

SGD / Manufacturer	Dynamic Display (color)	Digitized Voice Options	Synthesized Voice Options	Scanning Options	Auditory Scanning	ECU	Integrated Head Mouse	Integrated Eye Tracking	Dedicated Devices	PC Based
Tech Touch / *AMDI*	X	X	X	X	X				X	X
MercuryII/MiniMerc / *Assistive Technology, Inc.*	X	X	X	X	X	X			X	X
V/Vmax/Eye Max / *DynaVox*	X	X	X	X	X	X			X	X
ERICA / *Eye Response Technology*	X	X	X	X	X	X	X	X	X	X
Vanguard Plus/Vantage Plus / *Prentke Romich Company*	X	X	X	X	X	X	X		X	
Pathfinder Plus / *Prentke Romich Company*	X	X	X	X		X	X		X	
TANGO / *Blinktwice*	X	X	X						X	
Say-it-SAM / *Words+*	X	X	X	X	X	X	X		X	X
Optimist 3HD / *Zygo Industries*	X	X	X	X	X	X			X	X
Say-it-SAM MyTobiIP10 / *TobiIATI*	X	X	X	X	X	X		X	X	X

HISTORY OF AAC 11

Table 1–3D. Text-to-Speech Devices

SGD Manufacturer	Abbreviation Expansion	Word Prediction	Synthesized Voice	Digitized Voice	ECU	Scanning Options
Link *Assistive Technology*	X	X	X			
Dynawrite/ *DynaVox*	X	X	X	X	X	X
Convertible *Words+*	X	X	X	X	X	X
LightWRITER(S)	X	X	X			X

The tables are organized by level of technology and provide information on the characteristic features of devices at each level. The list of devices at each level is by no means exhaustive and is provided only as a guide to clinicians for making decisions about selecting devices for their clinical settings. The devices listed represent the most recent models available from the major manufacturers of AAC devices. Given the speed of changes in technology, this listing will need annual updating. To some extent, decision making with regard to equipment acquisition by an institution for use by patients while in acute care will differ from the process used in prescription of devices for traditional AAC users. A model for a hospital-based assistive technology service is presented in Chapter 12.

Etiologies That May Benefit from AAC

A review of the literature reveals that AAC systems have been implemented across the life span and with individuals with a range of etiologies that required some form of assistance with communication. At the beginning, AAC was implemented with laryngectomy patients (Brown, 1954) as well as other patient populations that were entirely unable to produce speech. Since then a significant philosophical change has occurred and the candidate patient population has expanded to include individuals who might have some limited oral speech capabilities. This evolutionary change has led to today's practice where there are effectively no etiologies that are excluded from receiving some form of AAC services.

During the field's infancy, AAC practitioners thought only congenital conditions, such as cerebral palsy and mental retardation, were appropriate for AAC interventions. Advances in technology allowed a far wider range of customization in terms of content and access mode and as a consequence, clinicians were able to extend services to individuals with acquired communication problems. Clinicians now serve individuals with far more complex etiologies. These include individuals with short and long-term communication problems that may result from disease or trauma. (Higdon & Higdon, 2004).

For a list of possible etiologies that may benefit from AAC interventions see Table 1-4.

ASHA's Stand on AAC

ASHA promulgated its first position statement regarding AAC in 1981 (Position Statement on Nonspeech Communication, ASHA, 1981), recognizing AAC as an

Table 1-4. Conditions That May Benefit from AAC Intervention	
Etiologies That May Benefit from AAC Intervention	*Research Citations**
Amyotrophic Lateral Sclerosis	Ball, Beukelman, & Bardach (2007) Beukelman, Fager, Ball, & Dietz (2007)
Aphasia	Jacob, Drew, Ogletree, & Pierce (2004) King, Alarcon, & Rogers (2007) Lasker, Garrett, & Fox (2007)
Autism	Mirenda (2003)
Brainstem Stroke	Costello, (2000) Culp, Beukelman, & Fager, (2007)
Burn Victims	Hurtig & Downey, (2005)
Cerebral Palsy	Beukelman & Mirenda (2005)
Dementia	Bourgeois & Hickey (2007)
Guillain-Barré	Beukelman & Garrett (1988)
Head & Neck Cancer	Sullivan, Gaebler, & Ball (2007)
Mental Retardation	Miller, Light, & Schlosser (2006) Wilkinson, & Hennig (2007)
Mental Retardation: Severe to Profound	Romski & Sevcik, (1988 &1996)
Progressive/Degenerative Diseases (Multiple Sclerosis, Huntington's Disease, Parkinson's Disease)	Honsinger, (1989) Yorkston & Beukelman (2007)
Respiratory Insufficiency	Happ, (2001)
Spinal Cord Injury	Britton & Baarslag-Benson, (2007)
Traumatic Brain Injury	Beukelman, Fager, Ball, & Dietz (2007) Fager, Doyle, & Karantounis (2007)

**Note:* The citations listed are offered as a reference point. The list is by no means exhaustive.

appropriate treatment option for nonspeaking individuals. Today AAC is viewed as a system by ASHA (ASHA, 2004). ASHA now recognizes the use of AAC for both temporary and permanent communication impairments. ASHA's current position stipulates "zero" exclusion candidacy for AAC. Thus, all individuals who cannot use normal communication channels are potential candidates for AAC. The speech-language pathologist's task is not to evaluate the individual to determine whether he or she is a candidate for AAC, but rather to determine where the individual may fall on the communication continuum in order to provide some form of AAC (ASHA, 2004). AAC systems can complement an individual's current method(s) of communication or, in some instances, replace natural speech and/or negative behaviors. Thus, speech-language pathologists are challenged to view communication as a multimodal system that can vary from individual to individual (ASHA, 2004). And, although there are no standardized test batteries for AAC evaluations, there are guiding principles that all clinicians should follow. They include: a valid assessment of cognitive, sensory, perceptual, social, motor, reading/literacy, writing, and linguistic capabilities, and identification of barriers to participation. The goal of all AAC interventions should be to maximize the user's abilities to express their needs efficiently and effectively and allow for active participation across a range of environments. Thus, ASHA suggests the use of the participation model proposed by Beukelman and Mirenda (1988) to address and identify opportunities and barriers that may preclude participation noting that barriers to participation are not always physical, and may include policies, practices, attitudes, knowledge, and skills that preclude successful use of an AAC system. Consequently, AAC is universally viewed as being within the scope of practice for speech-language pathologists with roles and responsibilities being defined as:

- "Recognize and hold paramount the needs and interests of individuals who may benefit from AAC and assist them to communicate in ways they desire."
- "Implement a multimodal approach to enhance effective communication that is culturally and linguistically appropriate."
- "Acquire and maintain the knowledge and skills (ASHA, 2002) that are necessary to provide quality professional services."
- "Integrate perspectives, knowledge and skills of team members, especially those individuals who have AAC needs, their families, and significant others in developing functional and meaningful goals and objectives."
- "Assess, intervene, and evaluate progress and outcomes associated with AAC interventions using principles of evidence-based practice."
- "Facilitate individuals' uses of AAC to promote and maintain their quality of life. "
- "Advocate with and for individuals who can or already do benefit from AAC, their families, and significant others to address communication needs and ensuring rights to full communication access." (American Speech-Language-Hearing Association, 2005, p. 1)

It is in this spirit that we suggest rethinking the implementation of AAC in acute care settings with a variety of etiologies across the life span. Today's AAC philosophies and advances in current technology allow us to advocate and promote successful use of AAC systems with acutely ill patients at a time when the need for efficient and effective communication is paramount.

2 Challenges

Perhaps one of the reasons that the implementation of AAC in acute care settings has been problematic has been due to the many challenges the clinician may face. This may explain why the use of more high-end voice output devices has not been widely implemented in acute care settings. Only a modicum of research exists, in part because the traditional use of high-end AAC systems has been limited to individuals for whom oral language is no longer an option or whose oral communication attempts required repair. Clearly, the acutely ill patient is different from the "typical" AAC candidate who is in need of assistance due to congenital or acquired etiologies. These typical AAC candidates have included individuals with developmental disabilities, mental disabilities, and significant neuromotor involvement. Such individuals are typically served in outpatient settings (Beukelman & Mirenda, 2005; Zangari, Lloyd, & Vicker, 1994). The clinician's caseloads have not typically included the acutely ill patient, despite the fact that such individuals often cannot communicate and are unable to participate in their own care (Baker & Melby, 1996; Robillard, 1994).

Although the literature is filled with studies examining the use of AAC with more traditional candidates it is less extensive for studies of patients with temporary oral language impairment or patients who are acutely ill. In fact a review of the literature reveals only a limited of published accounts of AAC use with such patients (Downey & Hurtig, 2006). These studies are discussed in more detail in Chapter 3. The reason for such a dearth of research may be due to speech-language pathologists' (SLPs) continued belief that the implementation of AAC with acutely ill patients is extremely problematic.

Generally, SLPs tend to view the acutely ill patient as being too medically fragile and/or unstable. They often view a bedside evaluation as being impossible and may believe that the implementation of a high-end communication system is too time consuming and not a service that can be executed with any efficacy or efficiency. This conclusion is a result of the clinician's belief that there are barriers (see below) that are unique to the acutely ill patient and actually preclude the use of high-end AAC systems (Costello, 2000; Hurtig & Downey, 2005, 2006):

- The patient's overall cognitive status may result in an inability to process information due to his or her medical condition and/or medication(s);
- The patient's limited motor abilities;
- The patient's reduced sensory status, that is, temporary lack of access to hearing aids or glasses;

- The patient's state may require the need for restraints to avoid medical treatment interference.
- Lastly, it may be difficult to roll out an AAC service with acute care patients because of the pragmatic constraint that most hospitals do not have a sufficient inventory of equipment to provide AAC systems to all patients in need of them.

Although these are valid observations and are barriers to practice they are not insurmountable and are not significantly different from those that are noted to occur with the more traditional AAC patient. Beukelman and Mirenda's (1998) Participation Model suggests that there are two types of barriers common in AAC practice: opportunity barriers and access barriers. Clearly, the barriers identified by most clinicians as often insurmountable are either barriers of access or barriers of opportunity. The access barriers or operational barriers would include the patient's cognitive/linguistic status, sensory status, motor status, and physical or chemical restraint status. The lack of equipment may be due to policy issues or attitudes originating in either the hospital administration or in the department of Speech Pathology and are barriers of opportunity. Agreeing that all of these "challenge" exists, the path to understanding them and perhaps overcoming them will require us to take apart each of these challenges.

Access Challenges

The acute care patient's status may be continually in flux and as such the means of access may need to vary over the course of the use of an AAC system. Our experience is that the patient's status tends to change in more predictable directions for most patients, thus making our ability to provide those patients with some form of a functional AAC system somewhat more straightforward. Even in the case of the patient whose status regresses, the obvious steps involve simplifying the system to allow for continued motivation to use the communication system/device and to, at the very least, maintain the basic function of access to the nurse call system. The key element to maintaining a communication system in spite of patient status changes is addressed in later chapters.

The one observation that is repeatedly overlooked and clearly helps to bridge effective AAC practice in the acute care setting is the fact that many of the patients in this setting tend to present with normal intelligence and intact language abilities. As we noted earlier, the potential challenges of implementing AAC in acute care that are often cited are based on traditional AAC practice with children for whom language development is delayed for a variety of reasons. Traditional implementation of an AAC system with a developing child tends to be described as a "process" and thus implies a long implementation time line. We agree that this statement is true for children who are in the "process of acquiring language" but believe that it is the process of language acquisition that is time intensive rather than the implementation of the AAC system. Most acutely ill patients tend to have intact language systems; thus, the need to assist them in understanding the linguistic principles entailed in the use of an AAC device or directing them in their use of the device may not be a significant challenge. In our experience with adult and pediatric patients, the learning curve for successful use of an AAC device is short and not very steep.

The concern regarding effective bedside evaluation is less disheartening once we recognize that our patients will most likely present with an intact language system and that the greater challenge is operational access from a motor function standpoint. Although such access can appear to be a tremendous barrier it is can be readily addressed with the right equipment and bedside mounting hardware, both of which are discussed more comprehensively in Chapter 7.

Opportunity Challenges

Lastly, the perceived barrier resulting from the lack of a sufficient supply of equipment is an obstacle that is a real barrier of opportunity. The supply problem may stem from some combination of administrative policy, practice patterns, facilitator attitudes, as well as knowledge and/or skill with implementing AAC. Unlike traditional AAC implementation where devices are prescribed and purchased for a particular user, acute care implementations will require a radically different model for device acquisition. It is our belief that this opportunity barrier may perhaps be the most challenging to overcome. Given how few facilities currently provide AAC in acute care, the attitudinal or policy factors may contribute the most to the opportunity barriers. These attitudes may stem from past research which suggested that high end devices are not the AAC preference of acutely ill patients (Fried-Oken, Howard, & Stewart, 1991). Although this may have been the case 16 years ago, we do not believe it to be true now. Current advances in microprocessor technology have had huge impact on the quality of all our lives (Maxwell, 2000) and the field of AAC has benefited from those advances. The nature of the AAC devices that are available today both in terms of functionality as well as size and cost present a very different set of options from those that were available in the early 1990s. Many of these advances have markedly eliminated what might have been perceived as operational barriers in the past. More advanced and customizable selection methods exist in today's high-end systems and as such make access to AAC possible for individuals with extremely restricted motor function. Attitude barriers toward computers and computer use are diminishing for all segments of our society. Computers and computer use has become more commonplace; most of us cannot go to the store, go to work, pump gas, or get money from an automated teller without encountering some form of touch screen or dynamic display. This fact cannot be understated and has not gone unnoticed by manufacturers of AAC systems. More and more high-end device manufacturers are choosing to implement their systems on platforms that run Windows XP or Windows CE operating systems (e.g., Assistive Technologies, Words+, Dyna-Vox), which have become familiar platforms for AAC users and the individuals in their support networks. Only a few years ago it would have been rare to see a PC at the bedside in an intensive care unit. Now patients and staff can have access to computing and the Internet at the bedside. Just as "My Space" and "Face Book" provide for interaction and information exchange in the general population, applications like "Care-Pages" provide hospital patients and their friends and family with a means to communicate and share information. This rethinking of what equipment can be at the bedside should go a long way to removing some of those attitudes that created some of the opportunity barriers.

But perhaps the most difficult of the opportunity barriers involves the attitudes and fears of clinicians to have to deal with difficult situations including "end of life" decision making. It is more common for clinicians to believe that their interventions will lead to better more productive lives and that provision of AAC moves patients up on some quality of life continuum. There is a tendency to assume that our interventions will fix the problem and lead to a better quality of life. Of course, we often fall into the trap of defining quality of life from our healthy person's perspective. The following is presented as an illustrative case:

Early in Hurtig's involvement designing assistive technology, he was asked to design a computer system for a woman with advanced ALS who was bedridden and who required ventilatory support. The only voluntary movement that she was capable of consistently making was a small grasping pressure force that she could generate with each hand. An atypical complicating factor was that she could not see. She had lost control of movement of her eyelids and as a result her corneas deteriorated and she was left locked in, incapable of speaking or seeing. At that point in time there were no AAC speech-generating devices on the market that could be adapted for her use. The system that Hurtig put together consisted of a first generation PC with an external text-to-speech circuit. He wrote a computer application for her to use that would generate text strings that would be passed to the text-to-speech circuit. The way she controlled the application was via two small microswitches that were held in each palm with elastic straps. The switches were connected to two of the parallel port input lines. The computer program sensed the state of those two switches and treated a closure of the right-hand switch as a Morse code dot and a closure of the left-hand switch as a Morse code dash. The program then converted the Morse code sequences to the characters in the text stream that was sent to the text-to-speech circuit. The patient was a highly intelligent and extremely motivated woman who was able to master use of Morse code in just a couple of days. She began to use the system to effectively communicate with caregivers and her family. With the system, she was capable of directing her care and participating in a wide range of conversations with family and friends. Most remarkably, from the very first day, she made requests for modifications that would enhance her communications.

From the outset, Hurtig began to work on communication rate enhancement. The patient worked to create a fairly large set of abbreviations (several hundred) that we used to generate an automatic abbreviation expansion table that the software application could use. After a couple of weeks, the patient indicated that she wanted to write messages to people off-line, so that she could send them notes and speed up face-to-face interactions. With some programming changes, she was able with *abbreviation commands* to save and retrieve text files as well as route them to a printer. As with the earlier modifications she rapidly mastered the additional sequence of commands. On an almost daily basis, Hurtig received printouts with requests for additional abbreviations. Her hospice care staff reported that she was quickly transformed from a very depressed individual who could only express frustration with tears to an individual who was actively engaged with her caregivers, family and friends. We felt really proud for having made such a dramatic change in her quality of life. Then one day, Hurtig received a note that indicated how grateful she was for having been given an effective means to communicate and that this had enabled her to make her needs and wishes known and to have meaningful end-of-life relationship-closing chats with her loved ones. The note ended indicating that she had said all that she needed to and that she had given instructions that she wished to be withdrawn from life support. Hurtig's first reaction to that note was one of utter devastation. For weeks he thought that he had failed because the end result was not a happy one. He had naively thought that he had succeeded in restoring the communication that the ALS had deprived her of and that the only good end was one in which she progressively did more and more. As time passed, Hurtig began to realize that it was her goals, not his, that were the most important. He had focused too much on building a system and giving her what she wanted. What her last note taught him was that the system had given her not only the ability to talk but, more importantly, the ability to assert her autonomy.

If we do not question our attitudes concerning what AAC is about or who we think can or cannot benefit from assistive technology, we will raise a barrier that will keep many individuals from achieving a higher quality of life from their particular perspective.

Although it is apparent that there are both access and opportunity barriers which appear to have precluded the use of high-end AAC systems with the acute care population, we want to argue that these are not barriers that cannot be eliminated. Clinicians need to monitor patient status closely through more consistent contact with nursing and medical staff, as well as with frequent re-evaluation for the appropriateness of some form of AAC intervention. The importance of leading the charge in educating the medical and nursing professions to the necessity of implementing communication options for those who experience temporary or permanent loss of speech is crucial for two reasons:

1. The Joint Commission on Accreditation of Healthcare Organizations (JCAHO) as of January 1st, 2006 now mandates all hospitals to identify the communication status of each of their patients (JC requirement {IM.6.2}, 2005); and

2. The National Institute on Disability and Rehabilitation Research, NIDRR, (Carlson & Ehrlich, 2005) has noted that the technologic advances our society has seen during the past decade suggest that this union of technologic breakthroughs and our society's belief in the empowerment of people with disabilities has intensified the need for a wide range of disability and rehabilitation research. The NIDRR suggests that research not be limited to the development of new technologies and that it also include examining innovative ideas regarding interventions and policies that will further advance the quality of life for people with disabilities, which includes the acutely ill population.

It was meeting the challenge of overcoming access and opportunity barriers that led us to re-examine the use of high-end AAC systems in acute care settings. Although some of the barriers persist, it has become evident that they are surmountable.

3 The Impact of Assistive Technology (AT) in Acute Care Settings

The impact that assistive technology can have on the "acutely ill patient" may be no different that than that of the "traditional" AAC patient. AT provides has the potential of reducing any frustration and/or anxiety the patient may be experiencing. Several research studies clearly identify the "powerlessness" that is experienced by the patient with impaired verbal communication due to oral intubation and suggest that this feeling is shared by the patient's communication partners as well (Fowler, 1997; Stovsky, Rudy, & Dragonette, 1988). The need to empower the critically ill patient is paramount and may be a factor in the patient's rate of improvement. Happ (2001) recommends considering the acutely ill patient's impaired communication and communication related responses along with the mental health status and the severity of their diagnosis. The literature is consistent in stating that there is a significant relationship between the patients' perceived state of responsiveness and the degree of positive communication by the patient's nurse. Nurses tend to have more positive communication encounters with those patients whom they perceive to be more responsive (Ashworth, 1980; Happ, 2001; Leathart, 1994). This point was clearly evident in Ashworth's study (1980) of communication difficulties between nurses and intubated patients. Ashworth observed the communicative interactions between nurses and patients on 5 intensive care units in England. Her investigation identified some key factors that influenced communication between 39 intubated patients and 115 nurses caring for those patients. Her findings suggested that 71% of the all communication was considered to be task-related and short in duration (less than one minute). She characterized these task-related encounters to be made up mostly of commands and questions associated with procedures related to the physical care of the patient.

Ashworth's findings were confirmed in similar studies conducted by Saylor and Stuart (1985) and Leathart (1994). The Saylor and Stuart study was a small-scale study of nurses who were permanently assigned to intensive care units and whose patients were intubated and conscious. Leathart (1994) designed an exploratory study to determine the state of communication between conscious, intubated, and orientated patients, and intensive care nurses. In particular, Leathart was interested in determining whether nurses are able to identify the needs and problems of their patients. Although her findings were consistent with Ashworth's, clearly the heterogeneity of her patient population was not comparable to the earlier studies. Leathart (1994) suggested that intensive care nurses understand that they need to communicate with their patients as much as possible; but in practice, the nurses have discovered that by minimizing their communication with patients they can reduce their own anxiety. This is an interesting fact and one that again speaks to the need to find ways to enhance communication options for patients so as to reduce both the patients' and nurses' level of anxiety.

Leathart (1994) also identified another potential problem with the state of the literature in this area. She suggested that Saylor and Stuart's (1985) findings must be interpreted cautiously because the design of the study may have induced a form of Hawthorne effect where the subjects' knowledge that they were participating in a study could have influenced the outcome. Thus, the subjects may respond to questions or perform in an atypical manner resulting in subject bias and possibly misleading results (Treece & Treece, 1977). Leathart (1994) indicated that subjects in Saylor and Stuart's study may have given certain responses because they knew the study was about communicating with patients and responded not in terms of actual practice but in terms of what they believed the investigators wanted. In any case, one can draw the tentative conclusion from Saylor and Stuart's study that nurses can identify the "preferred" issues and strategies that may impact on communicating with their patients regardless of what they personally felt and actually implemented with their patients.

Additional studies (Benner, 1984; Bergbom-Enberg & Haljamae, 1993) have suggested that the amount and quality of nurse-patient communication may also be a function of the nurse's level of experience in the intensive care units. Bergbom-Enberg and Haljamae hypothesized that more advanced nurses, nurses with more than 5 years of experience, are more familiar with the technical tasks involved with patient care and as such can better reflect on the gestalt of the situation. In such situations the nurses are not overwhelmed by technical tasks and as such are afforded more time to establish a relationship with the patient.

Traditional care of acutely ill patients with communication needs in the past has used several supplemental low-tech communication options (Fried-Oken et al., 1991; Happ, 2001). These options have included the use of simple preprinted communication boards, pen and pencil options, as well as gesturing and attempts to mouth words. The effectiveness of these approaches has been inconsistent, and all require the full attention of the listener/communication partner. Consequently, the burden of communication is on the listener. Thus, the perception of the patient's level of alertness and the patient's ability to communicate depends on the nurse's ability to make out the patient's intentions. Supplementing the patient's ability to communicate when he or she experiences impaired verbal communication is appropriate as a strategy to reduce communication breakdown and the burden on the nurse. This argument for supplementing communication becomes even more compelling when we note that nurses do not typically receive training in interpreting gestures and lip reading which are both necessary to interpret the nonverbal communication used by patients (Happ, 2001). This lack of systematic training is most likely a contributing factor for the increased anxiety that nurses may experience when dealing with the verbally impaired patient.

When intubated patients gesture that they want to talk, by raising a hand toward their mouths, that gesture is often misinterpreted as an attempt to self-extubate. A negative outcome of that misinterpretation of that gesture is placing the patient in physical restraints.

Imagine this situation from the patient's perspective. You indicate you want to communicate and what happens is that you are "punished" by having your hands put in restraints. This turn of events will not do much for building a positive relationship with your caregivers.

Another possible contributing factor causing great anxiety for both parties may be the patient's inability to verbalize that he/she requires assistance. In an intensive care setting, this may be a factor which causes grave concern not only for the patient but also for members of the patient's family. It is hard to deal with a loved one in distress who has no means of communicating that distress. This concern is enhanced by the patient's complex medical state which may be life threatening. In such cases, family members may be reluctant to leave the patient alone, compromising their own well-being. This is most often the case with pediatric patients. Parents, although completely exhausted, refuse to leave or sleep due to their concern that their child will require assistance and no one will be there to interpret the child's efforts to get help. Access to a viable nurse call is every patient's right and is, perhaps, the most important form of communication a patient can have. Making a nurse call accessible can be a huge comfort to both the family and the patient in complex medical situations. This would allow family members and care providers to leave the bedside knowing that if the patient has needs or becomes distressed that he or she would be able to alert nursing personnel. With fairly simple low-tech methods or with some of today's higher tech options, it is fairly easy to adapt the conventional nurse call so that all patients can activate them easily (see Chapters 5, 6, and 7).

Although limited research regarding the use of high-tech AAC systems with acutely ill patients is available, the use of AAC in a medical setting is not completely new. For well over a decade clinicians have used some form of AAC in acute care settings. It is more common to see the use of low-tech options at the bedside. Often acutely ill patients have been provided either basic communication boards or simple pen and paper options to aid in their communication efforts. In some cases clinicians have introduced the use of an electrolarynx with the acutely ill patients who are not orally intubated. The routine use of these lower tech forms of AAC has been characterized by Mitsuda, Baarslag-Benson, Hazel, and Therriault, (1992) who concluded that AAC teams in hospital settings must address the following to ensure successful implementation of AAC systems:

1. Understand the administration attitudes/barriers,
2. Understand the organizational attitudes/barriers, and
3. Address personnel training needs.
4. Ensure the availability of equipment. That includes electronic options like a lightweight neck-type electrolarynx, or an oral-type electolarynx and other low-tech options such as alphabet, word, and picture boards, as well as, simple wipe boards. The clinician should have portable and mountable

message boards or eye gaze/pointing boards that can be used at the bedside.

Although the use of an electrolarynx and/or low-tech options have helped some patients, these forms of AAC continue to be of limited utility for patients with significant motor impairments. Intubated patients are limited in their ability to move the oral structures necessary for the successful use of an electrolarynx. Likewise, patients with limited or no limb movements are unable to hold the electrolarynx and activate it.

Many of these patients often face long hospitalizations followed by long-term rehabilitation. The need to medically stabilize the patient can often delay the start of rehabilitation for a considerable period. Meanwhile the patient's psychological well-being can easily become compromised. Again, imagine yourself as a nonverbal patient with much to say but no way to say it. If your hands don't work, the use of pen and pencil or a simple wipe board is of no help to you. It is typical that such a patient is faced with overwhelming fear and a sense of hopelessness (Happ et al., 2004).

Again, we would like to suggest that the limited use of high-tech AAC options in hospital settings is due to several access barriers described by Garrett et al. (2007) as practice barriers, equipment barriers, environmental barriers, and attitude barriers. Equipment barriers can spill over and become practice barriers. In the past, limits on technology and the high cost associated with high-tech systems also contributed to professional/administrational and organizational barriers. The technology may have had limited functionality and the staff may have been ill-prepared to program and implement the available AAC systems. Our experience has shown that recent advances in technology allow for increased successful use of AAC in acute care settings. Our ability to demonstrate the successful implementation of high-end AAC systems should aid the clinician in overcoming the access opportunity barrier of "attitude." We acknowledge personnel training is critical to successful implementation and address this vital issue in Chapter 12. It is highly likely that the lack of adequate personnel training will continue to perpetuate access opportunity barriers. How can nurses or other health care providers refer patients to speech-language pathology if they have not been provided training regarding the existence of augmentative/alternative communication options?

Garrett et al. (2007) suggest that environmental barriers are in place in the ICU which may preclude the use of higher tech AAC systems. However, this barrier can be overcome (see Chapter 7) by using IV poles (common equipment available on all ICUs) as a mounting platform for the AAC device thereby allowing for a multitude of positioning options for patients. The need for ease and flexibility of positional changes is paramount as ICU patients often are placed on inflated beds that continually change the patient's position. By incorporating equipment in a less obtrusive manner, we can remove potential resistance from health care professionals about introducing additional technology at the bedside. ICU health care providers work in an environment where they must deal with complex medical conditions, an array of high-end life-saving equipment and extremely emotional family members. Any additional stress added to this equation is especially undesirable.

REVIEW OF AAC IN ACUTE CARE SETTINGS

Although the literature on the use of high-end AAC options is sparse, there are four medical centers pioneering the use of AAC in acute care settings. They include: Costello (2000) at Boston's Children's Hospital; Happ et al. (2005) at the University of Pittsburgh Medical Center; Etchels et al. (2003) at the Ninewells Hospital in Dundee; and our work (Hurtig & Downey, 2005, 2006) on the implementation of high-end speech generating devices at the University of Iowa Hospitals and Clinics (UIHC). These four represent the genesis of implementation of AAC in acute care settings.

Costello (2000) developed a model for the use of AAC interventions for patients with planned admissions who would be in critical care units due to post-surgical management needs. He studied 43 patients ranging from 2.8 to 44 years of age who experienced temporary loss of speech secondary to intubation, tracheostomy, and/or mechanical ventilation. He outlined the details of preoperative and postoperative interventions as well as strategies for patient directed vocabulary selection and digital voice message banking, using a range of low- to high-end AAC devices (e.g., Step-by-Step, DynaVox). Costello conducted discharge interviews with patients and family members that revealed that the Boston Children's model successfully addressed the anticipated need to communicate via alternate means, as 100% of the participants denied feelings of frustration or stress due to their inability to speak during the postsurgical period when they did not have use of their natural voice.

Happ et al. (2005) investigated the use of voice output systems with patients following surgical procedures for head and neck cancer. She studied 10 patients with a mean age of 57 years who received electronic speech-generating devices, even though they retained functional writing abilities, following their surgical intervention. In addition to the option of using handwriting, she offered patients a choice of two different voice output devices: (a) the Message Mate, a multi-level communication aid that uses digitally recorded speech and offers the patient up to 32 messages per level and (b) the DynaMyte, a high-end communication device with unlimited vocabulary/message options, that was programmed to provide an on-screen keyboard for text-to-speech generation as well as environmental control (ECU) options. She reported that most of her patients preferred writing and gesturing to the voice output devices, but noted that voice output devices may be more practical for patients who want to construct complex messages in the immediate postoperative period. It is important to note that there appeared to be two potentially negative factors influencing this study.

First, the Message Mate limits the user's vocabulary and does not provide the user with environmental control options, which can be critical in empowering the patient and lead to the patient's "buy in" to use the designated communication system. Secondly, the configuration of the DynaMyte, while providing its users with an on-screen keyboard, is not as efficient as more standard text-to-speech devices such as the DynaWrite or LightWRITER. The DynaWrite and LightWRITER devices provide users with a standard keyboard allowing them to use actual keyboarding skills, as compared to the one-handed "hunt and peck" strategy that is the typical access mode for on-screen keyboards. Thus, Happ's device implementations may have been viewed by the patients as either being too limiting or too slow. This led to her conclusion that the barriers to successful implementation of high-end AAC systems would need to be addressed by design improvements, staff education, and individual assessment by a speech-language pathologist with expertise in AAC.

The ICU-Talk project (Etchels et al., 2003) was a collaborative effort of the Department of Applied Computing, the School of Nursing and Midwifery at Dundee University, the Department of Speech-Language Pathology and the Intensive Care Units at Ninewills Hospital, Dundee, to examine the communication problems of their patients. Their collaboration led to the birth of a prototype software system (ICU-Talk), which was designed specifically for their intubated patients who were alert and interested in communicating. They surveyed nurses who cared for 19 patients, 36 to 76 years of age, who used the ICU-Talk system. The patients involved in this study were unable to write. Their survey results indicated:

- 68% of the nursing staff indicated they needed to cue the patient to use ICU-Talk.
- 44% indicated that the patients used ICU-Talk with someone other than the nurse.
- 12% indicated that patients used ICU-Talk as the first means of communication.
- 44% indicated that ICU-Talk helped with patient care.
- 24% indicated that ICU-Talk did not interfere with their observation(s) or care of the patient.
- 72% indicated that the patients stopped using ICU-Talk and preferred other forms of communication.
- 76% indicated that they did not find it difficult to understand the patient when they used ICU-Talk.

Again, these findings highlight the need to examine the patient's needs and desire to communicate in acute care settings, as well as the nursing and medical staff's desire to provide the acutely ill patient with more effective and efficient communication options.

Hurtig and Downey (2005, 2006) have piloted the use of high-end communication systems (DynaVox, Assistive Technology Inc., Prentke-Romich) in all critical care units (Pediatric Intensive Care Unit [PICU], Surgical Intensive Care Unit [SICU], Medical Intensive Care Unit (MICU), Intermediate Pulmonary Care Unit [IPCU]) and step-down units at the University of Iowa Hospitals and Clinics (UIHC) with considerable success. Their work has focused on evaluating the benefits of providing a broad range of AAC options to patients who may have had compromised motor function. The majority of their patients desired enhanced communication or the ability to exercise environmental control during their hospital admission. They studied more than 200 patients ranging in age from toddlers to octogenarians. Their preliminary findings indicate that high-end assistive technology can be implemented with a variety of patients across the life span with various etiologies and prognoses. The Hurtig and Downey study contradicts earlier studies (Fried-Oken et al., 1991) which indicated that the use of high-end speech generating devices was not preferred by most acutely ill patients. These findings may reflect both the impact of technologic advances and more tailored programming of the devices to meet the needs of acutely ill patients.

The Hurtig and Downey protocol has been effectively used with trauma and burn victims, patients with cancer, neurodegenerative diseases, Guillian-Barré syndrome, organ failure, and transplant candidates all of whom have required ventilatory support. Given the diversity of the patients in the Iowa implementation, some patients were provided an introduction to AAC prior to admission and intubation whereas others (particularly trauma admissions) received their AAC systems once they were intubated. We consistently observed that providing environmental control unit (ECU) options can be the significant motivator to engage patients and to have them accept the AAC system and use its communication functions. Providing some level of ECU served as a starting point for the most challenging patients, including patients facing long-term disability. We noted that this also led to a "buy in" by nurses and physicians. Certainly, a patient who demonstrates the ability to use a device to communicate or control something in his or her environment will be viewed as being "more responsive."

Again, just imagine laying in bed with the overwhelming sense that life as you know it is over. This is often the feeling that motor vehicle accident victims experience. Their life has been changed in an instant, and they often experience a complete loss of control and can fairly quickly spiral down into deep depression. The use of environmental control units may not at first glance appear to be related to a patient's communication needs; it is, however, a powerful tool that can be used in the acute care setting to empower the patient and provide him or her with that "sense of self-control." ECUs can be used to provide the patient with a means to control any electronic device (e.g., a fan, a radio, a television). It has been our experience, at Iowa, that patients who initially refuse an AAC system will often agree to some form of ECU. As stated previously, improving the patient's "sense of self-control" can reduce the anxiety and frustration that the patient may be experiencing. Downey and Hurtig (2006) found that providing environmental controls is a necessary component of the overall AAC system and one that can be used as the motivator to engage patients, including the most challenging patients or patients facing long-term disability. The use of ECU, also, can alter the nurse's perception of the patient's level of responsiveness and, thereby, increase opportunities for positive communication between the nurse and the patient.

4 Assessment Protocol

Imagine how frustrating it must be for the patient to experience an array of examiners who constantly ask the patient to perform tasks that the patient is unable to complete. Such constant perceived failures, on the part of the patient, emphasize their immediate disability and may contribute to increased anxiety and depression. In the context of so much failure, a patient may not be willing to undertake any instrumental AAC/AT intervention.

The protocol used at Iowa includes screening of the patients' sensory status, alertness level, motor abilities, cognitive-linguistic status, as well as their visual literacy and reading skills. The protocol is twofold: (a) interview of the patient's care staff and family members, and (b) a 5- to 10-minute bedside evaluation. Table 4–1 summarizes the fundamental questions one needs to address in such an assessment.

A preliminary review of the patient's sensory status is suggested as the starting point. Nursing staff and family members can provide the clinician with specific information regarding the patient's hearing and visual status. It is important not to assume that the patient does not wear glasses or use hearing aids simply because they are absent at the bedside. Sadly, there have been many cases where we have been the first to determine that the patient does wear glasses or uses hearing aids. It has been our experience that there are a number of reasons why glasses and/or hearing aids may be missing

Table 4–1. Questions to Be Addressed in Assessment

Is the patient alert and responsive?
Can one elicit a reliable yes/no response?
Is the patient aware of his/her condition (immediate and long-term)?
Can the patient use an unaided alternative communication system?
Does the patient understand the need for having an AAC system?
Can the patient understand how the AAC system works?
Does the patient understand the unique pragmatic constraints involved when using an AAC system?

(facial edema, patient's state of arousal, family member's fear of items becoming misplaced or the items may have been broken or lost when the trauma was sustained by the patient). This information is vital to ensure that the subsequent bedside evaluation is efficient and accurate.

The preliminary assessment continues with inquiry into the patient's ability to answer "yes/no" questions. Typically, the establishment of a patient's ability to answer such questions may have already been identified by the nursing staff or family members (Dowden, Honsinger, & Beukelman, 1986). It is important to capitalize on already existing forms of communication as long as they are functional for the caregivers and patient (Beukelman & Mirenda, 2005).

The preliminary assessment should conclude with a nursing summary of the status of the patient's motor functions. Nursing staff are often most familiar with a patient's range of motor skills. Physicians, physical therapists, and occupational therapists may also be good sources of information on the status of a patient's motor systems and the prognosis for improvement. Such information is vital to identifying reliable switch access sites if the patient has any form of compromised motor functions. The criticality of this information is that it leads the clinician to identify possible access sites quickly, thus reducing the patient's frustration by allowing the patient the opportunity to exhibit successful acts immediately.

In the absence of information from other caregivers, establishing a patient's ability to provide a consistent yes/no response is the first step to establishing any form of AAC/AT intervention. To begin with it will be necessary to get the patient to orient to the examiner. Because of the range in patients' states of arousal it may require a combination of visual, auditory and somatosensory stimulation to get a patient's attention. In doing this, it is essential that the level of stimulation be appropriate. When low stimulation levels may not be sufficient, one should not assume that one should automatically then shout and use vigorous somatosensory stimulation. Too strong a stimulation level may elicit a startle response with a variety of negative effects. It is essential that as one stimulates the patient that one attend carefully to any response by the patient. A patient may not open his eyes when asked to do so but may nevertheless be orienting toward the examiner with a subtle positional change. These positional changes may include:

- a shift in position/orientation like a tilting of the head
- a change in facial expression
- a change in tenseness of all or part of the body
- a slight movement of a limb.

In addition to answering the question, "Is the patient responsive?" one must make a determination of what sensory input channels are most suitable. If a patient is visually impaired or has difficulty keeping her eyes open using a visual display may not be effective. Likewise if a patient is deaf or hearing impaired use of auditory prompts may be equally ineffective. We have encountered many patients who for a variety of reasons have not been able to open their eyes or keep their eyes open for even a brief interval. Nevertheless, we have been able to use visual stimulation with some of these patients by assisting them by manually lifting their eyelids for brief periods.

Having established the ability to arouse a patient and have the patient orient to the examiner the next step is to identify one area of the body the patient can volitionally control. Often, clinicians stop when they have found one volitional gesture. One should systematically explore a range of options as a patient may need to use more than one depending on the particular circumstances and whether they are using a low-, mid-, or high-tech AAC/AT system. A fairly brief examination should allow the clinician to determine how many of the following the patient is capable of producing voluntarily (Video clip 4-1).

- Nod head (up/down)
- Tilt head (left/right)
- Eye blink (once/twice or squeeze shut)
- Gaze shift (up/down/left/right)
- Move tongue (stick out or place in right/left cheek)
- Shoulder shrug (right/left)
- Squeeze hand (right/left)
- Roll arm in or out (right/left)
- Bend and extend leg (right/left)
- Extend foot (right/left)
- Point with hand with or without tool
- Touch fingers of examiner's hand in sequence

Care should be taken to determine which of these movements are positionally independent and which require assistance from gravity. For example, when determining whether a patient can flex and extend a limb it is necessary to do so over the range of positions a patient may find herself. For example when a patient is sitting up she may appear to be able to flex and extend an arm but when supine she may not be able to extend the arm. Thus, there may be no true extension but the release of the biceps and gravity give the impression of extension. In such a case the use of a switch that would be activated by extension of the limb would not be appropriate for such a patient. Some might suggest that if the patient spends considerable time sitting up that such a switch setup be used; however, this would require an alternative for when the patient is supine. In most acute care situations, we have found that if the patient is uncertain about the location of the switch and what gesture is necessary to activate the switch, it is less likely that the patient will be successful in consistently using the switch.

When working in acute care settings, there are many reasons why it might not be possible, at a particular point in time, to identify a reliable response from a patient. One should not assume that one failure to elicit a response will rule out implementing an AAC/AT intervention. Failure at a particular point may be the result of the patient's current state of arousal which may be a consequence of either the admitting condition or administered medications which might impact both physical and cognitive functions. When an assessment yields a finding that a patient is unresponsive or cannot produce a volitional response, the approach to treatment often proceeds, unfortunately, as if the patient is in a chronic irreversible state. Julia Tavalaro (1997), who suffered a massive stroke and was thought to be vegetative, lay in a hospital for years before a clinician recognized that she was capable of making a volitional response. She went on to becoming a successful AAC user who wrote a memoir about her experiences and eventually was able to leave the hospital.

Jean-Dominique Bauby, the author of *The Diving Bell and the Butterfly* (1997) suffered a massive stroke that left him "locked in" and incapable of producing any gesture other than a gaze shift. Again, the recognition of the volitional gesture allowed him not only to provide a yes/no response to allow him to participate in his care, but it also provided a means for him to dictate his touching memoir. In this case, his clinician would orally go through the alphabet (in frequency order) until he shifted his gaze to indicate that that was the letter he wanted. So, laboriously, letter by letter and word by word, he provided his readers with an insight about how one's perspective on what constitutes quality of life shifts as one finds oneself incapable of talking, eating or moving. Had there not been any periodic reassessments in either of these cases, these two patients would have continued to be trapped in their "broken" bodies with no way to actively participate in their care, to interact with friends and loved ones, or to write books. Not everyone can write as touchingly and insightfully as Tavalaro and Bauby, but like them we all have needs and feelings that we need to express. In addition to talent these two individuals demonstrated a force of will that allowed them to write and communicate even when the only means at their disposal required every ounce of energy and sustained attention as well as tremendous demands on memory.

We have seen this similar will power in many of our AAC cases. Many individuals with ALS choose to use AAC devices that allow them to generate novel messages letter by letter even though phrase based systems would be physically easier. Recently, a client with cerebral palsy, seen in our clinic, wrote a brief paragraph to let us know what his goals for therapy were. He used his high-tech AAC device (Prentke-Romich, Pathfinder) in "spell mode" to compose that paragraph. There are many factors in his case that work against efficient use of his communication device, yet he spent almost 5 continuous hours composing that brief message. In large part, he is significantly hampered by poor positioning and device access problems. Hopefully, better positioning to allow easier access to his device as well as work on communication strategies will allow him to channel his energies and enhance his productivity. Just as with chronic patients, working with acute care patients requires dynamic assessment so that as a patient's responsiveness changes or as the patient demonstrates increased motor function an appropriate intervention can be implemented.

Once a volitional movement has been identified so that a patient can consistently provide a response to a yes/no question (Video clip 4-2), one can begin to systematically assess the patient's level of alertness. This can be done with a set of simple questions for which the appropriate response is known to the clinician conducting the assessment (Video clip 4-3).

- Is your name _____?
- Are your eyes blue?
- Are you _____ years old?
- Is your spouse/child/parent's name _____?
- Do you live in the State of _____?
- Is _____ the President of the United States?
- Is today Friday?

These questions allow an assessment of whether the patient is oriented in time and place. Care should be taken to provide a context for asking these questions. Imagine if you were the patient and someone came to your bed and asked you if you were Tom Jones when your name was Adam Smith. You might think that the hospital was not well organized and people didn't keep track of which patient was in which room. That would not be a confidence building interaction.

Our rule of thumb is that a patient may be considered alert and responsive if he or she provides at least three correct responses. Care must be taken to be aware of the patient's medical state and medications when attempting this assessment. For many patients it may be necessary to attempt the assessment repeatedly over a period of hours or days. Being able to begin an AAC intervention as soon as a patient is able to, will not only impact the patient's care but also address the concomitant psychological issues that stem from both the medical condition and the inability to use normal modes of communication.

Having established that a patient can provide a reliable response to simple yes/no questions, it is then possible to use that response in more relevant communicative interactions. Having a sense that the patient is aware of his or her condition is a critical prerequisite to engaging the patient in discussions concerning both short-term and long-term care. To that end, being able to use the reliable and volitional response, one can probe the extent to which the patient understands:

- His/her current physical state
- His/her mobility limitations
- His/her limitations on normal modes of communication
- His/her prospects for recovery of function or long term disability
- His/her understanding the need for assistive technology for environmental control
- His/her understanding the need for AAC to communicate.

Using the identified volitional gesture, the nurse can begin to use yes/no questions with the patient as part of the care plan (Video clip 4-4).

The next step would be to assess the patient's ability to follow simple instructions and demonstrate the ability to use the identified volitional gesture to make choices from an array that are made available on a simple low-tech communication board or on some form of AAC device.

One may begin with a single option (e.g., "get my nurse") and determine whether the patient can indicate that they want to communicate the specified option. If the patient is capable of making a pointing gesture to effect a direct selection then one can proceed to position the boards where the patient can see them and effectively use the pointing gesture. If the patient can only generate a yes/no gesture then the examiner should point to the option on the board and ask the patient if the option should be selected. If the patient appears to understand and can reliably indicate the choice then one can progress to a board with two options and then, depending on the patient's performance, progress to boards with larger arrays. If there is an opportunity to give the patient the ability to request or directly achieve environmental control (ECU) one can construct single and multiple step instructions (e.g., turn on the TV; turn on the TV and turn on the fan). For the patient who can make direct selections this step is straight forward (Video clip 4-5). For the patient who can only generate a simple gesture one must introduce the concept of scanning and instruct the patient to generate the gesture when the appropriate choice is indicated in the scanning. If a low-tech board is used, then the examiner should slowly move a finger across the array while watching for the patient to make the required response (Video clip 4-6). If an electronic device is used and the patient can activate a switch, then the device's scanning option can be activated (Video clip 4-7). If the patient can handle longer arrays it may be possible to introduce the options in a two-dimensional grid pattern (Figure 4-1, button grid).

To facilitate the use of these larger arrays, it will be necessary to introduce a nonserial scanning pattern for those patients who cannot use direct selection. Typically a row-column pattern is used (Figure 4-2, row/column scheme). It is essential that a patient can demonstrate that they understand how the scanning pattern works if one is to provide the patient with a significant number of options.

Because there will always be some physical limitations to the number of items that can be displayed on a single page/screen it will also be necessary to determine whether the patient can understand the navigation across pages (Video clip 4-8). Again, one may want to start with a limited number of rows and columns and progress to larger and larger arrays including alphabet/keyboard layouts (Video clip 4-9).

As with the other elements of the assessment protocol, one should repeat elements of the assessment to insure the reliability of the patient's responses and understanding of the organization of the communication system.

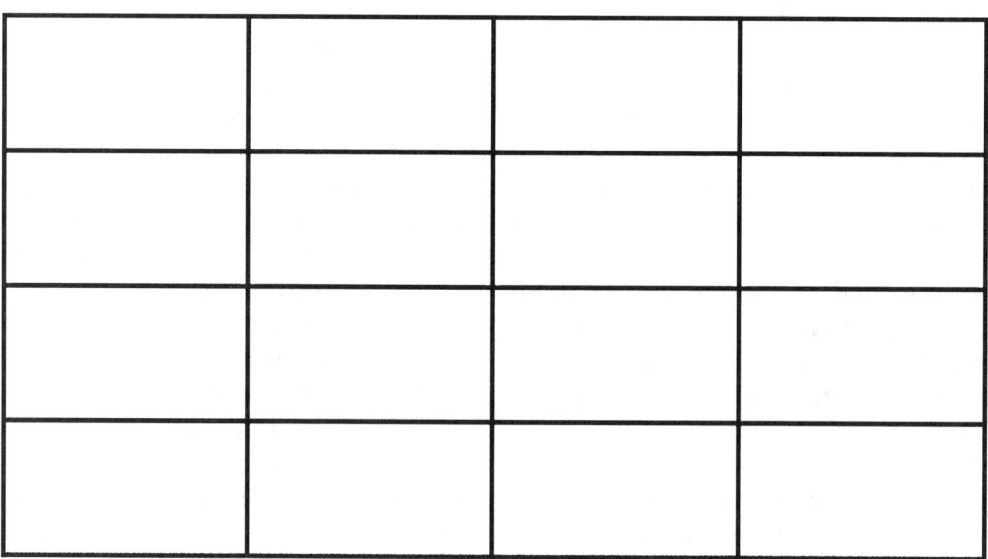

Figure 4-1. Button grid.

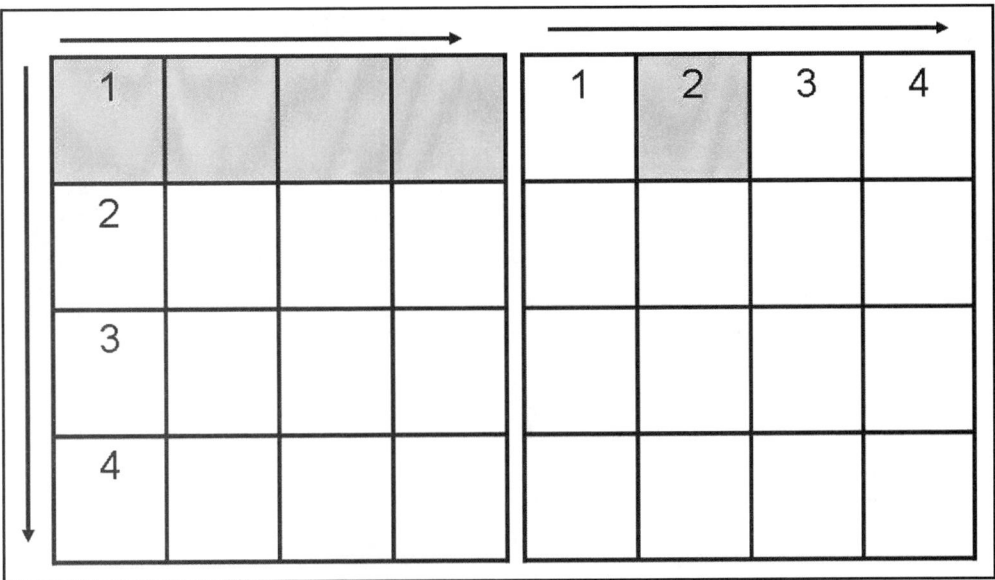

Figure 4–2. Row-column scanning scheme.

VIDEOS FOR THIS CHAPTER

Video clip 4–1. Identifying voluntary movement.

Video clip 4–2. Yes-no response—hand squeeze.

Video clip 4–3. Yes-no response—eye gaze.

Video clip 4–4. Yes-no response—used in managing care.

Video clip 4–5. Environmental control via direct selection.

Video clip 4–6. Caregiver manual scanning.

Video clip 4–7. High-tech device—auto scanning.

Video clip 4–8. High-tech multiple page-set AAC system.

Video clip 4–9. Using a high-tech on-screen keyboard.

5 Switches as the First Step to Establishing Communication

The first step to establishing communication is getting the attention of a communication partner. When we are in earshot and in the line of sight of someone we wish to communicate with, we can use sounds and gestures to alert them that we need something or that we want to communicate. Hospitalized and bedridden patient may need to get the help of medical staff who are not at the bedside; thus, they may not able to use the conventional means of initiating communication. For the hospitalized patient, being able to summon the nurse is an essential need. JC requires that each patient have access to an operational nurse call system. It is very common to see signs posted at the bedside to remind patients to use the nurse call rather than try to do something on their own and potentially fall. There are many alternatives that have been implemented in hospitals around the United States. They range from simple mechanical switches that plug into the headwall (Figure 5-1) and that are wired to the nurses station (Figure 5-2). When the patient activates the switch, a light illuminates outside the patient's room (Figure 5-3) and an audible alarm goes off at the nursing station (Figure 5-2). The call light remains illuminated until it is cancelled by the nurse on a panel in the patient's room (Figure 5-4). In settings where there is an intercom

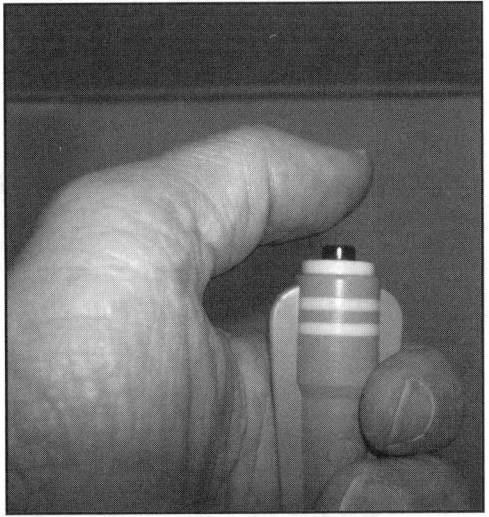

Figure 5-1. Push button nurse call.

that links patients' rooms to the nursing station, nurses may respond to patients' calls from the nursing station. In such settings, the nurse call may be integrated into a pendant that includes an intercom and controls for the bed, room lighting, and a TV (Figure 5-5). In some settings, these functions may also be incorporated into the bed rail (Figure 5-6).

The standard nurse call systems assume that a patient can activate the freestanding mechanical switches or the buttons on the pendants or on the bed rail and that they can hear and respond to the nurse over the call system intercom.

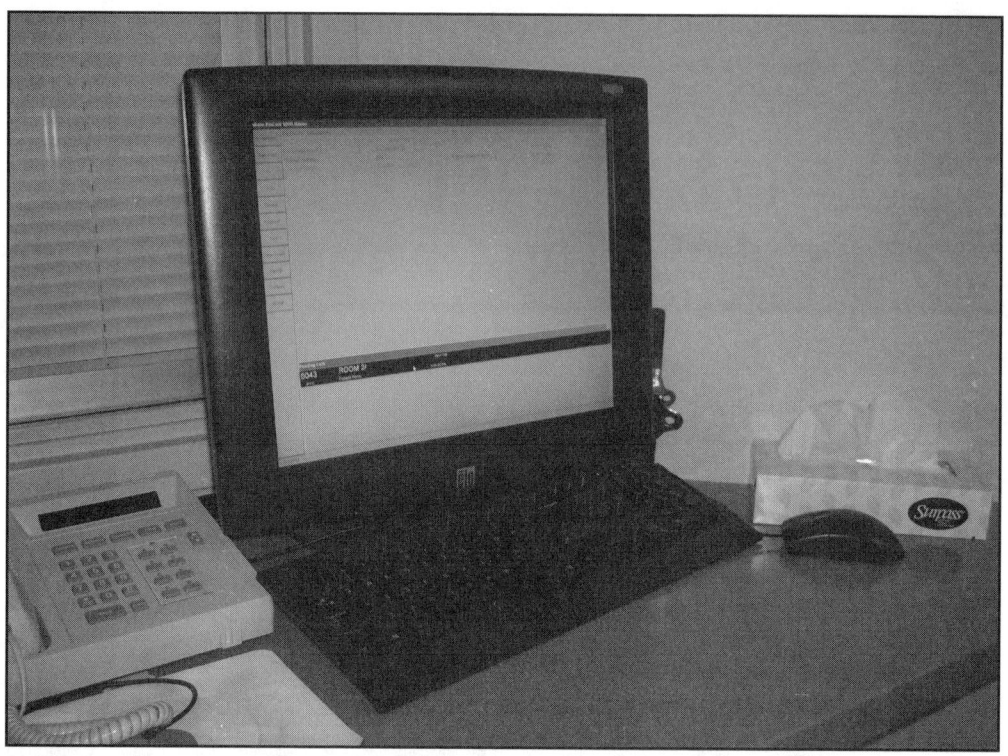

Figure 5–2. Nurse station call enunciator.

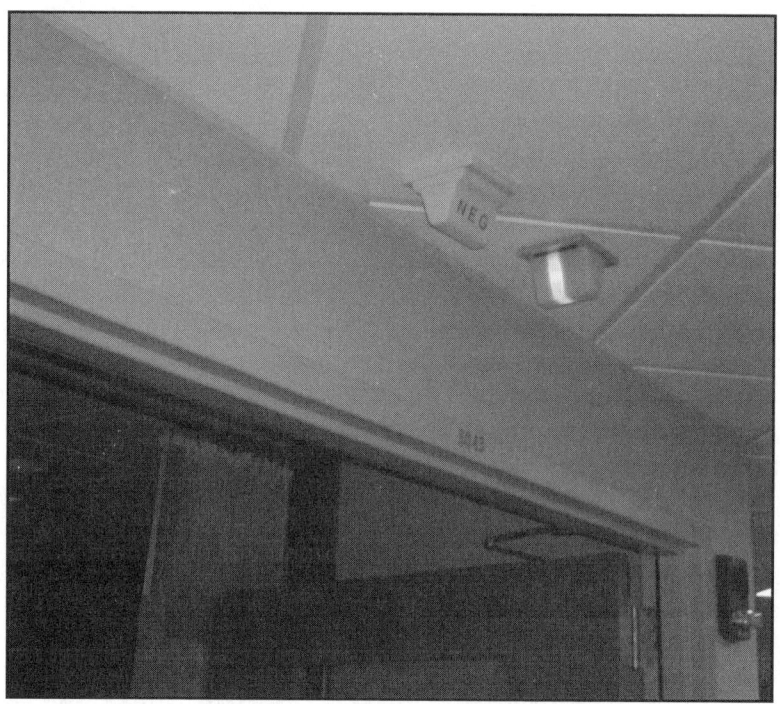

Figure 5–3. Nurse call door illuminator.

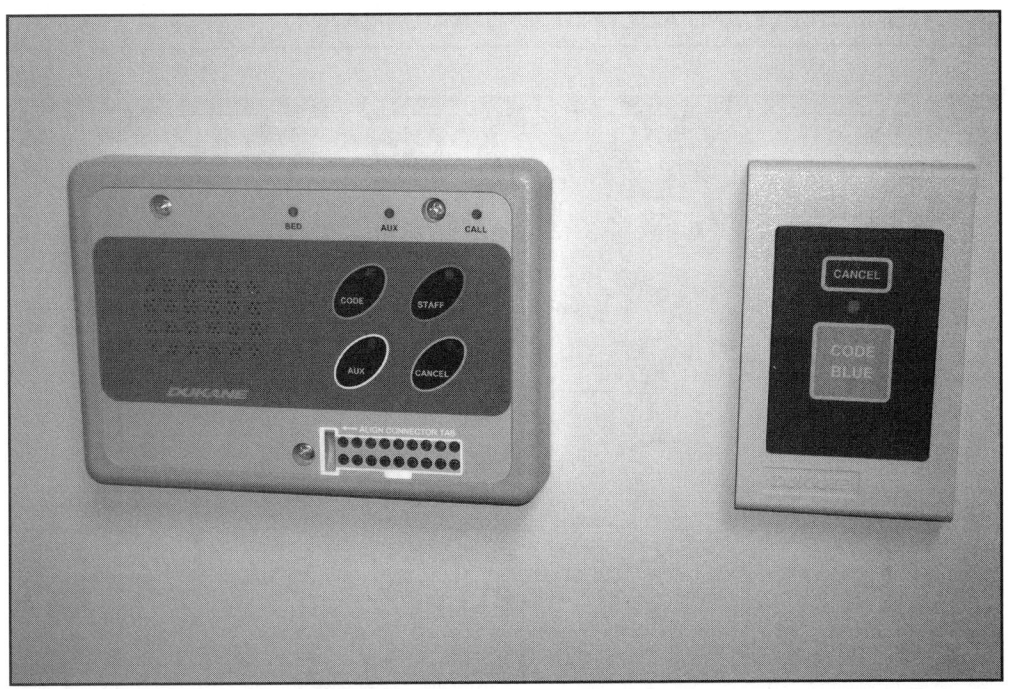

Figure 5–4. Nurse call panel on head wall in patient's room.

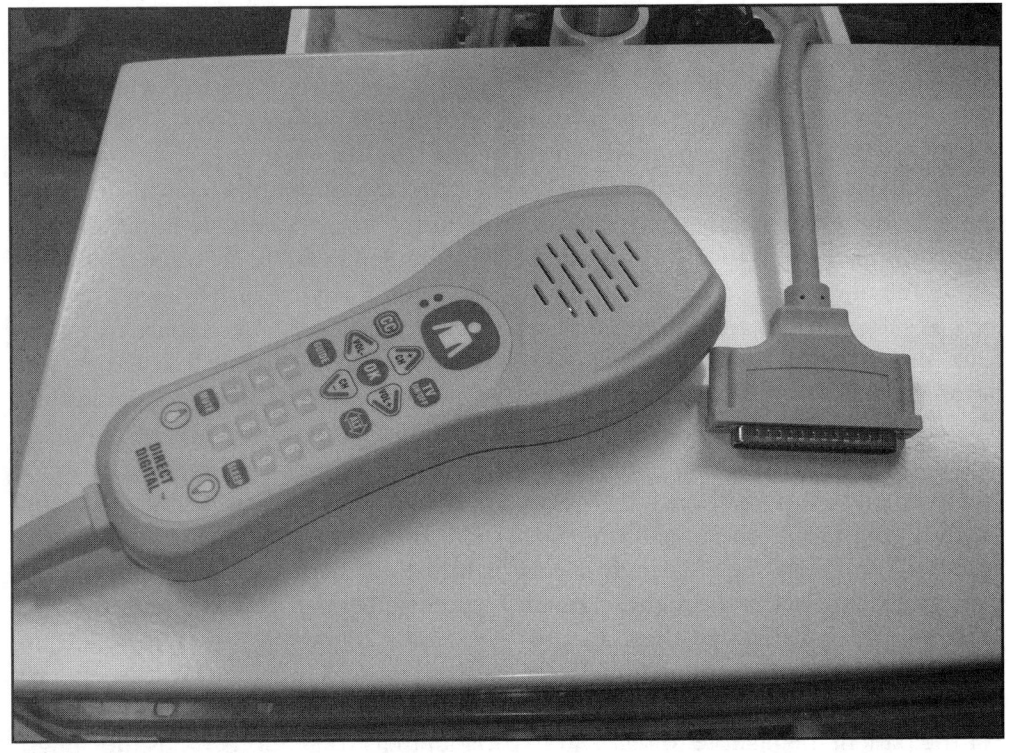

Figure 5–5. Nurse call pendant.

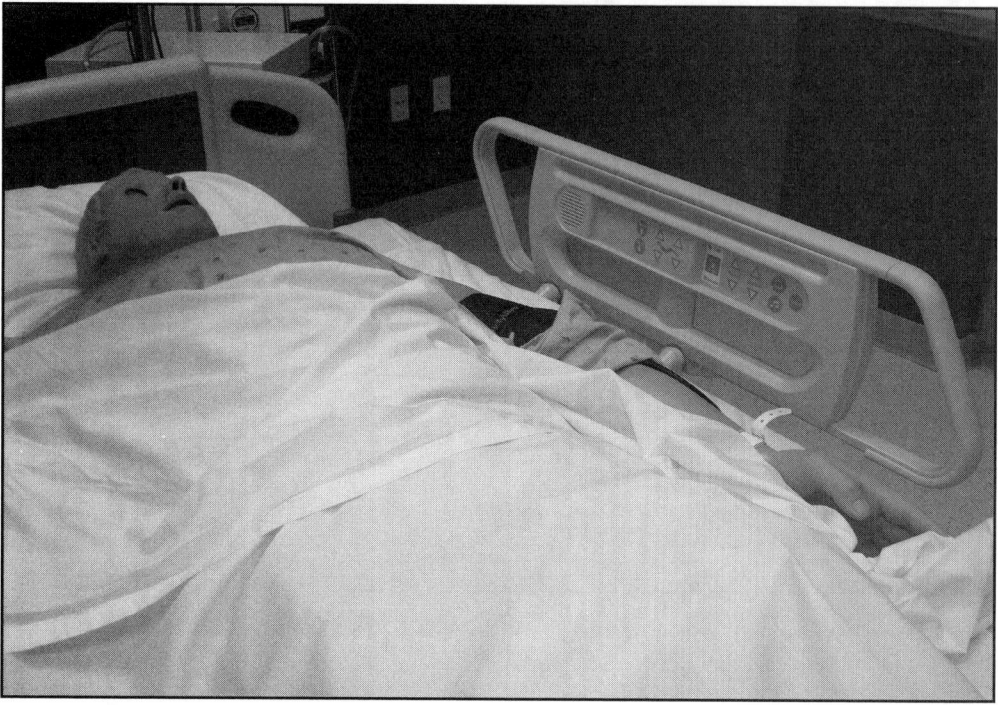

Figure 5–6. Bed rail nurse call button.

For the patient with limited sensory or motor abilities and who may not be able to speak, these systems pose a serious challenge. Such patients are anxious about being left alone and may attempt dangerous maneuvers to attract the attention of the nurses. Likewise, family members of such patients are also hesitant to leave the room for fear that their loved ones might not be able to summon help if needed. Situations such as these can lead to the development of an unhealthy codependency relationship, which may not be conducive to the long-term rehabilitation of the patient. For family members to be of assistance in the care of patients, it is essential that they get adequate rest and nutrition and that they can attend to their affairs outside the hospital. For the patient, being able to rest and to have some solitude may also be critical.

This may be particularly important to adolescents for whom "privacy" is perhaps most highly valued.

Because of the mechanical simplicity of nurse call systems, it is difficult for able bodied individuals to see how a simple switch may be difficult for a patient to access. Nevertheless there are many patients who are unable to use nurse call systems in their standard configurations. The most common cause of failure to access the nurse call is less related to the patient's abilities than to the placement of the switch or call pendant. Often, after some bedside treatment or after the patient has been repositioned, the staff or family members forget to place the switch or call pendant within the patient's reach. In such scenarios, when the patient has some motor skills they might attempt a dangerous maneuver to reach the switch. Alternatively, they may resort to shouting for the nurse. The latter strategy may unintentionally violate politeness conventions, disturb other patients, and result in a less than cordial relationship between the patient and the staff.

Some patients discover less disturbing alternative means of signaling for help. These may involve pushing something off the bed tray or the bed itself. These are not terribly effective as the sound may not carry, and once the item has been dropped, it cannot be retrieved to be used again. Like the call pendant, the nurse on coming into the room may place the object out of reach so that "it would not be dropped again." This is often the case when the object that was dropped was a urinal or telephone. Some patients have been known to ask for a bell or a rattle (e.g., beads in a specimen cup) that they might use as an alternative. In all such cases, the key to access is the care that nurses and family members take to make sure that whatever the patient uses is within reach.

Some patients on monitored units and who might be on ventilators discover that small positional changes can set off alarms. A small head position change can shift the position of the endotracheal tube and break the seal of the inflated cuff, which will set off a ventilator alarm. Agitated patients have been known to pull on the vent line and break the connection to the endotracheal tube or tracheostomy in order to set off the alarm to get the attention of medical staff. The risk of self-extubation is that such behavior creates often results in the patient being put into physical restraints and/or sedated. In many cases, the gesturing toward or tugging at the vent line is not an attempt to extubate, but the only means available to a patient who is merely trying to get attention.

Some hospital beds are equipped with sensors that detect if the patient attempts to get out of bed and then signal the nursing station. Compliant patients nevertheless have discovered that some positional changes, short of getting off the bed, will also set off such alarms. Patients' use of positional changes to use the alarms as an alternative nurse call system may be misinterpreted. Like the risk of self-extubation, the risk of leaving the bed may result in the use of physical or chemical restraints. Patients whose blood oxygen levels are being monitored with a pulse-oximeter quickly learn that if the sensor on their finger or toe is shifted slightly, the oxymeter alarm is activated and can be used to summon the nurse. Unfortunately, this can also be misinterpreted as equipment failure and result in either a silencing of the alarm or a more secure taping of the sensor on the finger and toe.

The problems related to accessing the nurse call system that many patients face result from either the failure of staff and family to ensure that the nurse call switch is within reach of the patient or the patient's failure to activate the nurse call because of limited strength, limited mobility, or excessive tremor. The former problems can be addressed with adequate staff training and family orientation to the need of never leaving a patient without checking that he or she can access the nurse call and that the call system is properly functioning. As simple as this may seem, the inability to reach the nurse call continues to be a problem in most hospitals and care facilities. Addressing the latter problems requires access to alternative nurse call technology or the ability to make modifications to existing systems that will enable the physically challenged patient to use them effectively.

NURSE CALL SYSTEMS: ALTERNATIVES AND MODIFICATIONS

The key to a successful alternative nurse call system is the identification of a switch or switch technology that the patient can activate. The most common alternatives to the nurse call pendant utilize either a pull cord or a simple push-button switch.

- The pull cord is perhaps the original nurse call system. In its mechanical version, it was connected via a pulley system to ring a bell at the nurses' station. The principle is identical to that used in "maid and butler" call systems in upper class Victorian homes. The pull cord requires the patient to pull on the cord much the same way a pull cord on a lamp or ceiling fan is used. This approach requires the patient to be able to grasp the cord and pull with sufficient force to close the microswitch installed in the headwall that closes the call circuit at the nursing station. One can still see such pull cord calls installed in doctors' office examination rooms as well as in restrooms and bathrooms (Figure 5-7).
- Simple push-button switches are usually held in the hand and activated by depressing the push button with the thumb. Patients need to be able

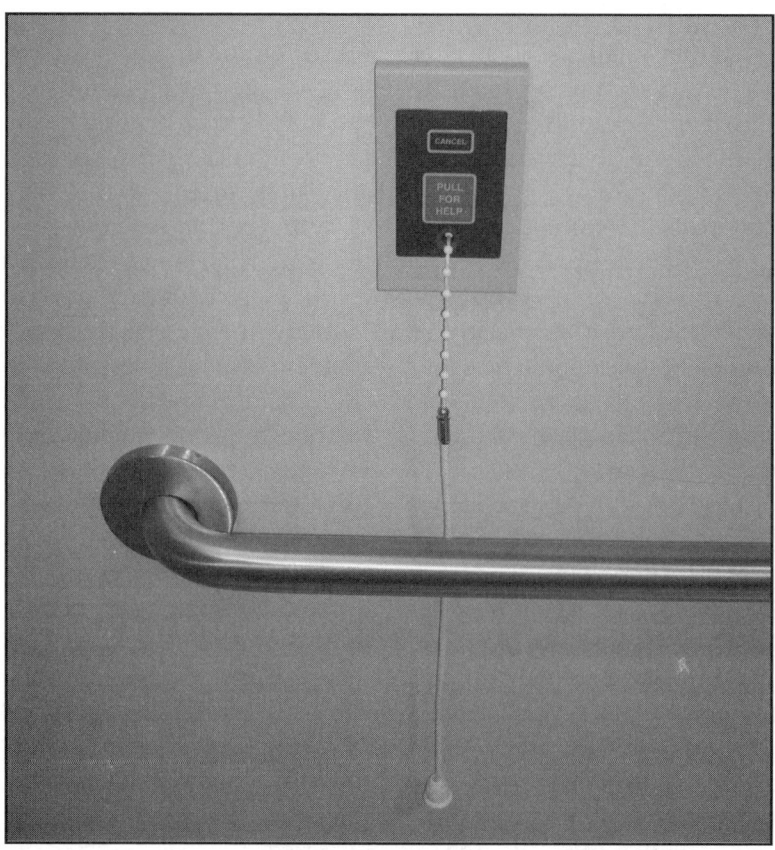

Figure 5–7. Nurse call pull cord.

to generate sufficient forces to press the button (450–470 g). Straps and or splints can be fashioned to hold the switch in the patient's hand (Figure 5-8) and keep it positioned where it can be activated with a simple movement of the thumb.

Two additional alternatives are commonly available for use in hospitals:

- One is a pneumatic bulb switch (Figure 5-9) that can be plugged directly into the headwall, assuming that an appropriate jack has been installed. This switch requires the patient to be able to squeeze the bulb at the end of the switch tubing (270–300 g). Like other nurse call systems, successful implementation requires the placement of the bulb where the patient can reach it. Clipping the cable to the bed sheet is the most common approach. When the patient is concerned about being able to reach for the bulb and when the patient lacks the motor skills to keep the bulb in the hand, the bulb can be secured in place on the patient's palm with a strap/splint or with tape (Figure 5-10). In a few cases, where the patient has no use of his or her hands, the bulb can be positioned so that the patient can grasp and squeeze the bulb with his or her lips.
- For patients who lack fine motor skills or the strength to use the pneumatic bulb switch, the use of a pressure plate switch (Figure 5-11A) should be considered. The standard nurse call pressure plate switch can be positioned so that any part of the body, that the patient can move and

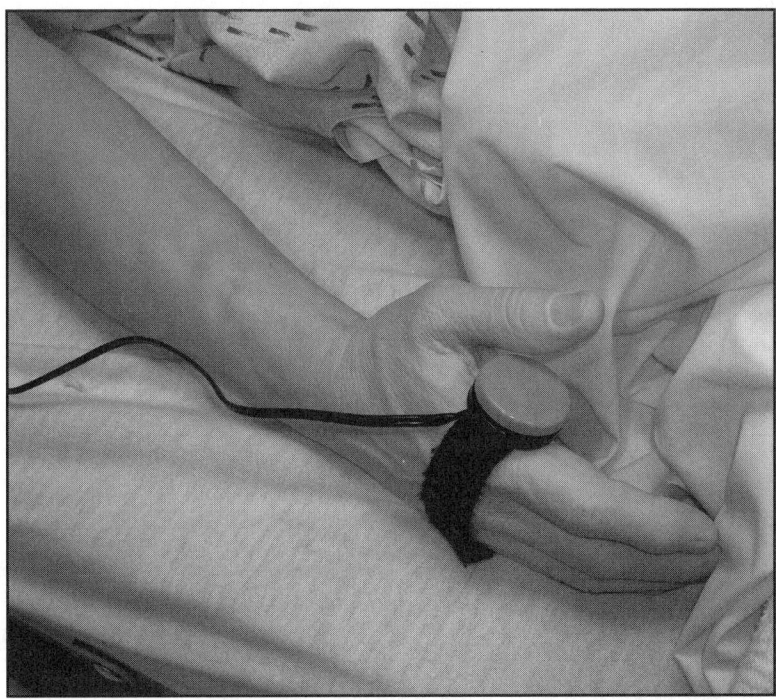

Figure 5–8. Hand strap switch.

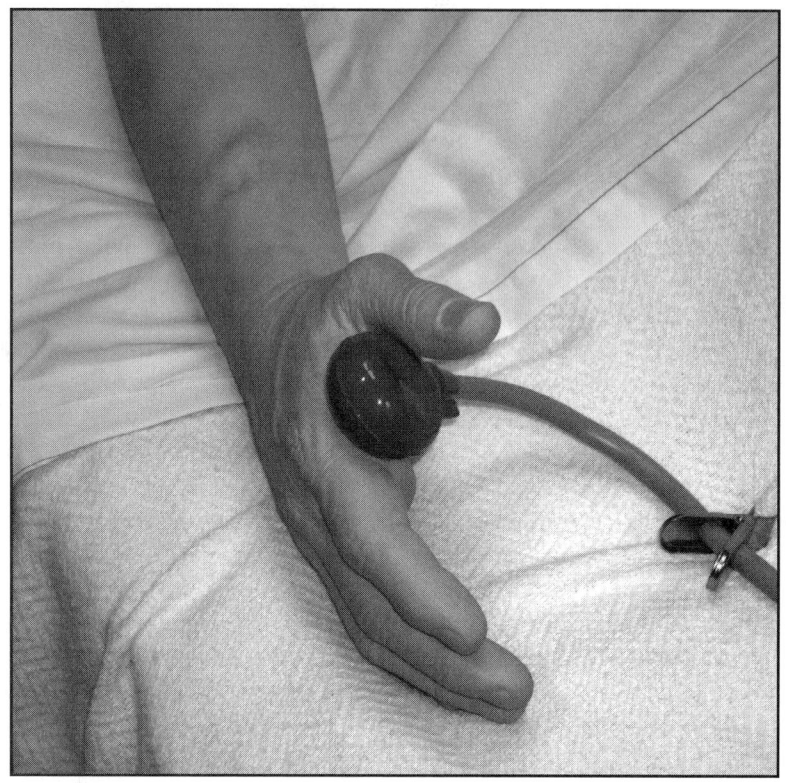

Figure 5–9. Pneumatic bulb.

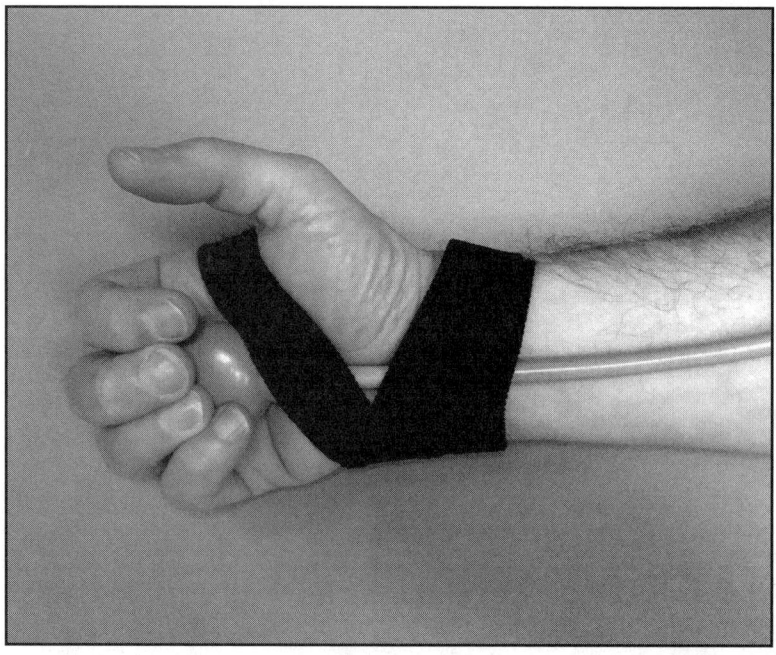

Figure 5–10. Bulb with hand strap.

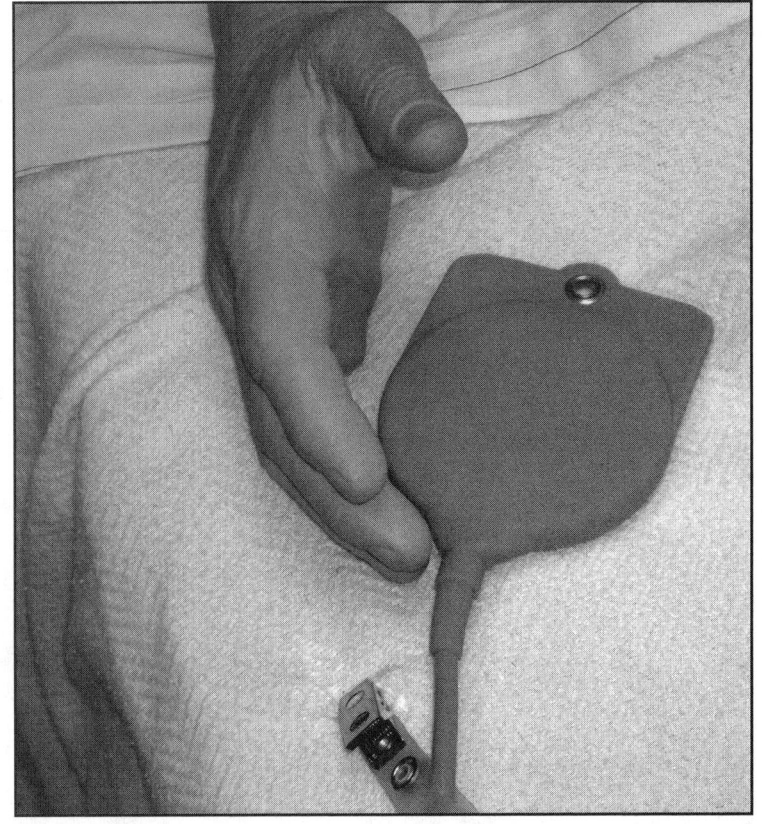

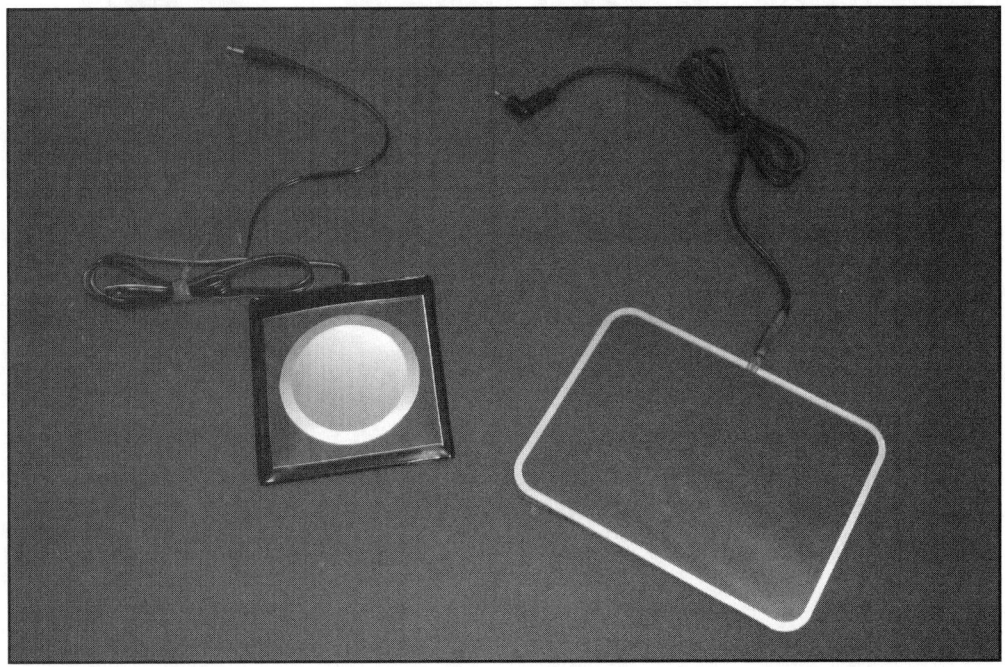

Figure 5–11. A. Pressure plate switch. **B.** Pressure plate switch.

exert a minimum of 300 to 700 grams of force with, can be used. Pneumatic versions of this switch may require anywhere from 900 to 1000 grams of force. For many patients these standard call switches require too much force and one should consider substituting pressure plate switches typically used with AAC systems, some of which only require 34 grams of force (Figure 5-11B). Key to the use of this option is proper positioning of the switch so that patients can use the arm, leg, or head to activate the switch (Figures 5-12A, 5-12B, and 5-12C).

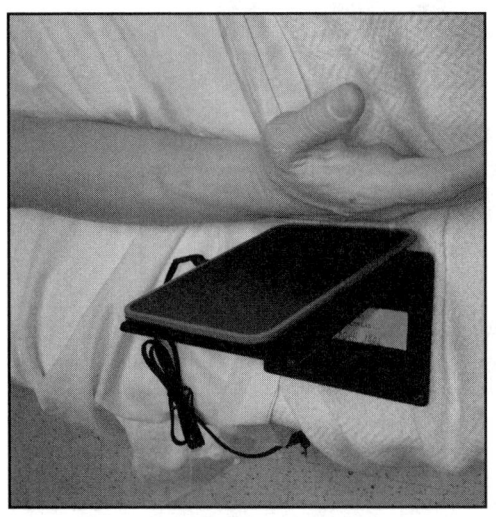

A

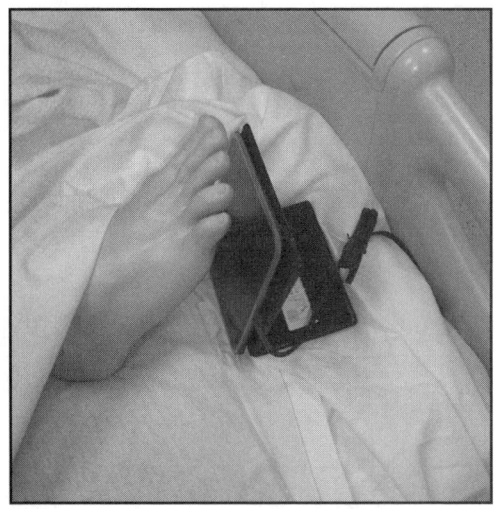

B

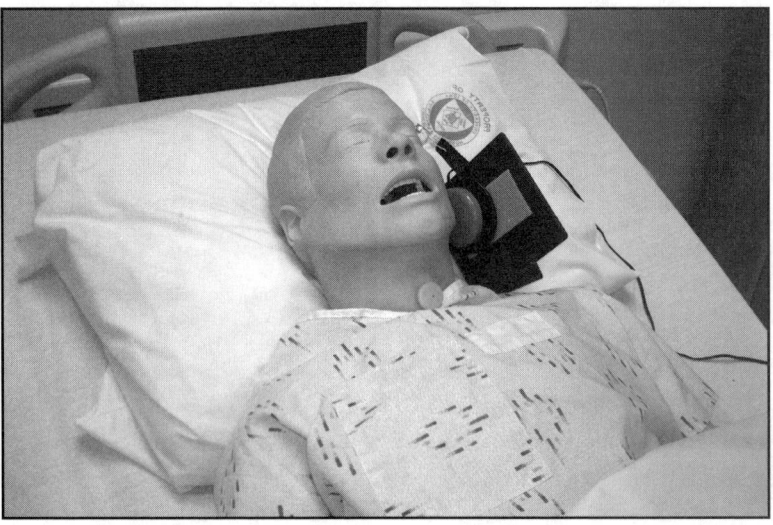

C

Figure 5–12. A. Arm switch activation. **B.** Foot switch activation. **C.** Head switch activation.

When none of the standard options discussed above can be used, alternative switch technologies that have been used in traditional AAC applications can be adapted to control the nurse call systems.

STANDARD SWITCHES

- Jelly Bean/Spec Switches: These are mechanical switches (Figure 5-13) that come in a range of sizes can be used much like the push button and pressure plate switches. These switches varying in the force and displacement required to activate them. These switches would be plugged into the headwall jack in place of the standard call switches. Like the conventional switches, proper placement for access is critical.
- Rocker Switches: These mechanical switches have a central fulcrum (Figure 5-14) so that a movement to one side or the other closes a different switch. Such switches allow the user to control two devices or a device that accepts dual inputs.
- Tongue Switch: This small switch (Figure 5-15) has a small coated lever that can be displaced by a movement of the tongue. This switch must be placed in close proximity to the mouth so that the tongue can reach the lever.
- Sip and Puff Switches: These switches (Figure 5-16) utilize either the mechanical pneumatic principle used in the pressure bulb switches or an electronic pressure sensing circuit. These switches can respond to both positive pressures (puffs) and negative pressures (sips), thereby allowing two alternative responses with a single switch. In these cases, the straw at the end of the tubing must be positioned so that the patient can grab it with his or her lips.

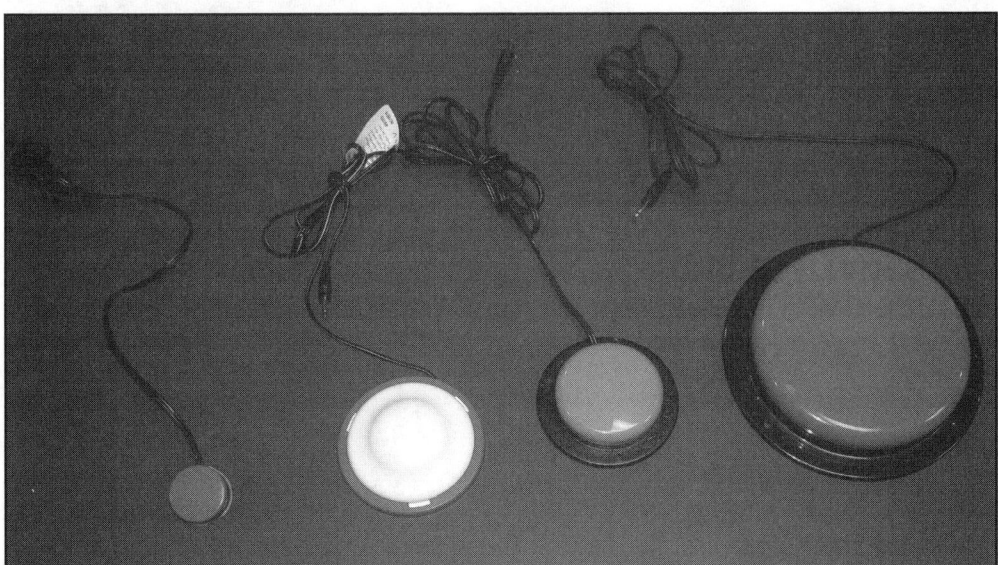

Figure 5–13. Jelly Bean/Spec switch.

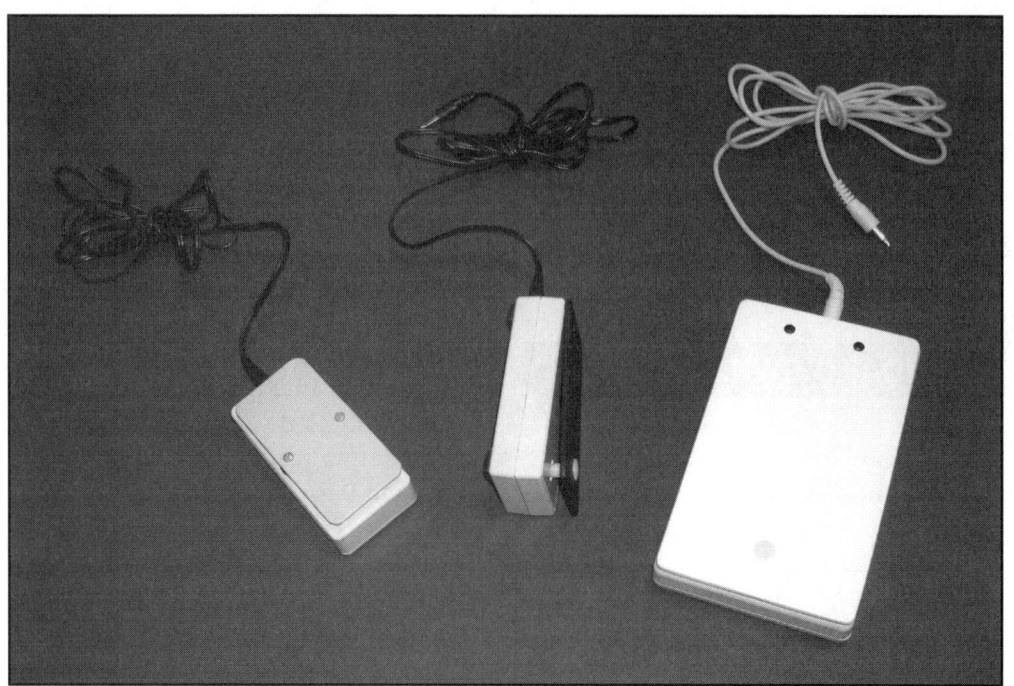

Figure 5–14. Rocker switch.

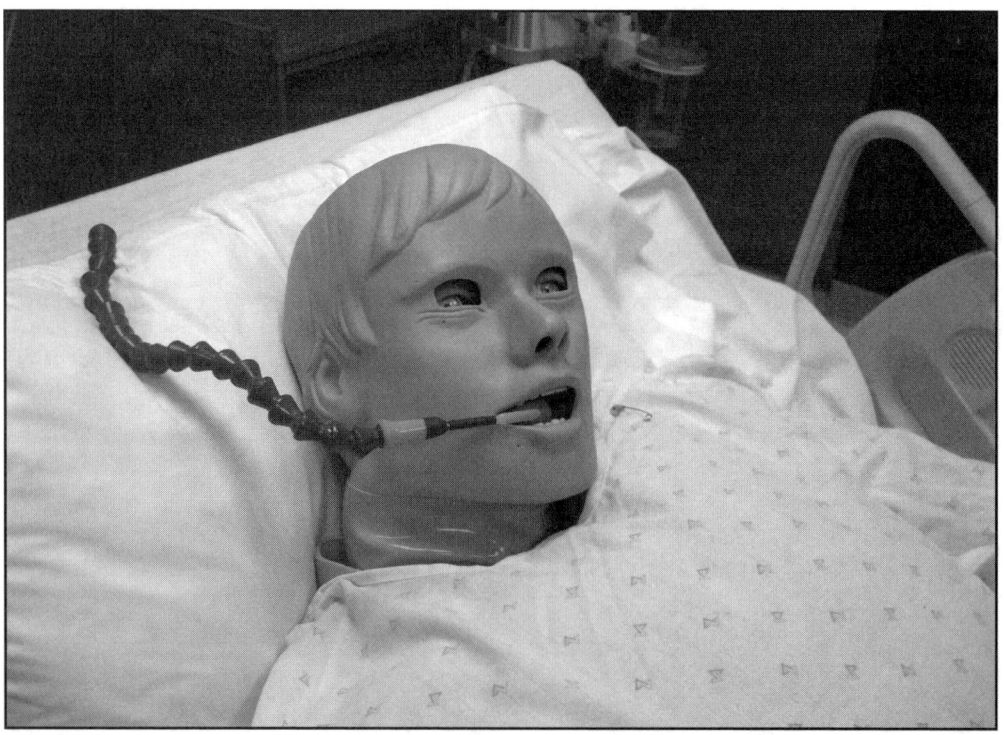

Figure 5–15. Tongue switch.

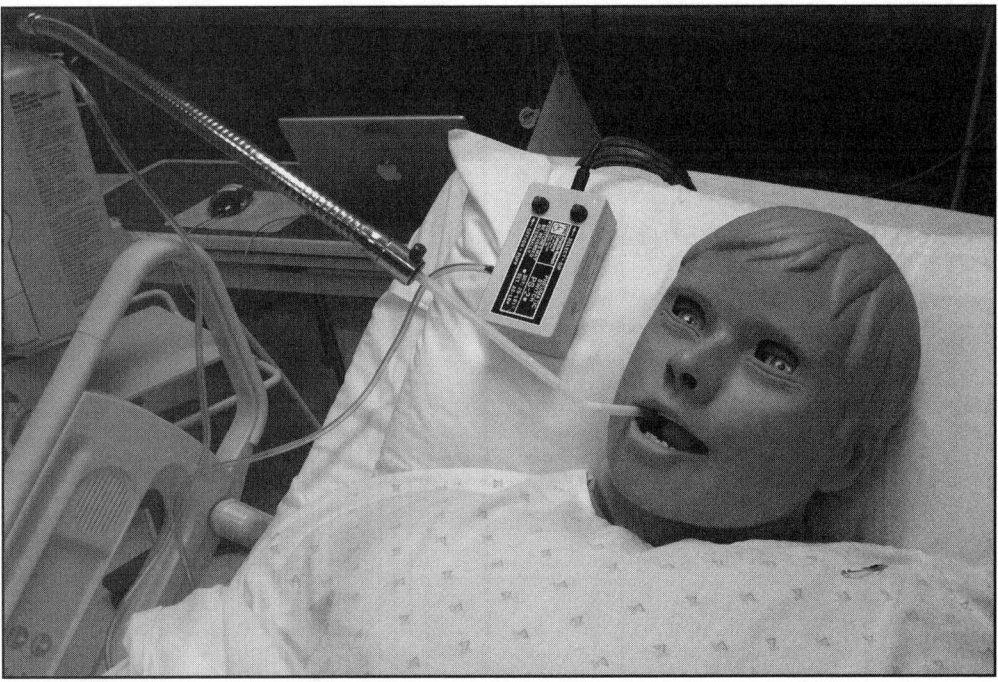

Figure 5–16. Sip and puff switch.

ADVANCED TECHNOLOGY SWITCHES

- P-Switch: This switch (Figures 5-17A and 5-17B) responds to small muscle movements. Its small circular transducer can be placed on the skin over the muscle that the patient can intentionally twitch to activate the switch. Common placements include the forehead where a rapid raising of the brow can be used or on the hand where a thumb movement can be used. This switch responds to the velocity rather than the displacement, so a slow movement will not activate the switch.
- Charge Transfer/Proximity Switch: These switches respond to the body's natural capacitance (Figure 5-18). They sense the capacitance and only require that some part of the body come in close proximity to the switch plate. No force is required to activate the switch.
- IR-Blink Switches: These switches utilize infrared (IR) light reflection to detect motion (Figures 5-19A and 5-19B). An infrared light source illuminates the target area and an infrared detector sense the reflection of the infrared light. When used as a blink switch, the change in reflectance associated with eyelid movement can be used to trigger the switch. The problem with most such switches is that they cannot distinguish the natural blink from the intentional gesture. Such switches can sometimes be adapted for use on other parts of the body. In this case,

50 AUGMENTATIVE AND ALTERNATIVE COMMUNICATION

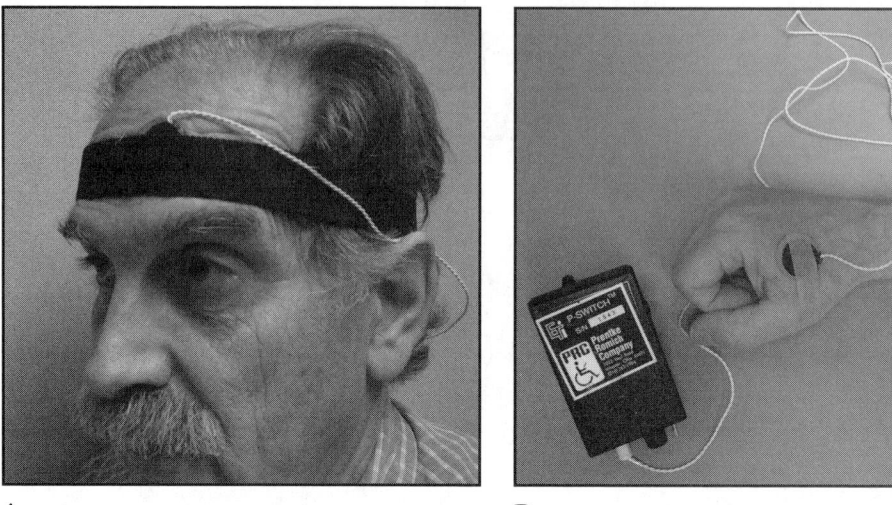

Figure 5–17. A. P-switch forehead activated. **B.** P-switch hand activated.

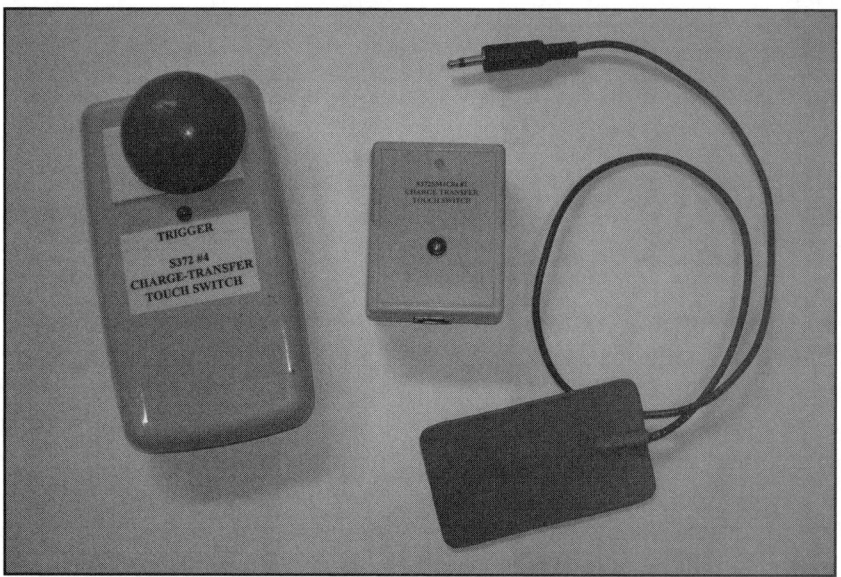

Figure 5–18. Charge transfer/proximity switch.

the voluntary movement by the patient changes the distance between the IR source and the body surface reflecting the light.
- Voice-Activated Switches: These types of switches utilize a Schmidt trigger circuitry that senses the voltage change from a microphone signal. The onset of a vocalization causes a spike in the voltage that can be used to trigger the switch. A head-mounted microphone or a

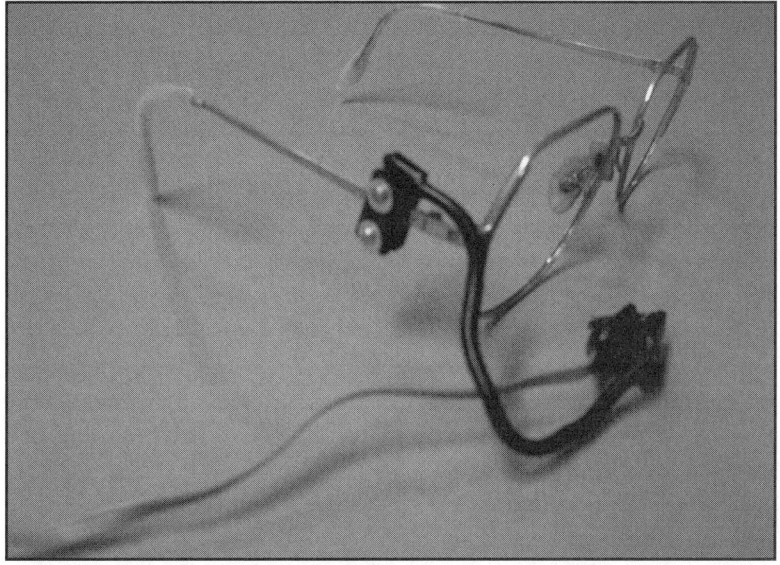

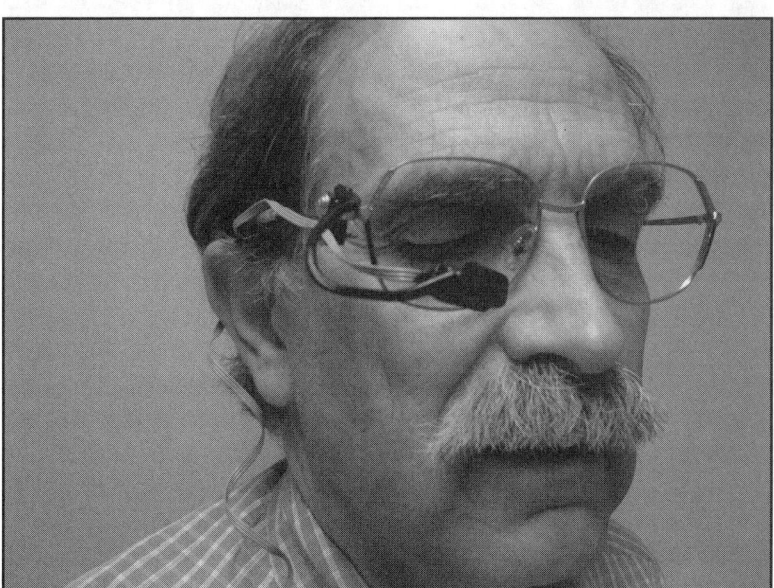

Figure 5–19. **A.** IR blink switch. **B.** IR blink switch.

throat microphone can be used (Figures 5-20A and 5-20B). These switches sometimes are used in settings where the patient can make an abrupt sound by banging on a hard surface like the bed rail. This kind of a configuration allows any physical gesture that the patient is capable of making to create the noise to trigger the switch. Of course, the limitation is that any abrupt noise in the patient's room will activate the switch.

52 AUGMENTATIVE AND ALTERNATIVE COMMUNICATION

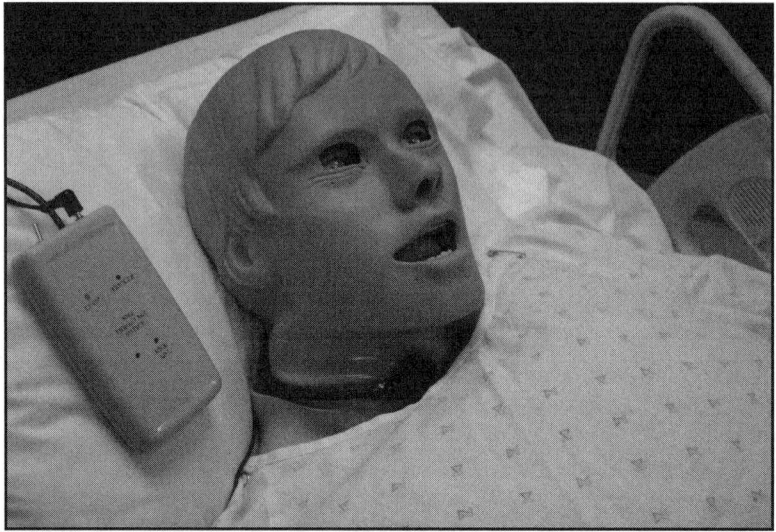

A

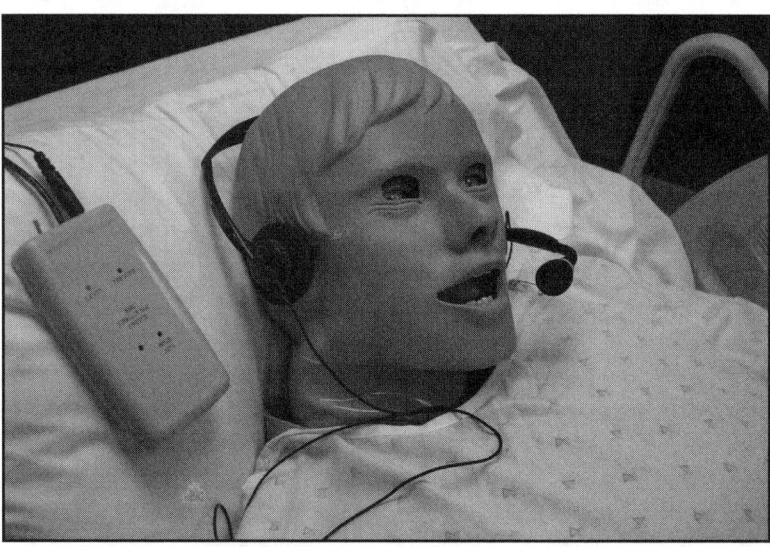

B

Figure 5–20. A. Voice-activated switch-throat microphone. **B.** Voice-activated switch-head mounted microphone.

- Speech Recognition Circuitry
  - Free-standing remotes with X-10 control options (Figure 5–21): Some universal remotes that are on the market allow the user to use voice commands to control a range of electronic devices including X-10 modules like the universal relay module that can be interfaced with standard nurse call circuits
  - Computer-based systems: PC-based systems using voice recognition software can be configured to control electronic devices using either an RF (radio frequency)- or an IR-control circuit that can

SWITCHES AS THE FIRST STEP TO ESTABLISHING COMMUNICATION 53

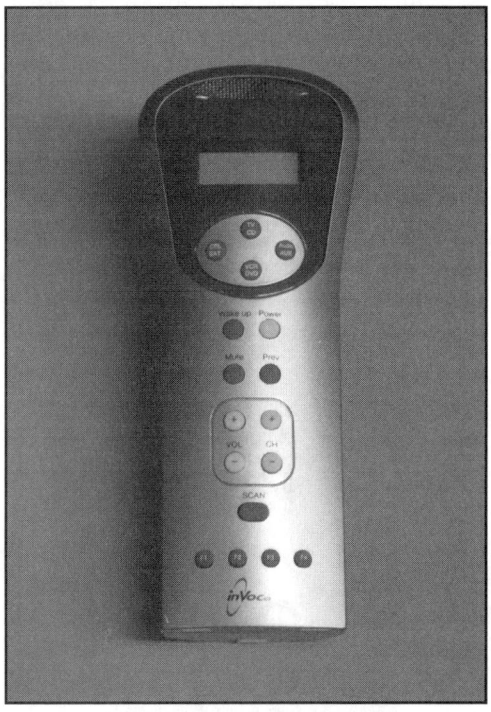

Figure 5–21. Voice-activated remote.

directly or through an X-10 system control a range of devices including the nurse call system. Windows XP now incorporates a voice recognition option. A number of home automation systems that are on the market provide "hands-free" control via X-10 modules.

■ Head Position Switches (Figure 5–22): These switches sense the patient's head position and can be interfaced with computers or AAC devices and function as mouse alternative. These switches either utilize a reflected IR signal or an RF signal picked up with multiple receivers mounted on a head band. The head movements are converted to the *x-y* movements of a conventional mouse. The head then can control the on-screen cursor. When used in conjunction with another switch, the patient has

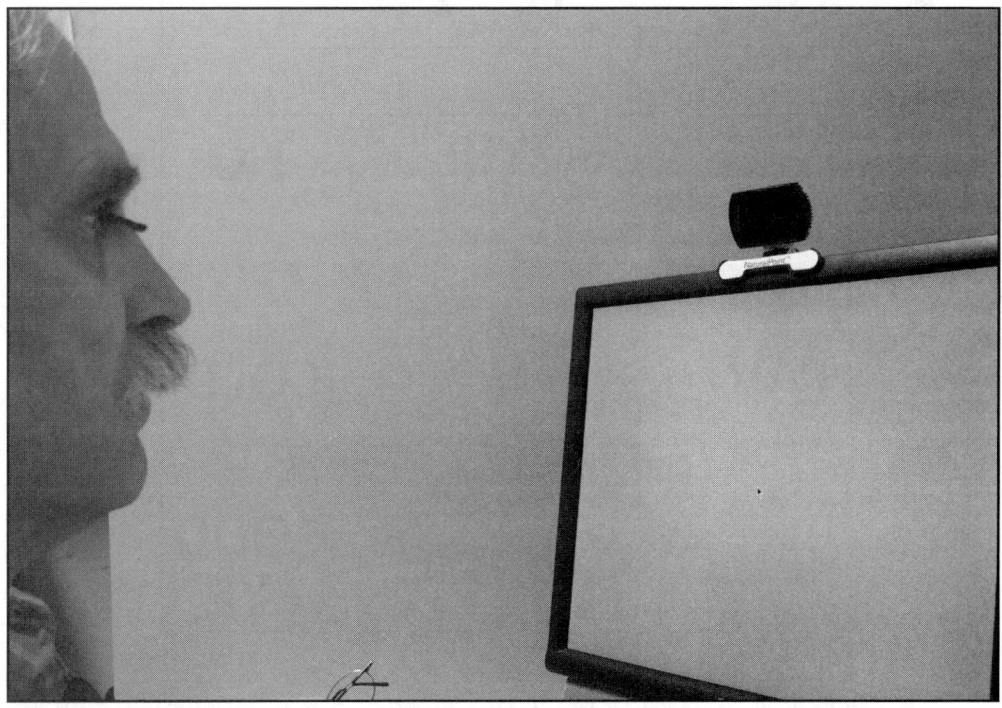

Figure 5–22. Head Tracker-SmartNAV.

a full mouse alternative with the other switch functioning as the mouse click. When no other switch activation is possible, the system software can be set to use a dwell function to serve as the mouse click. Thus, when the head is held steady for the specified dwell time, the software issues a mouse click.

- Eye Movement/Gaze Switches: In patients whose motor abilities are restricted to their extraocular muscles, eye gaze is the only voluntary gesture that can be utilized. In such patients, gaze shifts are often utilized to indicate a simple yes/no response. The use of a Plexiglas ETRAN board (Figures 5–23A and 5–23B) allows

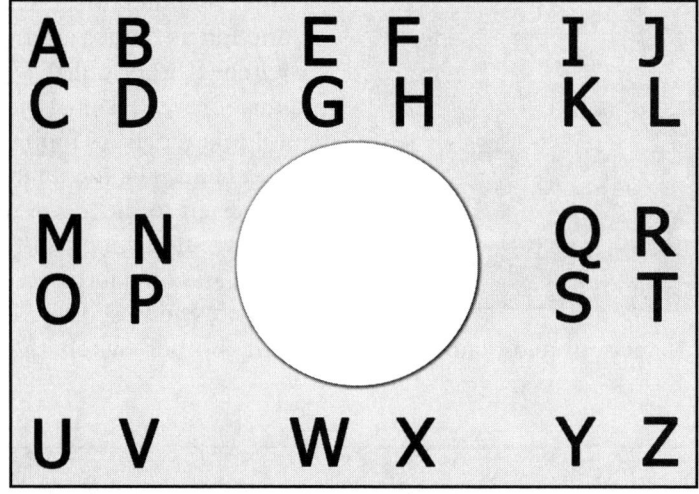

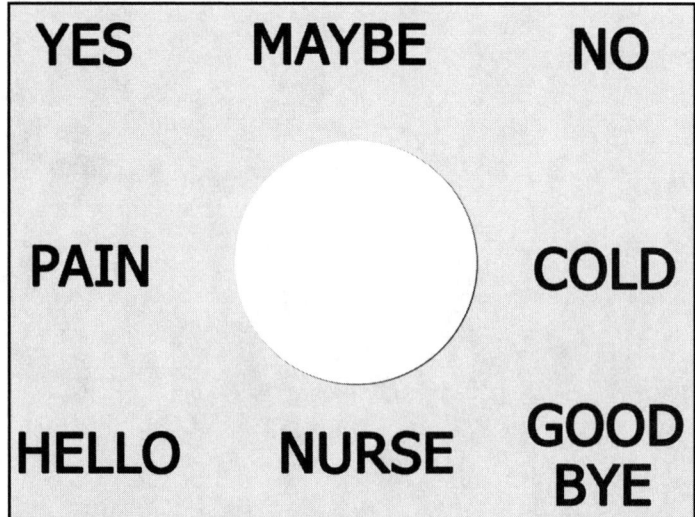

Figure 5–23. A. ETRAN—Gaze directed communication—alphabet. **B.** ETRAN—Gaze directed communication-phrases.

the patient to communicate with a trained partner by making selective gaze shifts to locations on the board on which either letters, whole words, or icons are displayed. When the ETRAN is laid out for spelling (see Figure 5-23A), the patient must make a series of directed gazes to identify the selected letter. For example, if the patient wanted to spell the word "dog," in order to select the first letter of the word, the patient would first look to the upper left and then to the lower right. This system requires training of both the patient and the communication partners. Another key to successful use is the positioning of the ETRAN (see Chapter 7, Figure 7-3).

Until recently, transducing eye movements required expensive and complex laboratory based systems that required a great deal of effort to keep calibrated and as such were not available for use with patients. Newer video-based approaches to eye-tracking (Figures 5-24A, 5-24B, and 5-24C) have reduced the size of the system and the calibration problems. These systems, like the head position systems, allow eye gaze to serve as the control of the computer cursor.

Having an assortment of switches available will ensure that patients with a range of physical challenges will be able to access nurse call systems, patient-controlled analgesic pumps (PCAs) as well as a range of AAC systems. However, because of more severe limitations of their motor

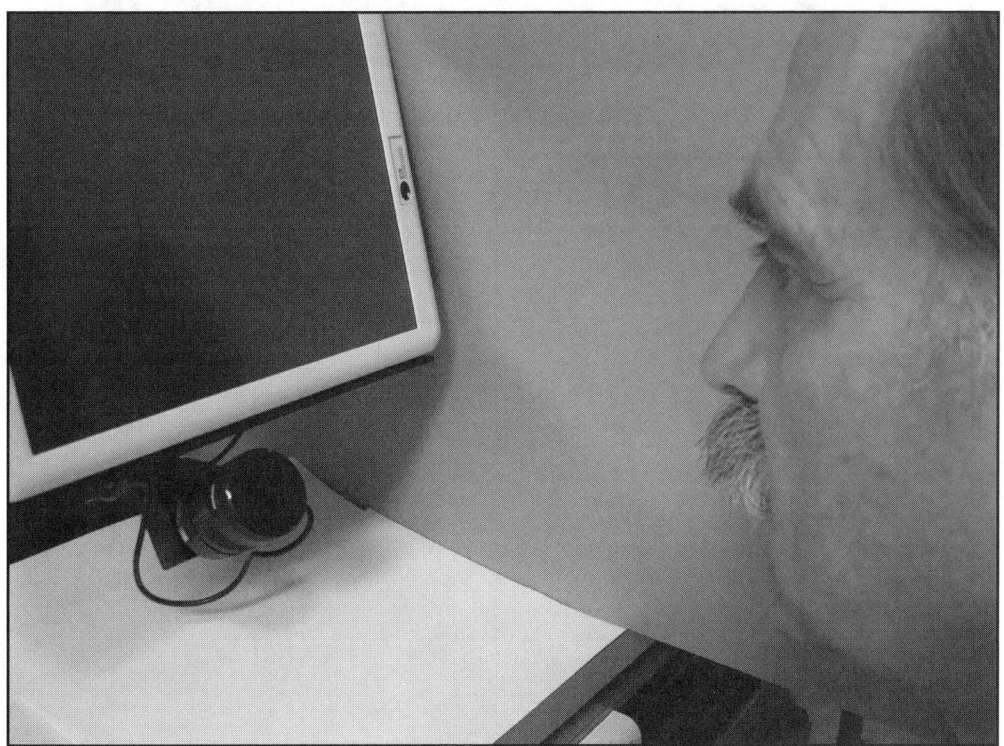

A

Figure 5–24. A. Video eye tracker—ERICA. *continues*

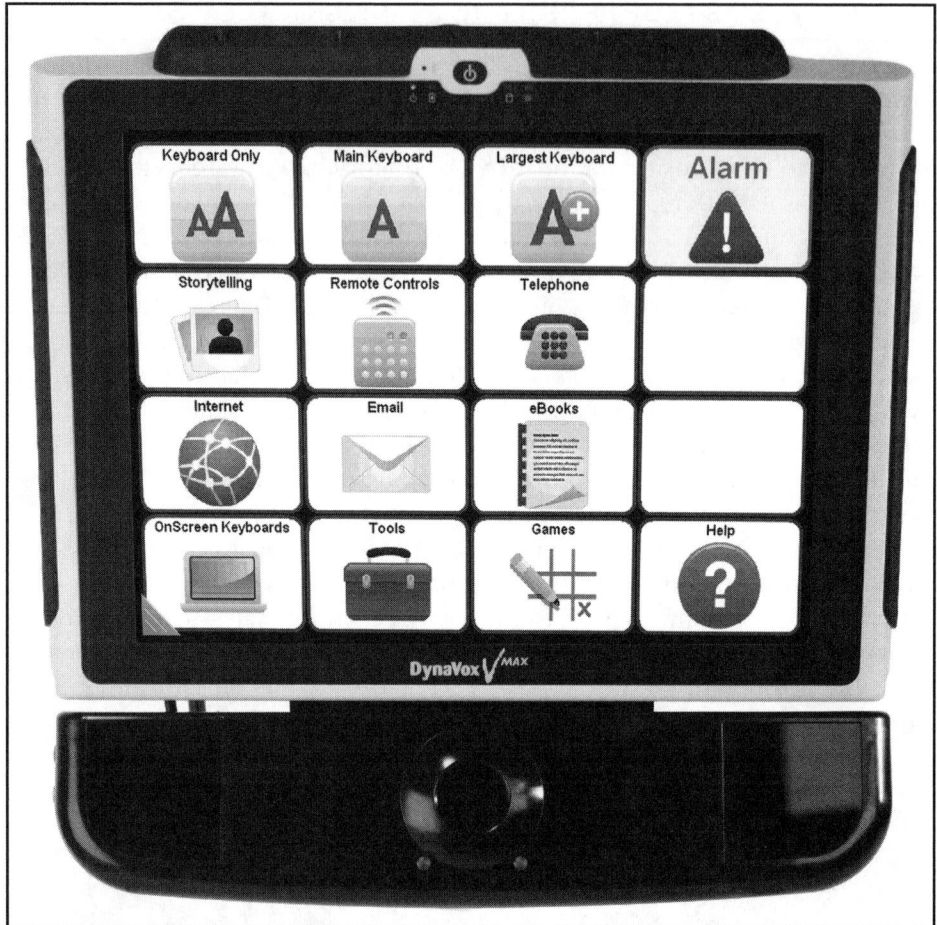

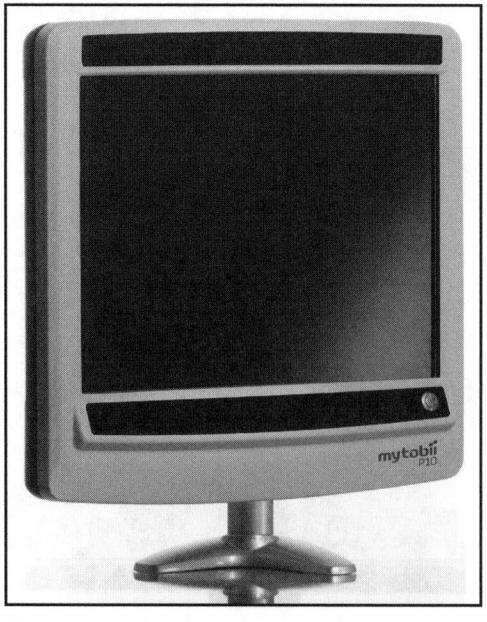

Figure 5–24. *continued* **B.** Video eye tracker—Dynavox EyeMax. **C.** Video eye tracker—MyTobii.

systems, some patients may need adaptations made to commercially available switches as well as to switch mounting systems that can keep the switches positioned so that patients can easily and reliably access them. These adaptations are addressed in Chapter 7.

IOWA SMART SWITCH

For patients whose voluntary movements are very limited and possibly obscured by tremor, most commercially available switches will either not detect the movement or be unintentionally activated by the tremor. The Iowa-Smart Switch (Figure 5-25) was developed to address the needs of such patients. To detect only the intentional gesture and not respond to tremor or unintentional gestures, the switch uses a small microprocessor to process the transducer signals based on the kinematics of the intentional gesture. The switch was designed to accept inputs from pressure transducers, charge transfer circuits, and infrared detector circuits. This wide range of transducers allows for use of the switch anywhere on the body where a reliable movement can be elicited.

Like conventional proximity switches, the charge transfer circuit requires only minimal displacement and no force to activate. It senses a capacitance change when some part of the body comes into proximity of the switch. We have successfully used such switches with traumatic injury patients who are quadriplegic, with patients with progressive neurodegenerative diseases, as well as with patients who may be temporarily incapacitated. Because such transducers are extremely sensitive, the Iowa Smart Switch can be programmed to respond only to patterns

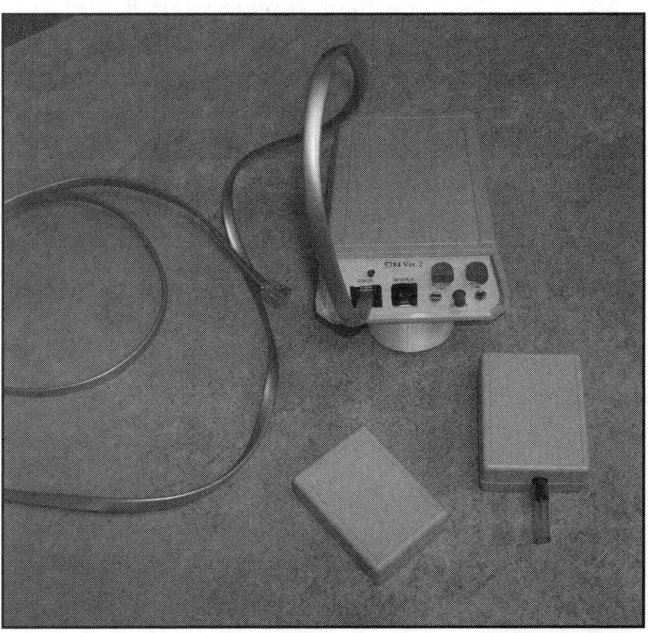

Figure 5-25. Iowa Smart Switch.

of transducer state changes that fit the temporal kinematic characteristics of the intentional gesture. By setting both a minimum and a maximum time for a transducer state change, we can effectively preclude a tremor from activating the switch. The beauty of this approach is that we can detect a low amplitude gesture that may be buried in a higher amplitude tremor.

The pressure transducer circuit can either be used to detect small changes in oral pressure with either an open straw or with a sealed bulb. It can also be used to detect small forces that can be generated by any part of the body that is positioned to compress a sealed bulb. The Iowa Smart Switch can be programmed to accept only a particular change in pressure that has a particular time course. Thus, a patient can keep a small pressure bulb in his or her mouth and only activate the switch by squeezing the bulb with a certain amount of force or hold that pressure change for a designated time interval.

Finally, we have been experimenting with an infrared (IR) transducer circuit that also requires minimal force and displacement. Thus, any gesture that can create a tissue displacement or movement that results in a change of reflected IR, is sufficient to activate the circuit. A common placement of such circuits is in proximity to the eyelids. In this setting, as the eyelid closes for a blink the amount of IR light reflected by the eyelid changes. In order to distinguish between an involuntary blink and an intentional wink, the Iowa Smart Switch can be programmed not to respond to the rapid sequence of reflectance changes associated with the natural high velocity blink or to the slow nonreversing reflectance change associated with drooping eyelids in a tired patient.

Thus, with the appropriate switch technology ranging from simple mechanical switches to microprocessor-based solutions like the Iowa Smart Switch, it should be possible to provide even the most physically limited patients with switch access as long as the assessment has identified a reliable voluntary gesture. Although solutions like the Iowa Smart Switch use the latest digital chip technology, they can only be successful implemented if the switch is mounted appropriately so that the patient's access to the switch transducer is maintained. Chapter 7 addresses the issues of finding an appropriate mounting system that will ensure that the patient has continuous access to the appropriate switch/transducer.

6 Iowa AAC Templates

Over the last decade, we have used some form of AAC with a wide range of patients at UIHC, from 3-year-olds to octogenarians. The etiologies that resulted in the patients' needing AAC included trauma, burn, stroke, cancer, cardiopulmonary, and neurodegenerative diseases. In some cases, patients simply lacked the ability to speak; in others they were also severely limited in other motor domains. Our experiences, with the approximately 200 patients who have participated in our research and development protocol, has led to the development of some default communication templates that we can implement with AAC systems over the range from low to high tech. Although we have tried to refine these templates so that they will have maximal utility for the widest range of patients, it should be noted that we view these only as convenient starting places for clinicians to use in orienting the patient to AAC systems and in designing a personalized AAC system that suits the specific needs of the patient. The companion DVD provides copies of template files that can be printed or accessed and edited with BoardMaker™ software as well as template pages that can be used with the high tech devices like the Dynavox V and Vmax. Although our implementation often uses a high-tech AAC system that incorporates a speech-generating device, the templates can and have been used as low-tech communication boards.

This chapter presents not only the content of the templates but also a strategy for moving a patient from a single action or phrase AAC solution to a multi-page hierarchically organized system that gives the patient a large set of communication options as well as options for environmental control. Some of the decisions about what form of template to use should be conditioned by whether the patient will be able to use direct selection or whether he or she will need to utilize a scan selection method. The level of complexity of the templates in terms of the number of elements per page and the row-column organization needs to be set based on the physical, cognitive, and psycho-affective state of the patient. For some of our patients who quickly grasp how to navigate through the templates and make selections, we can begin with the complete set of template pages, each of which contains many phrases or action options. For the most critically ill trauma patients, starting with the full set would be akin to starting a young child at the expert level on a video game. The failure to grasp the "rules" and the ensuing frustration would lead to a rejection of the game or in our case, use of the AAC system. The key is to not start with a potential failure but rather to build on success. A good dynamic assessment protocol should provide a good idea of the level of complexity at which to start a patient. If the patient appears to be able to attend and track information, we might demonstrate the complete system and then indicate that, like video games, it is prudent to start at a novice level and then progress as the patient masters controlling the system. In a number of cases, we have started a patient with a "one button" system that performs a simple function like summoning the nurse and over a period of a couple of hours moved the patient to a row- and column-based scanning system. The key is building on the patient's success at generating the volitional gesture necessary to make selections at the appropriate time. For patients who will need to use some sort of aided pointing device for direct access selections, or patients who will activate a switch to control a scan selection system, it is essential that they develop confidence that they can produce the appropriate motor response to produce the desired speech output or control of an environmental device (i.e., nurse call, TV).

ONE BUTTON TEMPLATE

Providing a patient with the means to access the nurse call, a PCA, or to control a fan or turn on the TV is often the first step in getting a patient to accept their situation. A scene in the recently released film based on Jean Dominique Bauby's memoir, *The Diving Bell and the Butterfly*, shows poignantly what failing to give a patient a means of using a volitional gesture to control the environment. Mr. Bauby suffered from locked-in-syndrome and the only voluntary gesture under his control was a gaze shift. The staff used that gesture when asking yes/no questions and also when using an auditory scanning through the alphabet to allow him to construct messages. However, when he was left alone in his room he had no means of summoning assistance. The scene in question has Mr. Bauby lying in bed watching a World Cup soccer match while an aide hangs a feeding bag for his tube feeding. As the aide proceeds to leave the room he switches off the TV. There Bauby was, left alone and deprived of one of the few pleasures he could still appreciate the way he did prior to his stroke. Had Mr. Bauby been fitted with a switch activated by his gaze shift, he might have been able to summon assistance or with an ECU controlled the TV on his own. At the time of his stroke in 1995 and treatment over the following year, blink switches were coming on the market and might have been tried had they been available to his clinicians. Unfortunately, he did not have that option. For our patients with as little motor control as Mr. Bauby had, as well as for those who can either point with a limb or use head movements or shifts in eye gaze, there are options to access assistance from people even when they are out of the line of sight.

We start with a single button template; most often the option is for summoning the nurse utilizing a link to the environmental control (ECU) function of an AAC device (see Chapter 9). Alternatively, in ICU cases where a nurse is always present, the button can be assigned one of a number of other functions. For some patients, it might be to produce a request to summon a family member, to request medication for pain, or to request oral or pulmonary suctioning. For other patients, we have assigned the button to an alternative ECU function, such as access to a patient-controlled analgesic pump (PCA) or to control the TV in the patient's room (see Chapter 8).

With just a single large button as a target, developing the necessary control to access the touch screen can begin at a very simple level. This works well with patients who have sufficient limb movement to touch the screen or control a track ball to move a cursor to a target, with patients who can use a head-mounted pointer to touch the screen, or patients who can use a head or eye mouse to move the on screen cursor (see Chapter 5).

TWO-THREE BUTTON TEMPLATES

When a patient can understand the relationship between a button on the template and the action it produces (e.g., speech or ECU), it is possible to introduce additional options to work on refinement of the pointing gesture for the patients who will be able to perform direct selection activation of the buttons or to introduce scanning for patients who can only produce a single or limited number of nondirectional gestures. Most mid- and high-tech AAC systems have a scanning function that sequences through the options available, with the patient making a selection of the desired item when it is highlighted. In a single switch scanning system, the device moves through the options using one of a number of scan patterns and at a specified scanning rate. For simple templates with a small number of items, a simple serial scanning pattern may be appropriate. One instructs the patient to look at the item desired and when it is highlighted the patient is told to activate his or her switch. For patients who have visual acuity issues or can not see, systems can be set for auditory scanning, which provide an auditory prompt as the system scans through the items. These auditory prompts can be delivered to the patient over a "private" speaker or ear-bud. When the number of items increases, it becomes necessary to optimize the scanning pattern so that it does not take too long for a patient to get to the desired item. Row/column and column/row patterns are among the most commonly used optimizing patterns, although block patterns (right/left, top/bottom, quadrant) can also be useful in certain applications (Video clip 6-1). In these cases, the system scan pattern proceeds by row, column, or block. When the row, column, or block of the desired item is highlighted, the patient activates his or her switch. This then sets the system to scan the items in the selected row, column, or block. The patient then activates the switch again when the desired item is highlighted. Although this means that a patient must activate the switch twice to obtain the desired action, the time saving of these scan patterns often outweighs the additional physical effort. If the patient can control two switches, one switch is used to step through items while the second switch is used to have the device perform the action assigned to the selected item.

Selecting the second or third option for the template should be based on those communication acts or ECU functions that have the greatest value for the patient. We have found that, for patients who are intubated or have a tracheostomy, being able to request suctioning is often a high priority. For patients with limited mobility, requests for repositioning have also been very important.

GRID-PATTERN BUTTON TEMPLATES

When patients demonstrate an understanding of scanning through two or three options, one can progress to grid-pattern templates. Care should be taken to not generate templates with too many rows or columns. A patient's ability to navigate through and effectively use larger templates will be a function of a variety of factors (sensory limitations, motor skills, ability to learn associations between button display and function). Figures 6–1A–D illustrate a possible progression from one to four button option communication pages. Using dynamic assessment, one can increase or decrease the available options to ensure effective use by the patient. Some patients may remain with a fairly simple template for extended periods. For other patients, the progression to more complex templates can be very rapid and one should be prepared to make system modifications fairly quickly. We recommend having a range of templates ready so that little effort and time would be required to progress a patient or, in cases where a patient's condition worsens, to easily simplify the template. The template generating strategy we have adopted at UIHC involved asking nurse managers on the inpatient units to work with us in generating core template items that may cover the typical needs and care requirements of patients on their units. Although particular items may not be applicable to a particular patient, having a starting template in which only one or two items need modification greatly reduces the time it takes to get the appropriate template set for a patient. Although reprogramming high-tech AAC devices can, with trained personnel, be done at the bedside, we need to try to keep the time required to do this to a minimum. In cases where the AAC solution entails a low-tech approach with communication boards, having premade boards allows for a very quick adjustment to fit the patient's needs. In order to make board creation and modification something that can be done on the inpatient units, we are planning to make the page templates available on a shared network drive that is accessible from all the units. A network deployment of the software used to generate the communication boards will allow clinicians and support staff to make customized boards, which should have broader appeal as their content would be tailored to the individual patient.

SIMPLE BUTTONS WITH LINKS TEMPLATE

When an individual has needs for a communication and an ECU repertoire that exceeds what can reasonably be placed on a single grid, one should consider a hierarchically organized set of templates. This can be accomplished with both high- and low-tech solutions. In the high-tech solutions, the function assigned to a button can be a link to open another page or pop-up window (Video clip 6–2, Figures 6–2A and 6–2B). Thus from a single "main" page, the user can access many other pages. The same functionality is accomplished in low-tech solutions where an index page with tabs can be used to with a multiple page communication book (Figure 6–3).

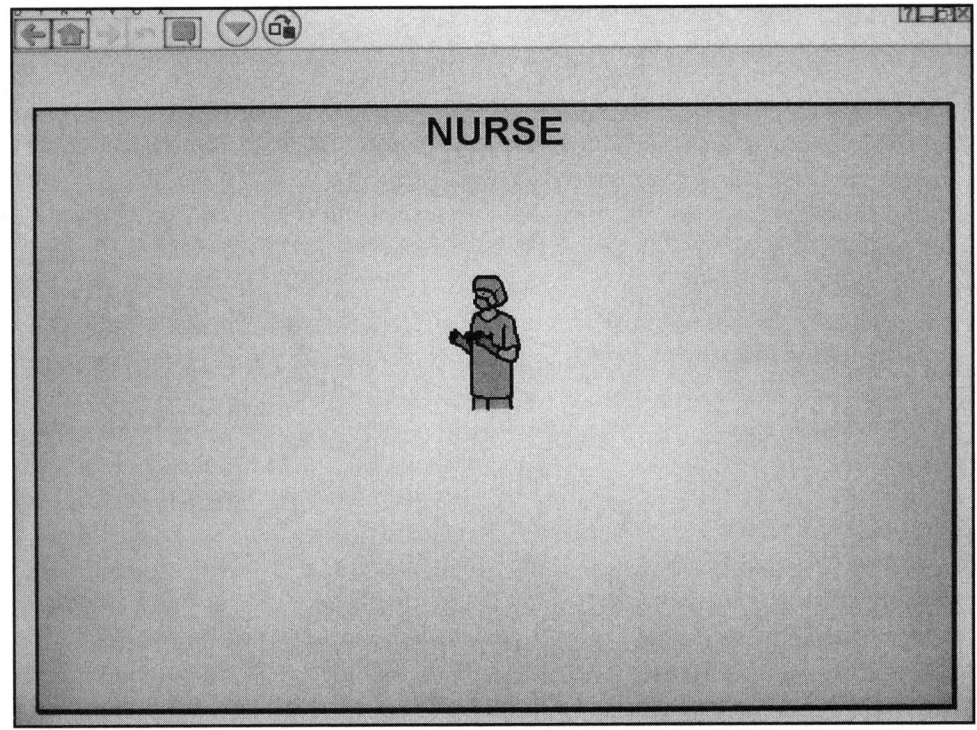

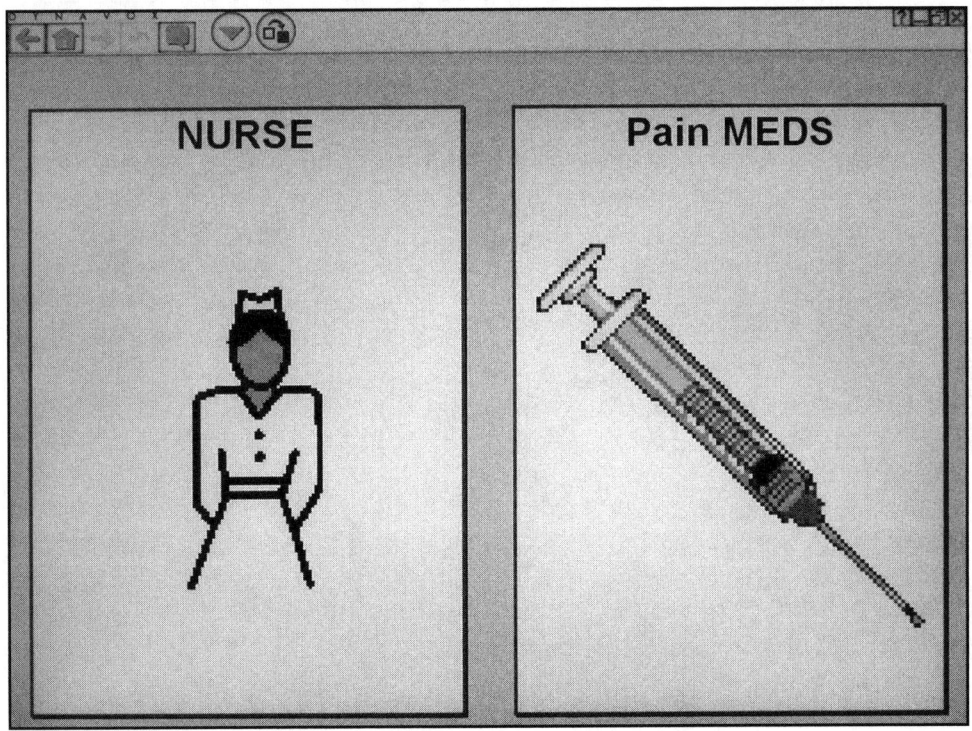

Figure 6–1. A. Single button page, **B.** Two button page *continues*

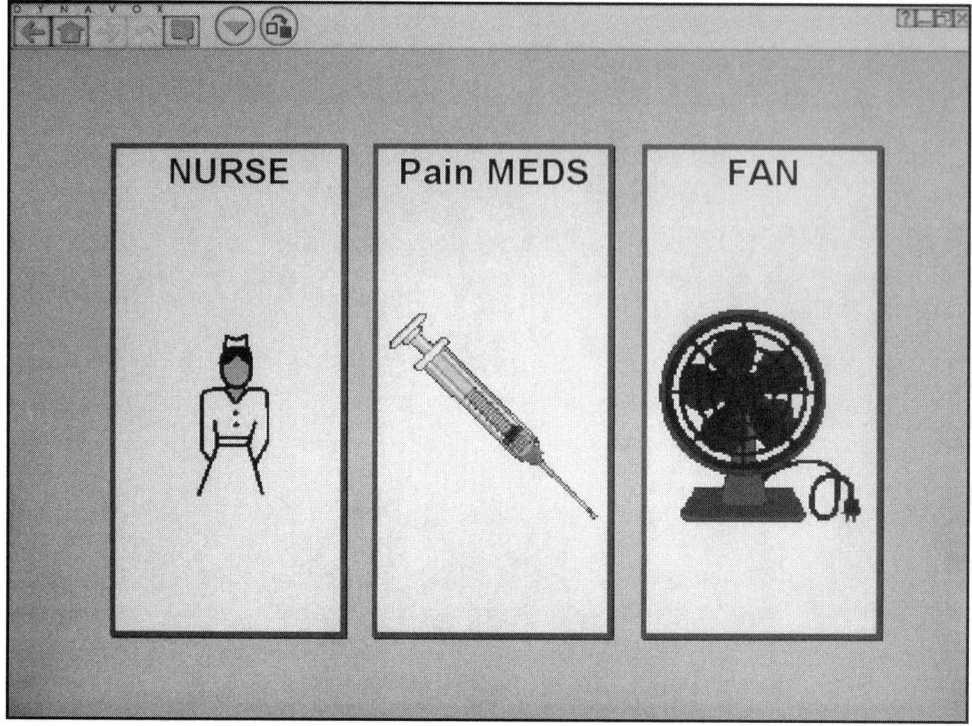

C

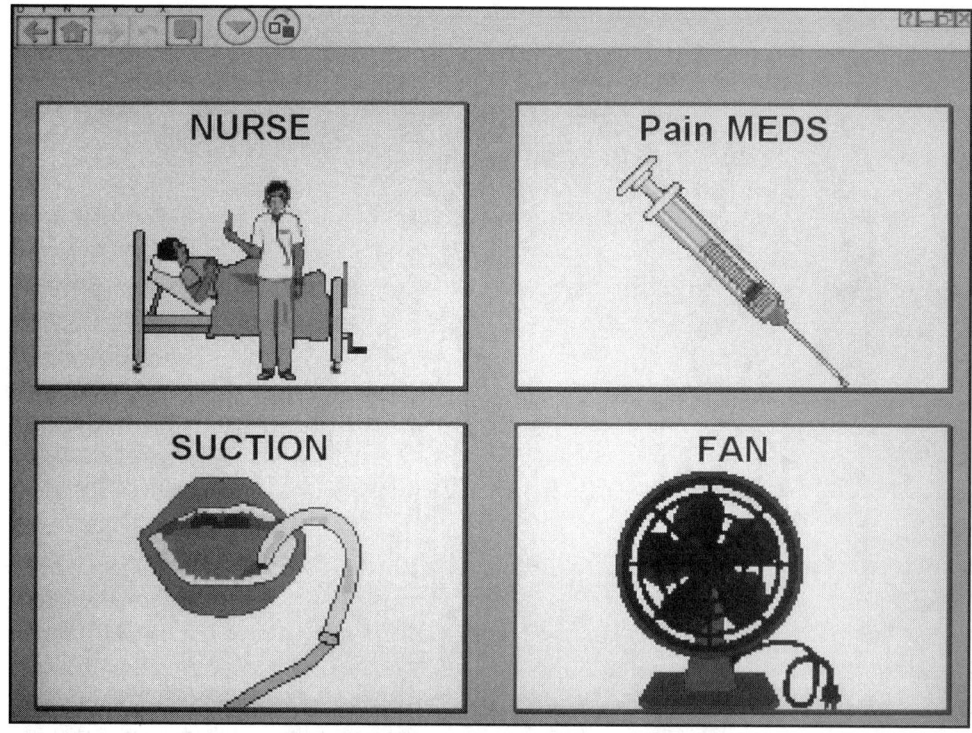

D

Figure 6–1. *continued* **C.** Three button page, **D.** Four button page.

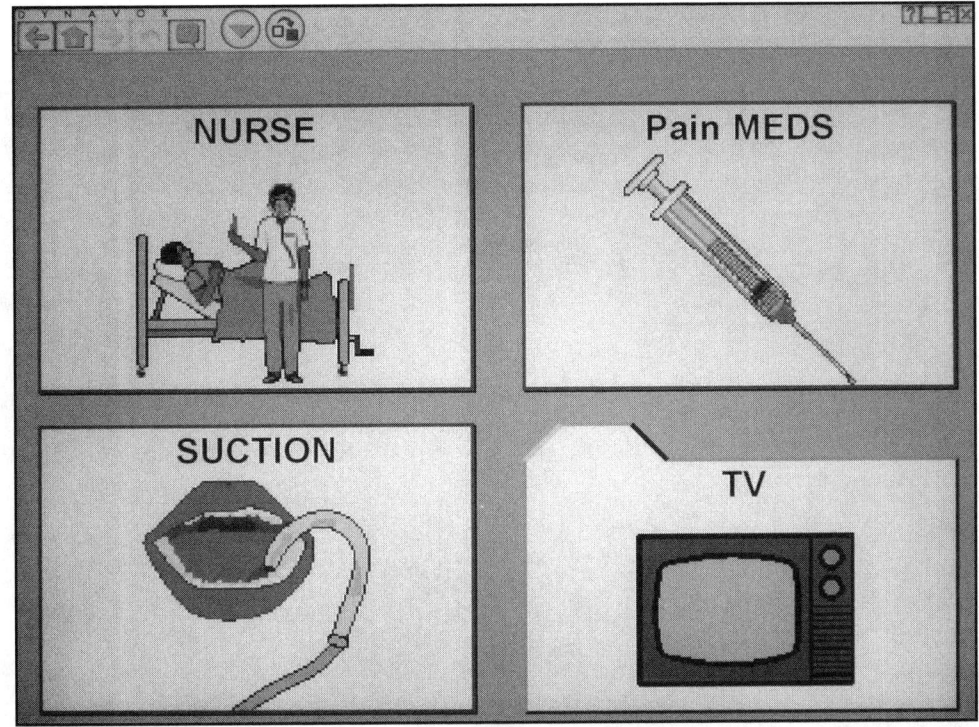

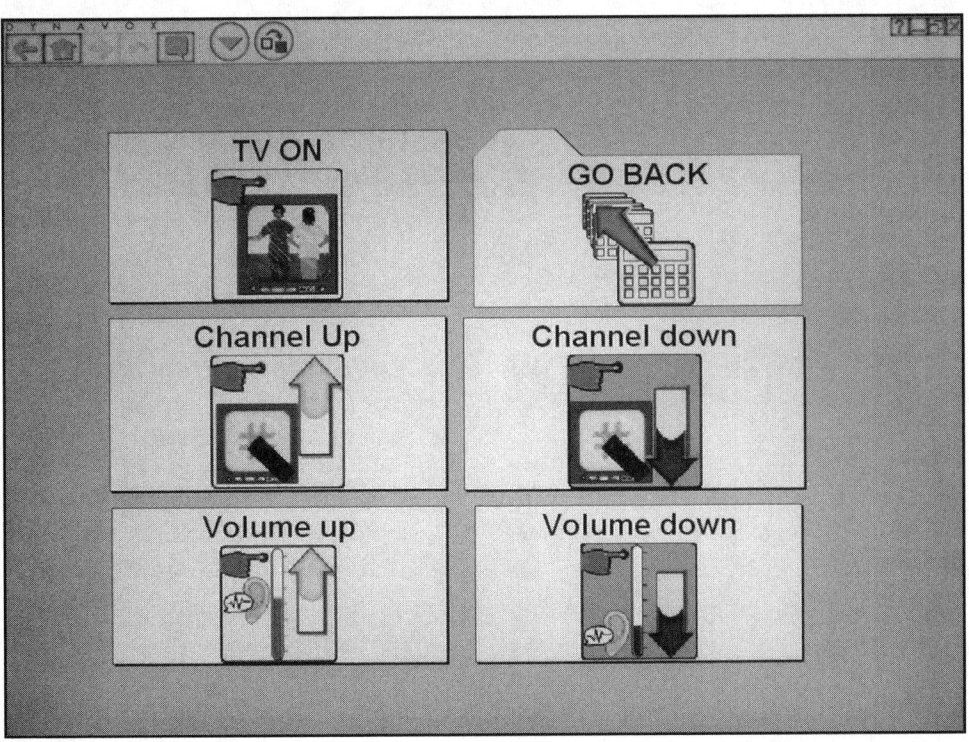

Figure 6–2. A. Four button array with a link button, **B.** Pop-up to control TV with a "Go back" link button.

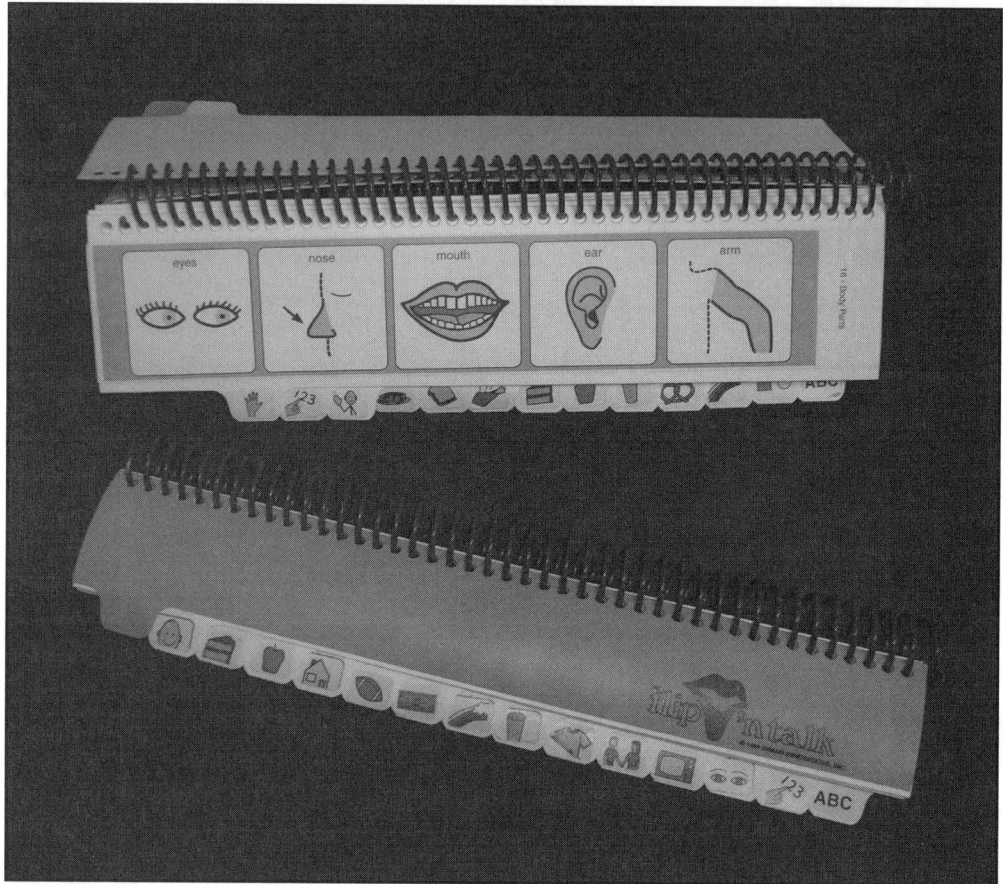

Figure 6–3. Communication book with tabs.

THE IOWA TEMPLATE

The full set of our default hierarchical page set has been implemented on a range of high-tech AAC devices (Dynavox, ATI, and Prentke Romich) that use dynamic displays that can be controlled either directly using a touch screen, a mouse or track ball, head or eye tracking, or in scanning mode with some form of switch control. The AAC device can be mounted on an IV pole on an adjustable arm to allow positioning of the device where the patient can see and access it (Figure 6–4).

Top Level Menu Page

The main or top level menu (Figure 6-5) is laid out as a 4×3 grid with a combination of direct action buttons and link buttons that provide access to additional pages. Direct action buttons are simple buttons that are associated with producing a particular voice output, ECU function or a combination of the two. The button in the upper right-hand side produces the message "Please get my nurse" and executes the ECU command to have the device send out IR signal that activates an X-10 relay module which is

IOWA AAC TEMPLATES   67

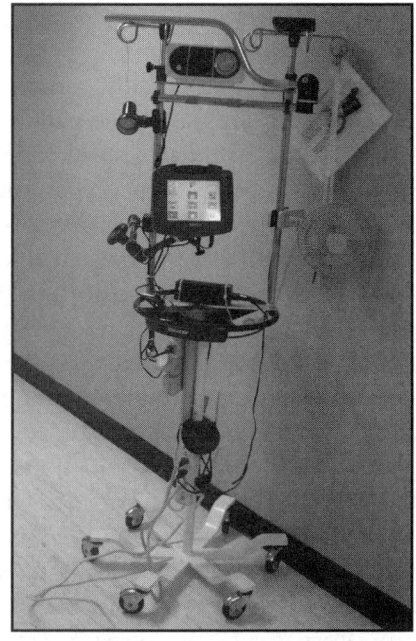

Figure 6–4. IV pole mounting.

connected to the nurse call system (Figure 6-6). Given the importance of pain management (see Chapter 8), we include a button on the top page that allows patients to produce the message "I need pain meds." Where appropriate, one can use an ECU command to control a second X-10 relay module that can be interfaced with a PCA (patient-controlled analgesic) pump that can deliver intravenous medications for pain.

Our experience has shown that patients are often concerned about knowing the date and the time. To that end, we also include a button on the top page that displays and produces the corresponding speech output of the day, date, and time. The remaining buttons on this page are links to a series of topically organized pages.

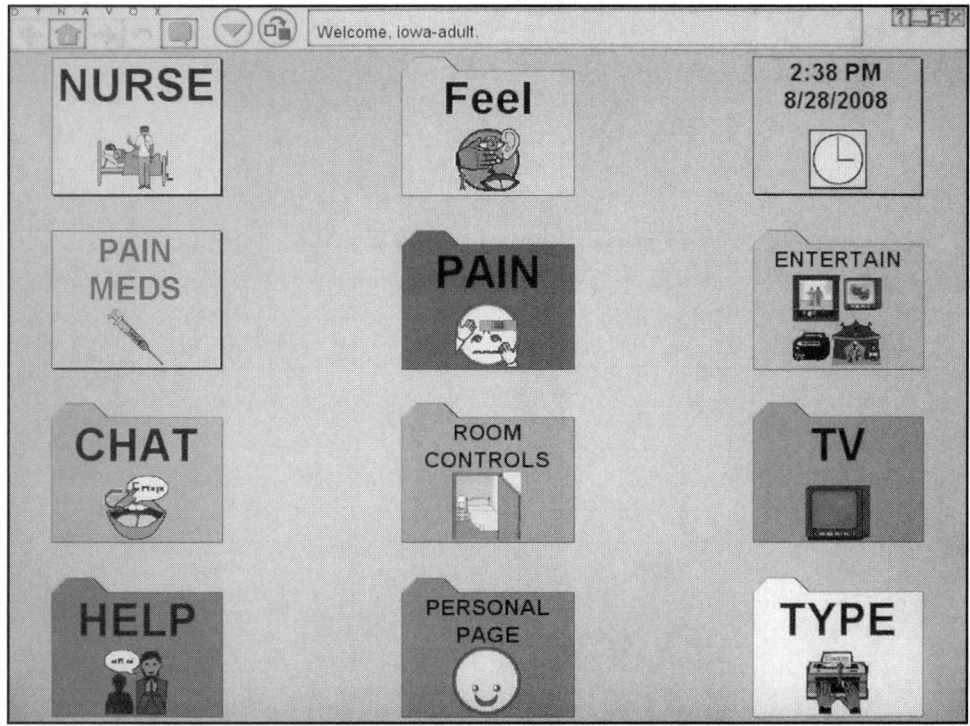

Figure 6–5. IOWA template—Main/top menu.

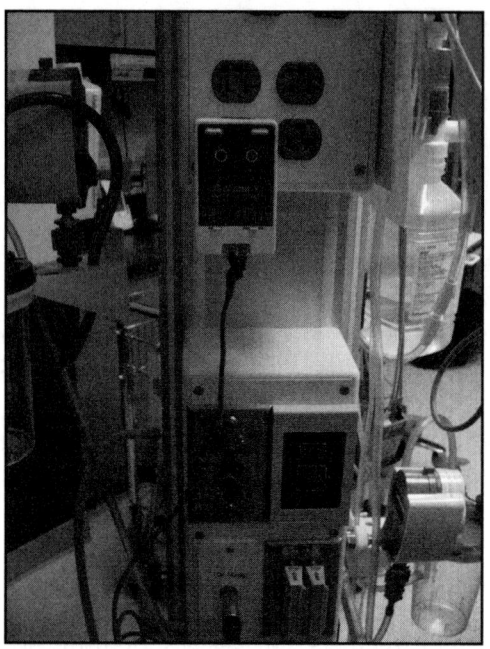

Figure 6–6. X-10 nurse relay.

Feelings Pop-up Page

Allowing a patient to quickly communicate how he or she feels physically and emotionally is an essential piece of patient-caregiver and patient-family communication. The Feelings Pop-up (Figure 6–7) provides a range of options that allow the patient to quickly indicate how he or she is feeling. The specific message options should be modified to suit the particular issues that the patient's etiology demands. One can set how the device responds to pop-up menu selections. In some cases, the pop-up can be set to "auto close" so that when the patient selects an option the pop-up automatically closes and the patient is returned to the main menu. Alternatively, the pop-up can remain open until a "Go back" button is

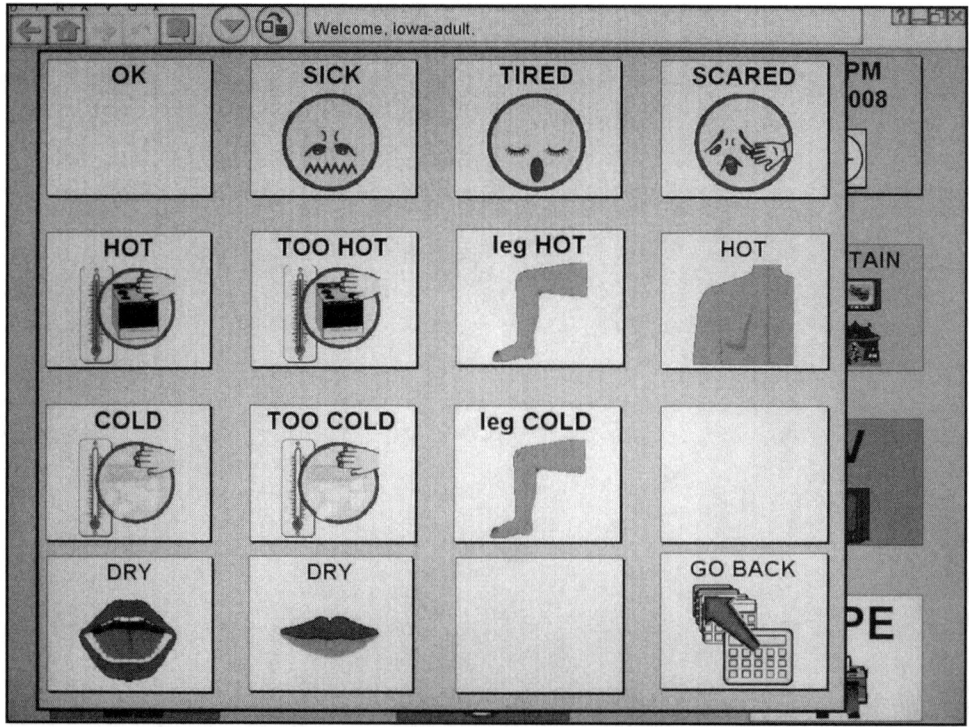

Figure 6–7. IOWA template—Feelings menu.

activated. In this mode, the patient can produce a series of messages about feelings in rapid succession without having to return to the main menu between utterances.

Pain Pop-Up Page

Effective pain management can be achieved if the patient can indicate the presence of pain, the locus of the pain and the magnitude of the pain. To that end, a link to a Pain Pop-up page (Figure 6–8) is provided on the Top-Level menu page. This pop-up contains buttons to indicate what part of the body is in pain as well as a link button to an embedded pop-up that provides access to the conventional 10-point pain scale (Figure 6–9).

Selecting the Pain Link button on the Top Level menu produces the phrase "I am uncomfortable" and then automatically links to the Pain Pop-up where selecting a body part produces a phrase of the format "my _____ hurts." If the pain scale is selected, then the system produces a phrase in the format "my pain is at level _____."

Entertainment Pop-Up Page

The Top-Level menu provides a link to the entertainment pop-up page (Figure 6–10), which provides the patient with the ability to request music, videos, or books on tape or select a computer game. In addition, when implemented on AAC devices that run on a Windows platform, buttons

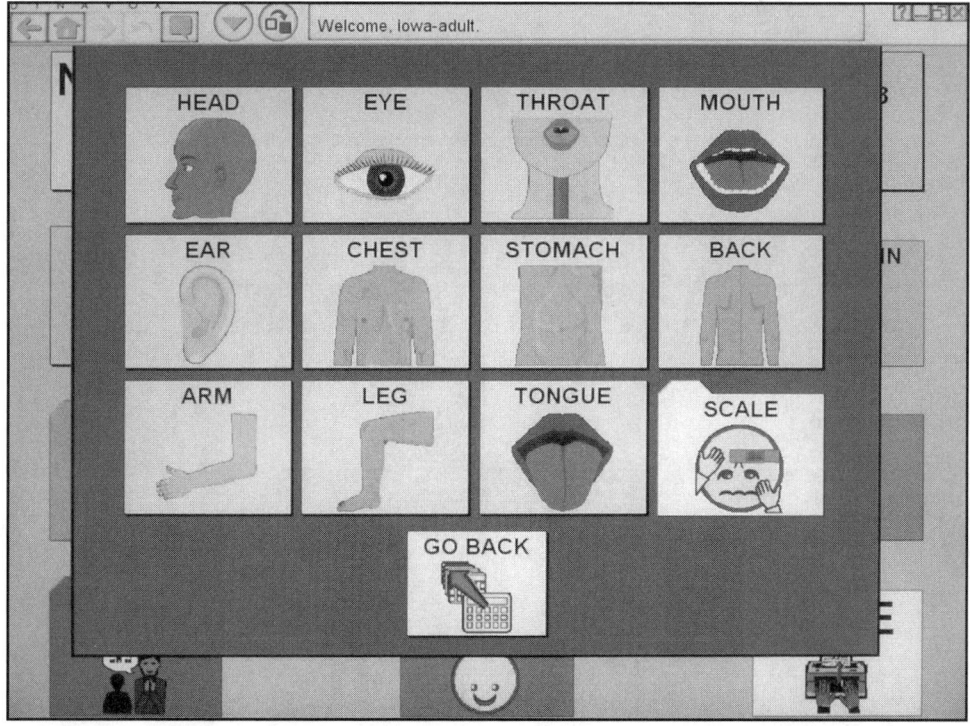

Figure 6–8. IOWA template—Pain menu.

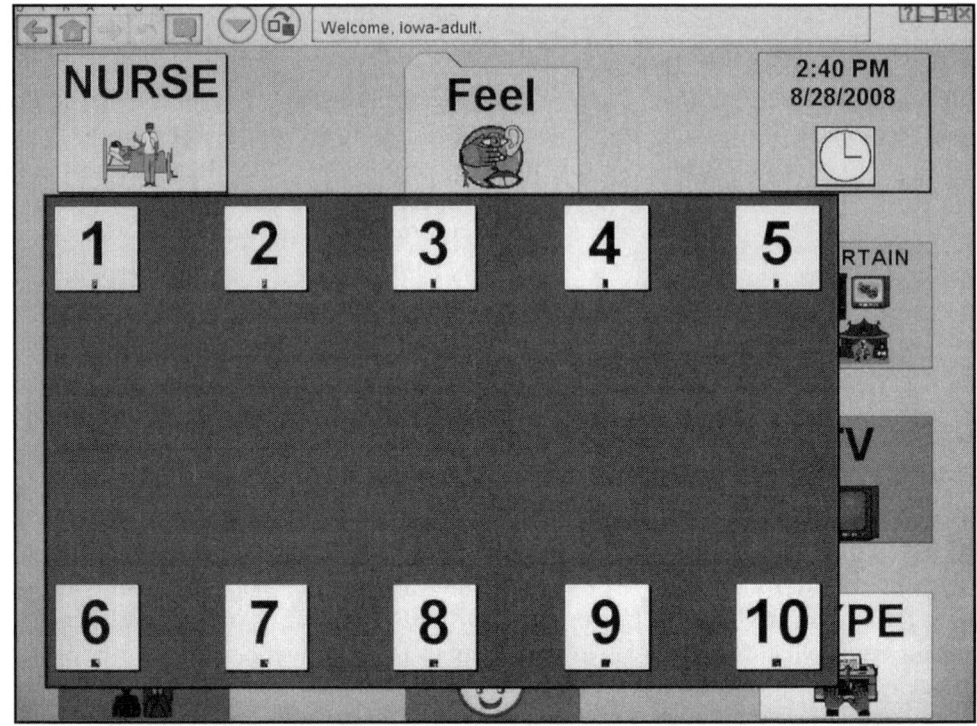

Figure 6–9. IOWA template—Pain scale pop-up.

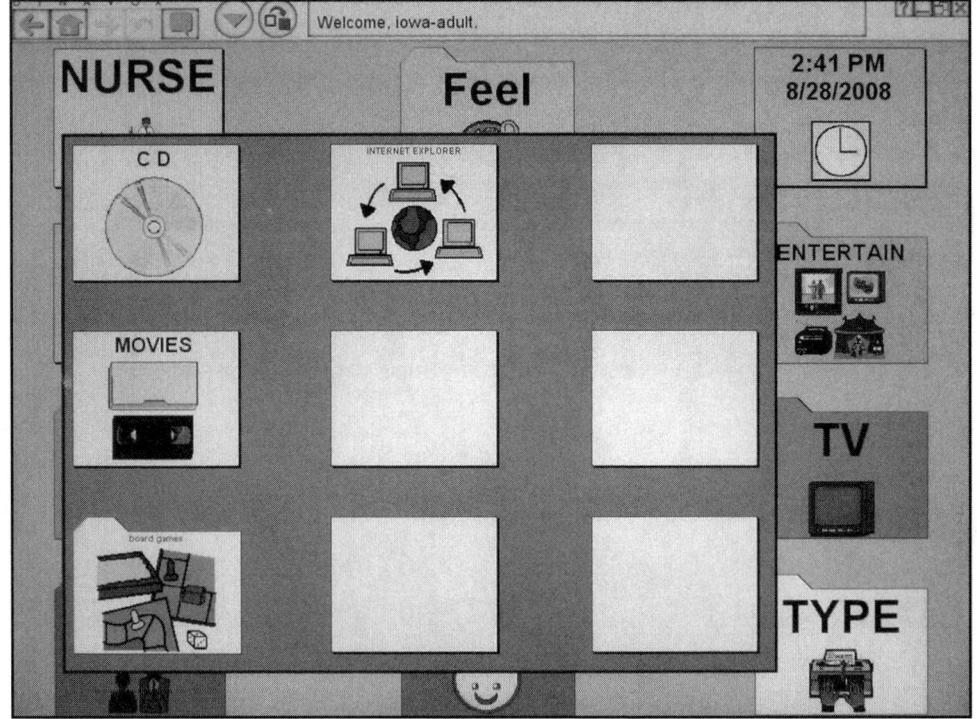

Figure 6–10. IOWA template—Entertainment options.

on this page can allow the patient to access any application installed on the device including games and an embedded or USB-controlled media player. Some devices have Ethernet ports to allow access to the Internet. In those cases, a link to launch an Internet Browser can also be added.

Chat Menu Page

From the Top-Level menu the user can access a Chat Menu page (Figure 6–11) that includes a set of basic conversation management options including greetings and questions. Because communication breakdown can occur, our patients have found it useful to have very quick ways of indicating that they or their conversational partners have not understood. We provide a generic "What?" and "That's not what I meant" to allow patients to get conversations back on track. Both children and adults have found having a phrase like "quit bothering me" extremely useful to curtail interactions and excessive attention by staff, family, and friends. The specific phrase associated with this button can be tailored to suit the patient's style preference. See Chapter 11, Cases B and E for a discussion of tailoring utterances to give patients their "personal" voice.

Medical Questions Pop-Up

Our patients have consistently indicated that knowing about their medical condition/prognosis is very important to them.

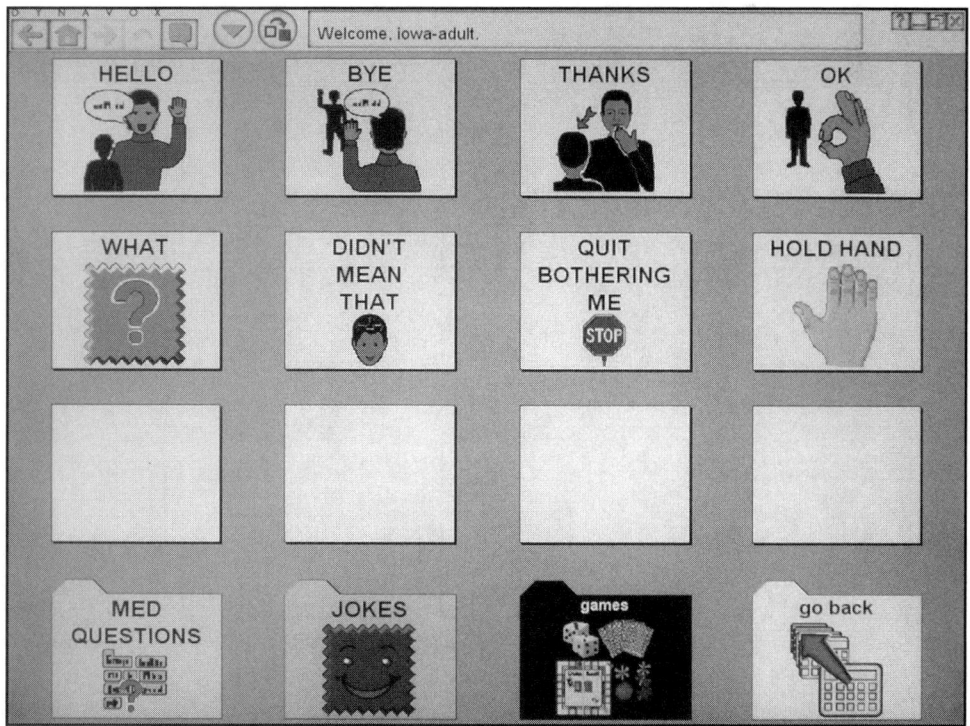

Figure 6–11. IOWA template—Chat menu.

For that reason we provide a link to a Medical Questions pop-up (Figure 6–12) on the Chat Menu page. This pop-up allows patients to inquire about how they are doing, how long they have been in the hospital, as well as when they will be able to come off the ventilator and have the nasogastric feeding tube removed.

Jokes Pop-up

We have also found that many patients, both adult and pediatric, feel the need to use humor to break the ice in interactions with caregivers and family. We let patients know about the option of having a Jokes Pop-up (Figure 6–13) and work at the bedside to add the specific jokes or humorous expressions that the patient would want to use. We continue to be struck that patients will often construct jokes that play on their current condition or the mental state of the nurses or family members (see Chapter 11, Case B).

Room-Control ECU Pop-Up

Providing patients with the ability to ask for lights, the TV, or a fan to be turned on and off provides patients some control of their environment. The Room Control pop-up (Figure 6–14) selections are associated with phrases such as "Please turn the _____ on" or "Please turn the _____ off" and each selection can also be associated with an ECU command that can activate X-10 modules that lights or a fan can be plugged into. If there is an

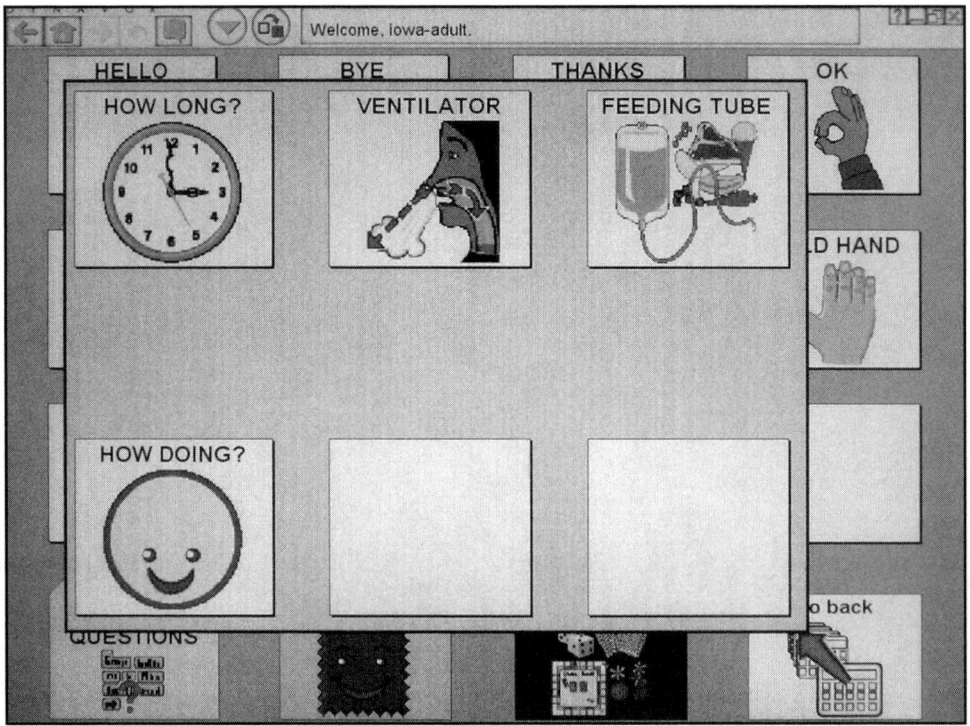

Figure 6–12. IOWA template—Medical questions.

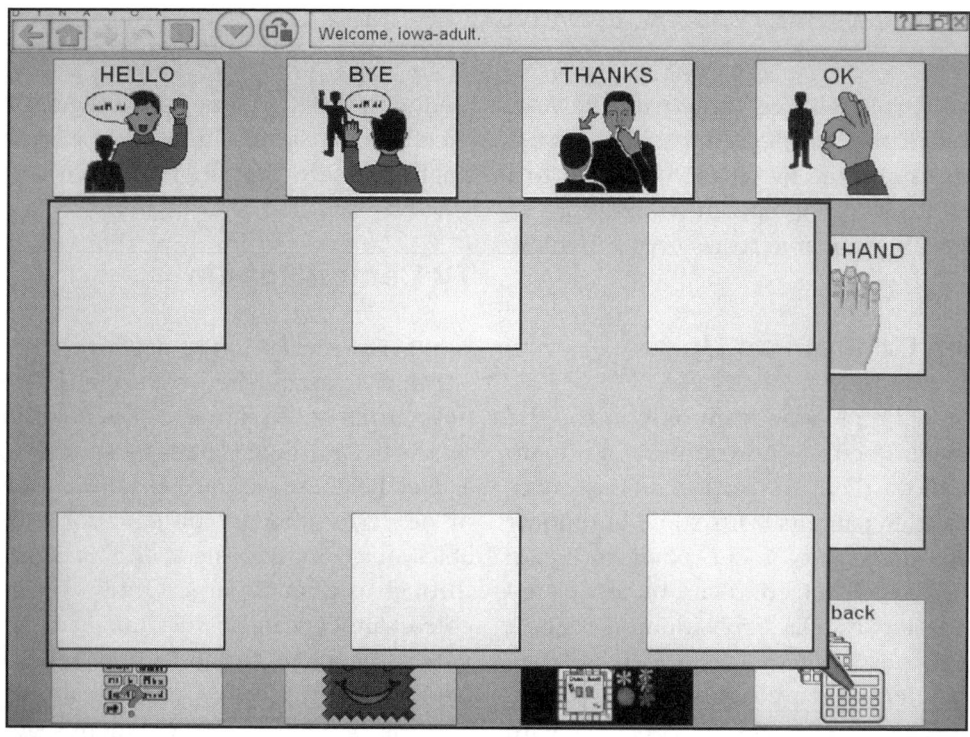

Figure 6–13. IOWA template—Jokes page.

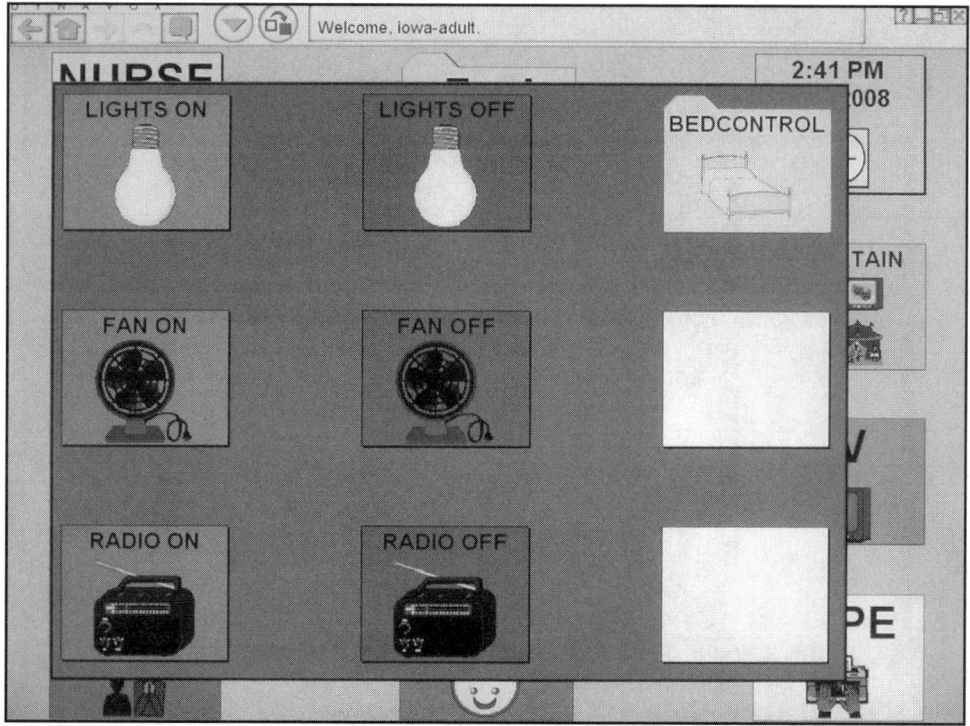

Figure 6–14. IOWA template—Room control.

IR-controlled TV in the room, the AAC device can transmit the appropriate IR signals to turn the TV on and off. A link to a Bed Control pop-up can be activated to allow the patient to request repositioning.

Bed Control Pop-Up

For patients who cannot control the standard bed position controls, a pop-up to allow them to ask for repositioning provides patients with some autonomy with regard to positional comfort (Figure 6–15). Each selection can be associated with a particular repositioning request (e.g., "raise my feet"). If an X-10 bed control interface is available, the functions of the selections can also be associated with the appropriate ECU commands associated with the X-10 functions assigned to each bed adjustment function (e.g., head up, head down, feet up, feet down).

TV Control Pop-Up

Control of the TV in the patient's room, is often accomplished by a limited set of controls on the nurse call pendant or on the bed rail (see Figures 5–5 and 5–6). Typically, these require a fair amount of dexterity and are difficult for even able-bodied individuals to use. Stepping through the much larger array of available channels can be very taxing as the patient needs to attend to both what is happening on the TV overhead and the controls, which are at the patient's side. If the TV can be controlled with an IR

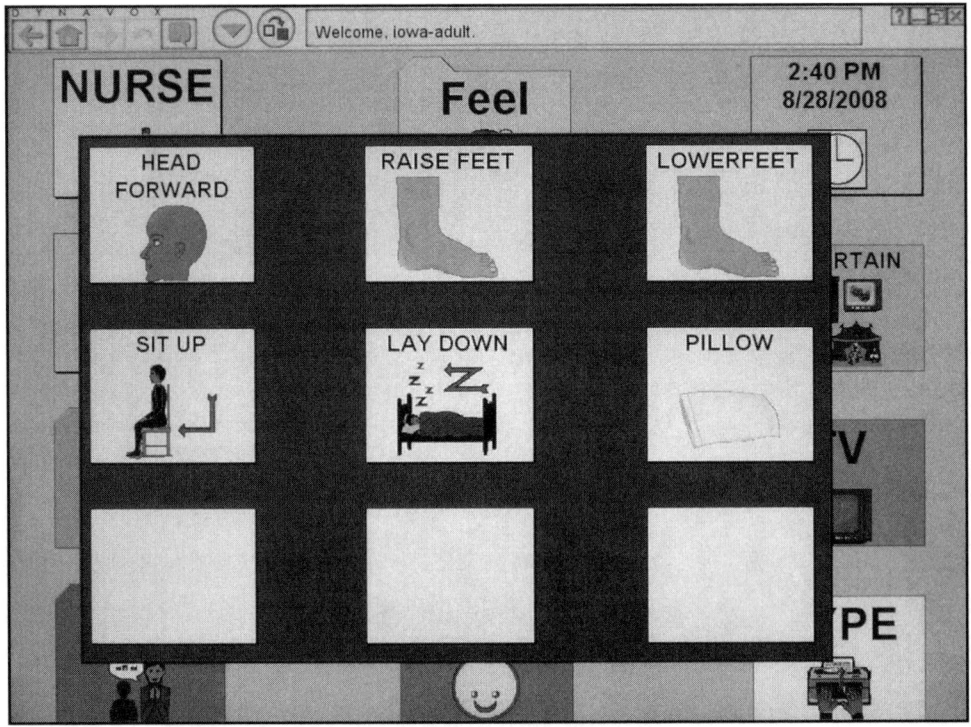

Figure 6–15. IOWA template—Bed control.

remote and if the AAC device is capable of learning or producing the appropriate IR codes, then a TV control pop-up (Figure 6–16) can be constructed that provides the patients with basic controls such as power on/off, channel up and down, volume up and down, channel recall, as well as specific codes for the particular channels that the patient wants to typically watch. Such a pop-up can also be used even when the IR control of the TV is not possible. In this case, each function can be associated with the appropriate phrase (e.g., "I want to watch the Discovery Channel"). Our experience has shown that control of the TV, like other ECU functions, provides a considerable degree of empowerment for the patient. It gives the patient some control his or her environment and how the patient chooses to spend his or her time. Recall the helplessness that Jean-Dominique Bauby described when the nursing aide turned off the soccer match he was watching on TV and he was left alone incapable of controlling the TV or summoning assistance.

Help Pop-Up

To provide patients with a range of requests for assistance the Help pop-up (Figure 6–17) is organized into a set of functional categories each of which has an associated pop-up. There are also a few direct function selections that allow patients to ask to be turned in bed, assisted with toileting, and to have their hands held. The **Get-Me** pop-up (Figure 6–18) provides the patient a way to ask for a range of people and things.

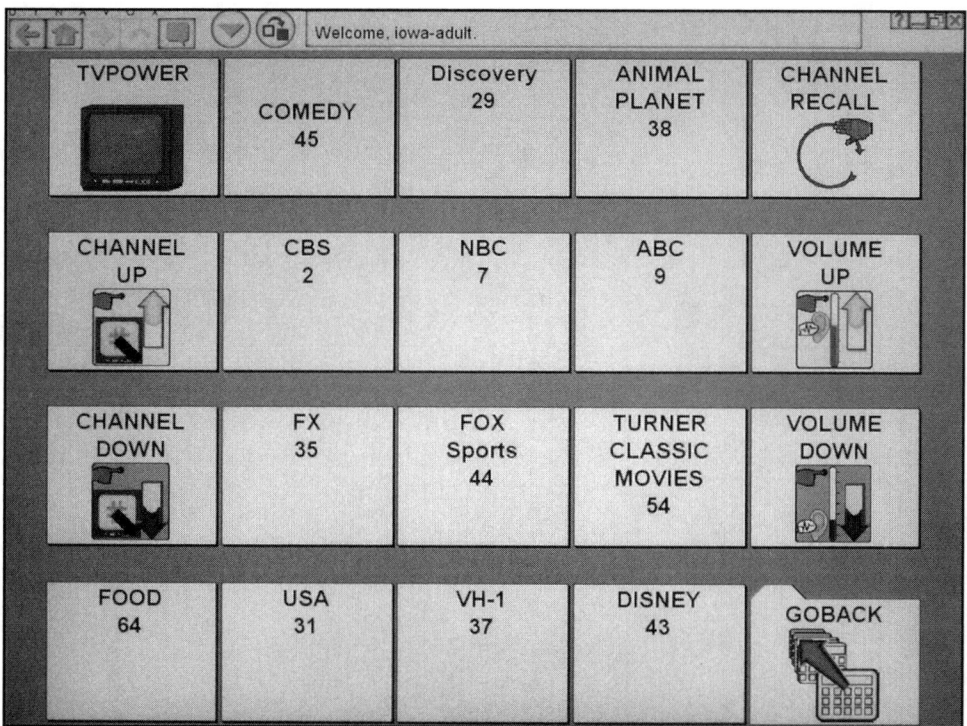

Figure 6–16. IOWA template—TV page.

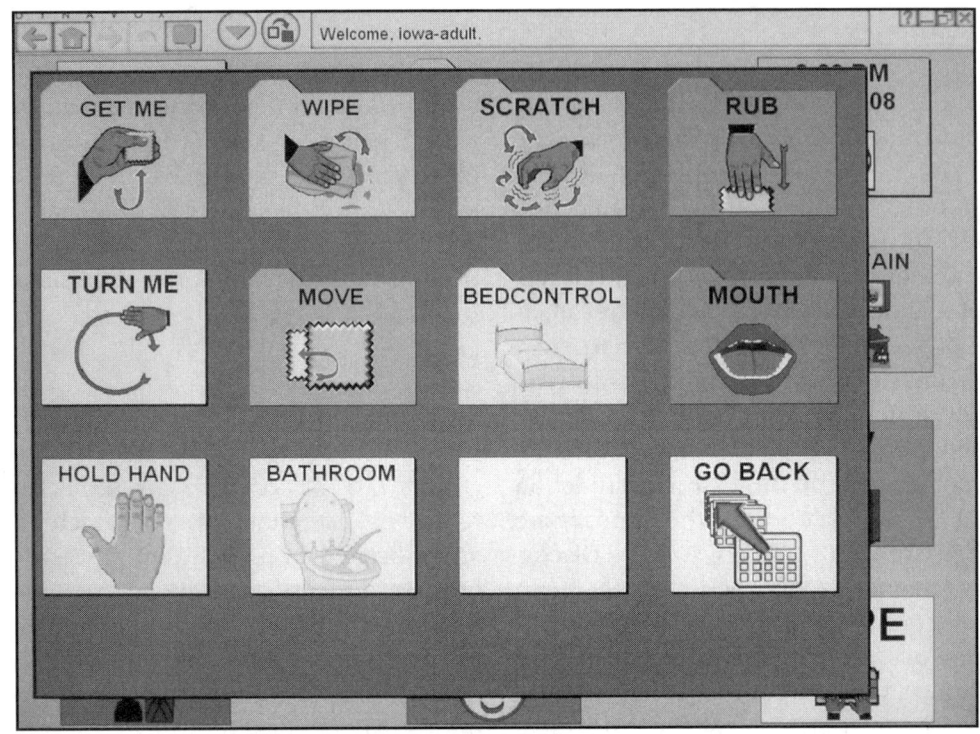

Figure 6–17. IOWA template—Help me page.

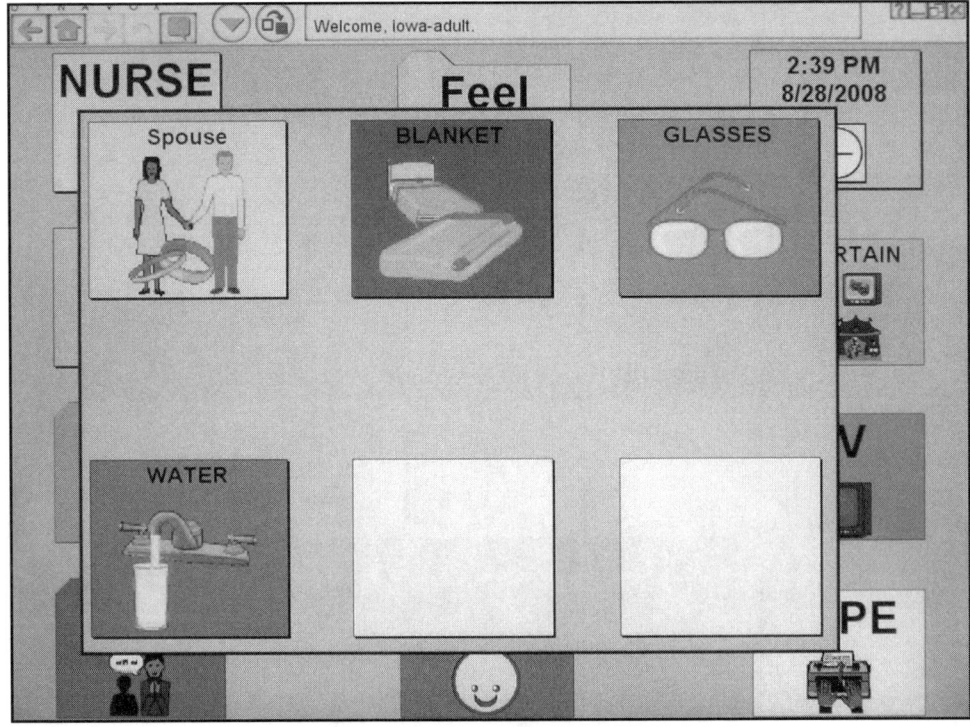

Figure 6–18. IOWA template—Get me page.

The **Scratch** and **Rub** options in the **Help** pop-up link to a **Body Parts** pop-up (Figure 6–19) and allow the patient to construct phrases such as "Scratch my ear" or "Rub my shoulder." The **Wipe** option in the **Help** pop-up links to a **Wipe My** pop-up (Figure 6–20). This pop-up allows the patient to request that some part of the patient's face be wiped. The **Mouth** option in the **Help** pop-up opens a **Mouth Cares** pop up (Figure 6–21) that allows the patient to request suctioning and other mouth care. We have found that providing a redundant access to the **Bed Control** pop-up from the **Help** pop-up is also useful in facilitating patients' ability to make requests.

Personal Pop-Up

The Top Level menu page provides a link to a Personal pop-up (Figure 6–22). This pop-up is populated with patient specific requests and utterances. We leave this category open to patient and caregiver choice. Patients often request questions or responses on particular topics of concern or interest. Some request content related to sporting events; many Iowans are into Big 10 sports. One patient who was a farmer wanted phrases to be able to talk about how the crops and livestock were doing. A pediatric patient wanted to be able to talk about school and friends. One patient wanted to be

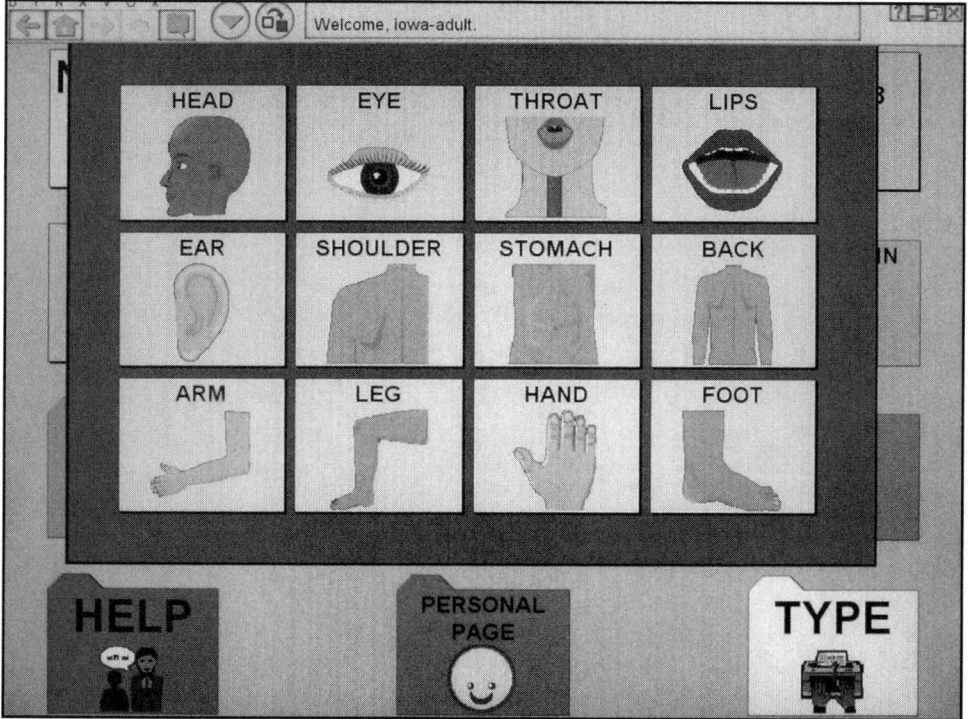

Figure 6–19. IOWA template—Body parts pop-up.

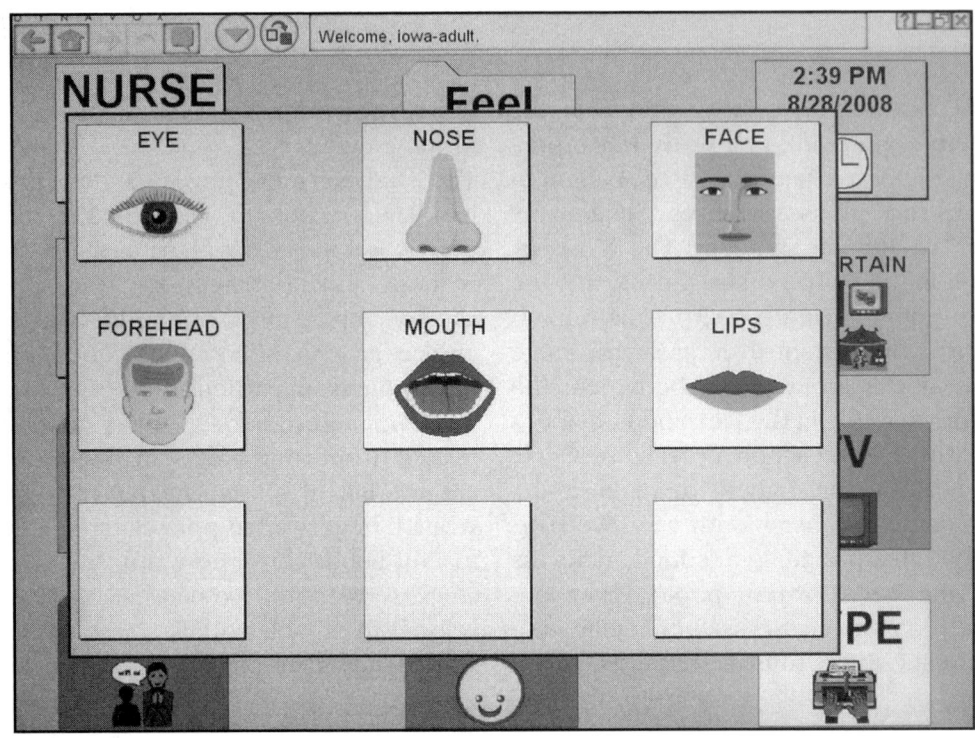

Figure 6–20. IOWA template—Wipe my page.

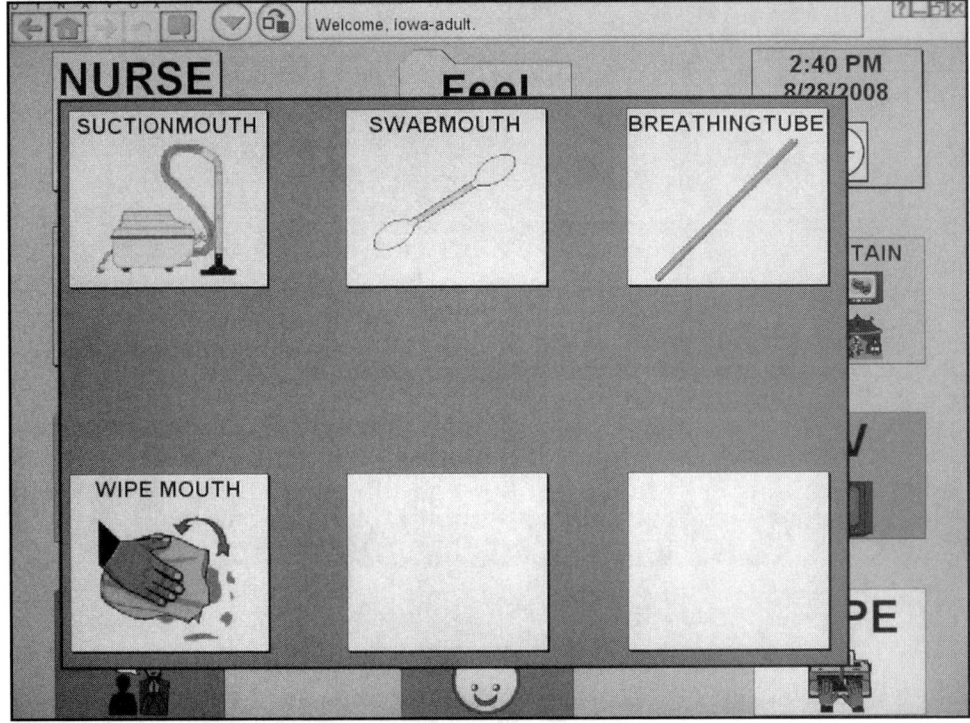

Figure 6–21. IOWA template—Mouth care page.

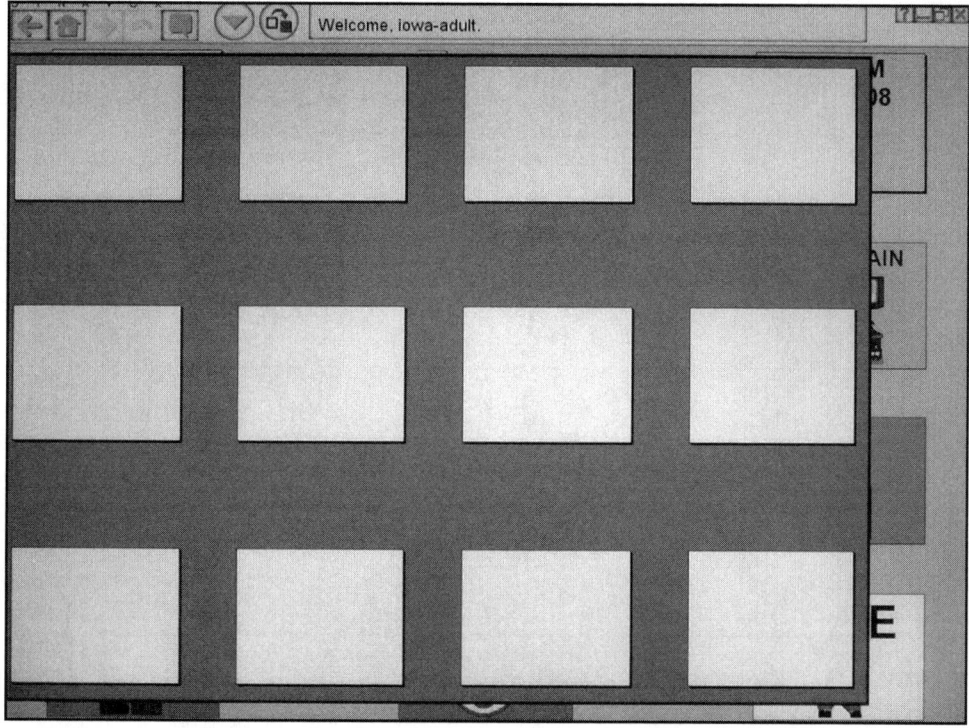

Figure 6–22. IOWA template—Personal page.

able to participate in tax return preparations. One elderly patient wanted to instruct her family about gifts for her many grandchildren.

Adding or changing items on all pages and pop-ups should be made to suit the particular needs of a patient and the form of the phrases should be consistent with the politeness level that fits the patient's personality. One factor that should be considered when selecting an AAC system is the ease with which changes to content can be made quickly at the bedside.

Novel Message Generation

We have been consistently struck by the fact that, regardless of the patient's physical limitations, patients want to be able to create novel message from scratch. To that end, we provide access to an on-screen key board (Figure 6-23) along with number (Figure 6-24) and punctuation (Figure 6-25) pop-ups. The patient selects one key at a time and constructs the intended message in the message window that is part of the keyboard page layout. A speak all button allows the constructed message to be spoken. Thus, the patient can construct the message and then play it out to the appropriate person. The page also includes command function buttons (e.g., save file and load file) that allow the patient to save the message for later use. Some AAC systems (i.e., Dynavox V) provide an easy way of saving of messages to menu buttons that can then be directly accessed without needing to search through a file directory.

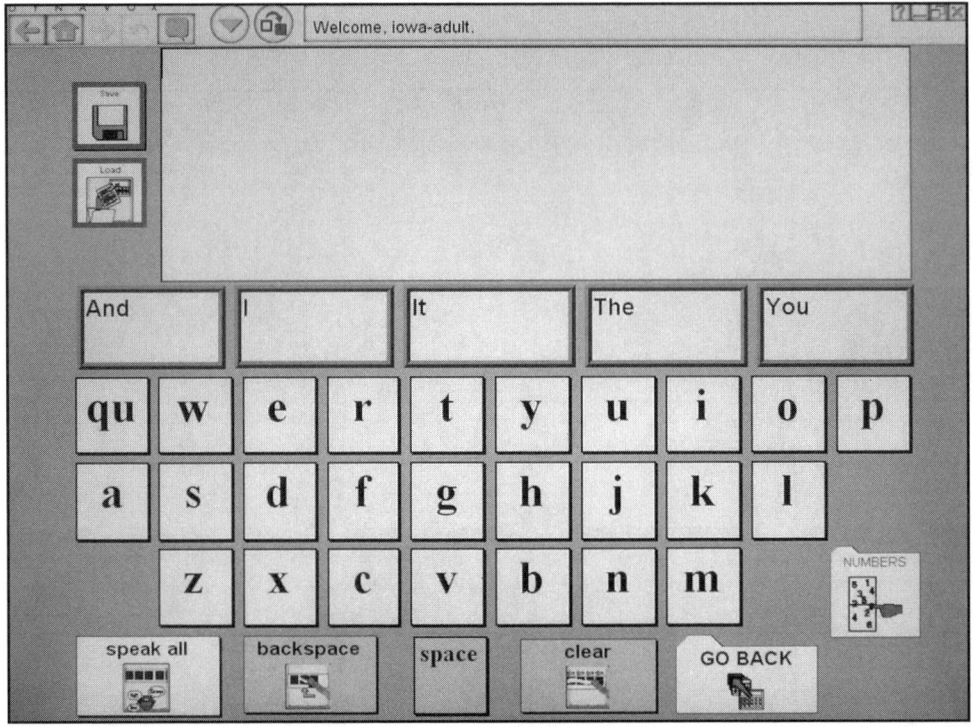

Figure 6–23. IOWA template—QWERTY keyboard.

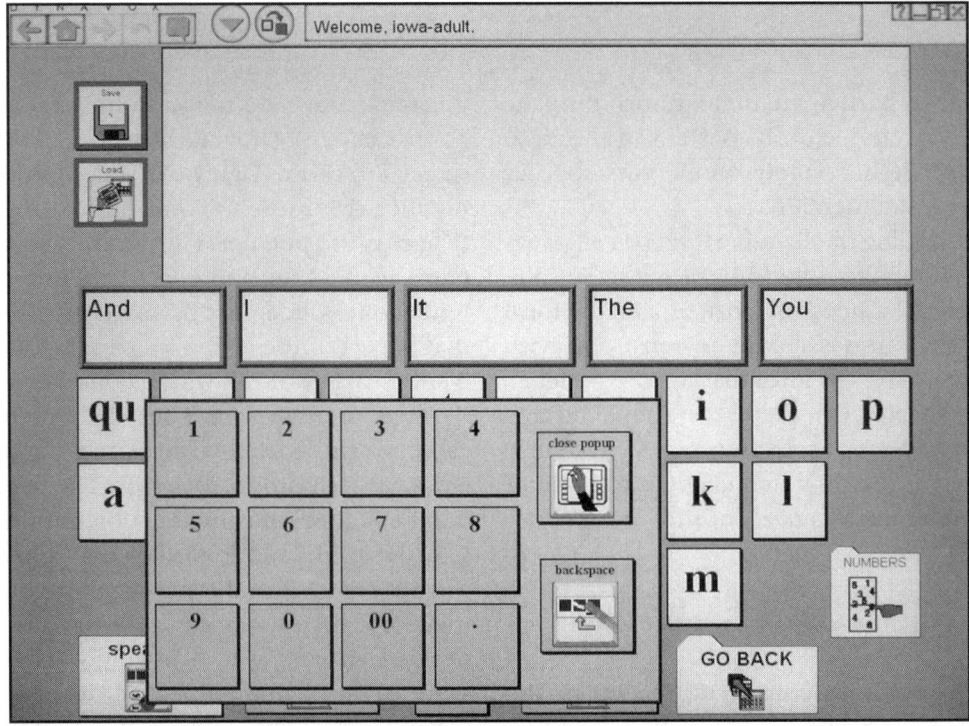

Figure 6–24. IOWA template—Number pop-up.

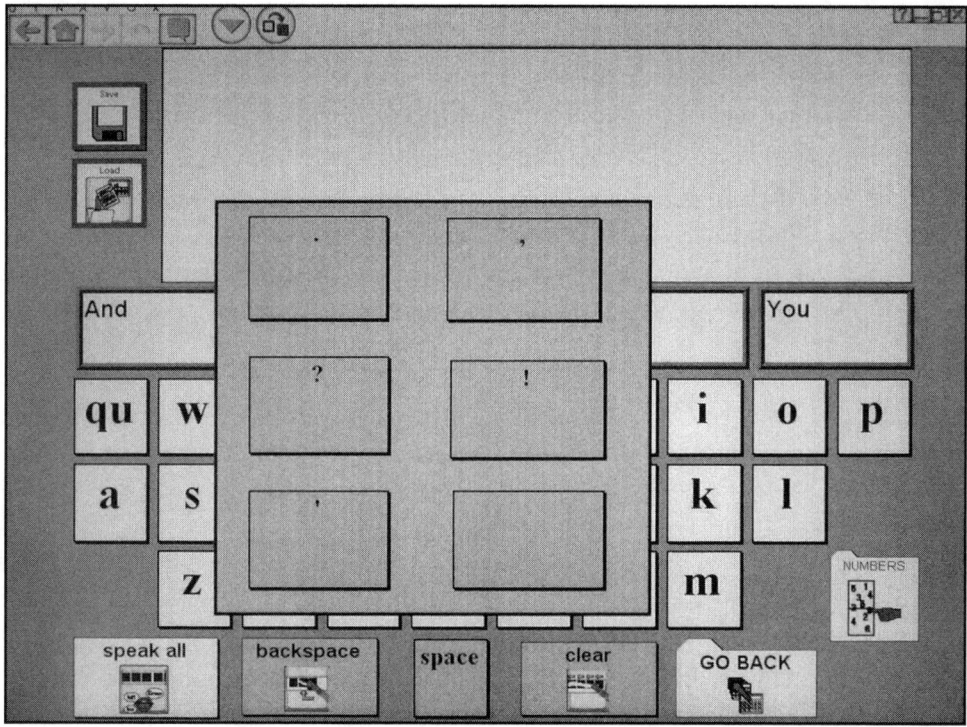

Figure 6–25. IOWA template—Punctuation pop-up.

Rate Enhancement Strategies

Because typing one key at a time is very slow and laborious in a direct select mode and even more taxing in a scanning mode, it is critical that one consider adding rate enhancement strategies. These strategies include rate enhancing keyboard layouts, word prediction, and abbreviation expansion.

For most patients who have done some typing prior to their hospitalization, the QWERTY keyboard (Figure 6-23) is the most often selected keyboard. These patients prefer this layout because it is the one they have experience with. They know where every key is.

To use a keyboard in serial scanning mode would not be practical. Using a scan pattern, like row/column scanning, would certainly reduce the time to get to the desired key. However, accidental selection of the wrong row would lead to a considerable wait before the correct row could be selected. To avoid the delay resulting from selecting the wrong row, we have constructed a keyboard template with a bailout button after the first button in each row (Figure 6-26). The function associated with these bailout buttons is to terminate the scanning on the selected row, thereby eliminating the delay that would result from having to scan the entire row.

For patients with no prior keyboard experience, the most commonly preferred keyboard is one which has the keys laid out in alphabetic order (Figure 6-27).

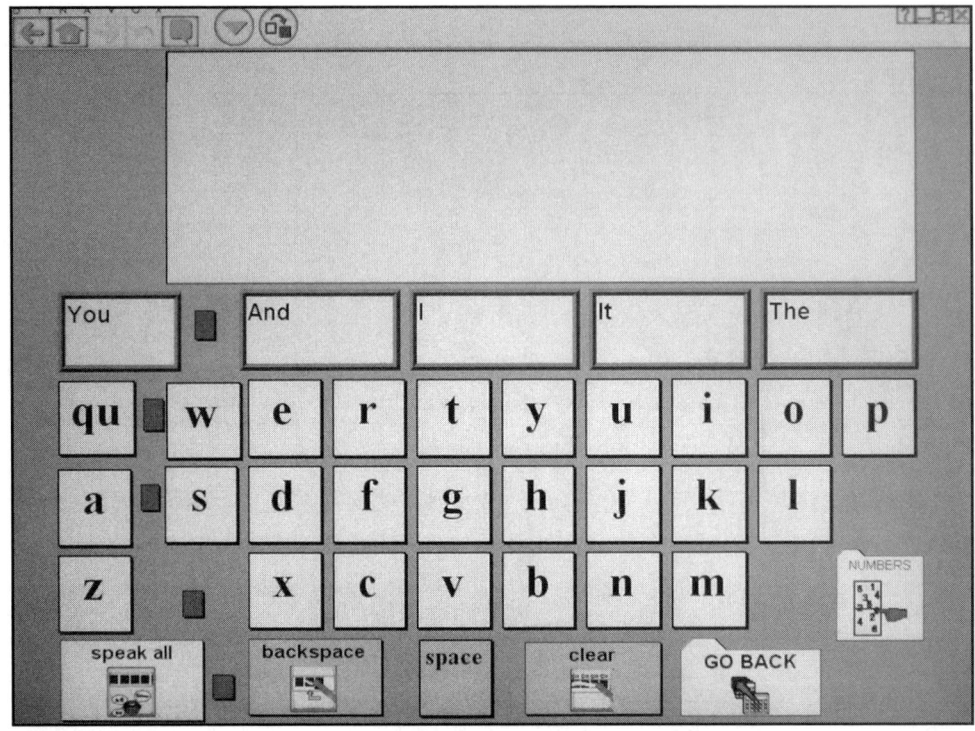

Figure 6–26. IOWA template-QWERTY keyboard—With bailout buttons.

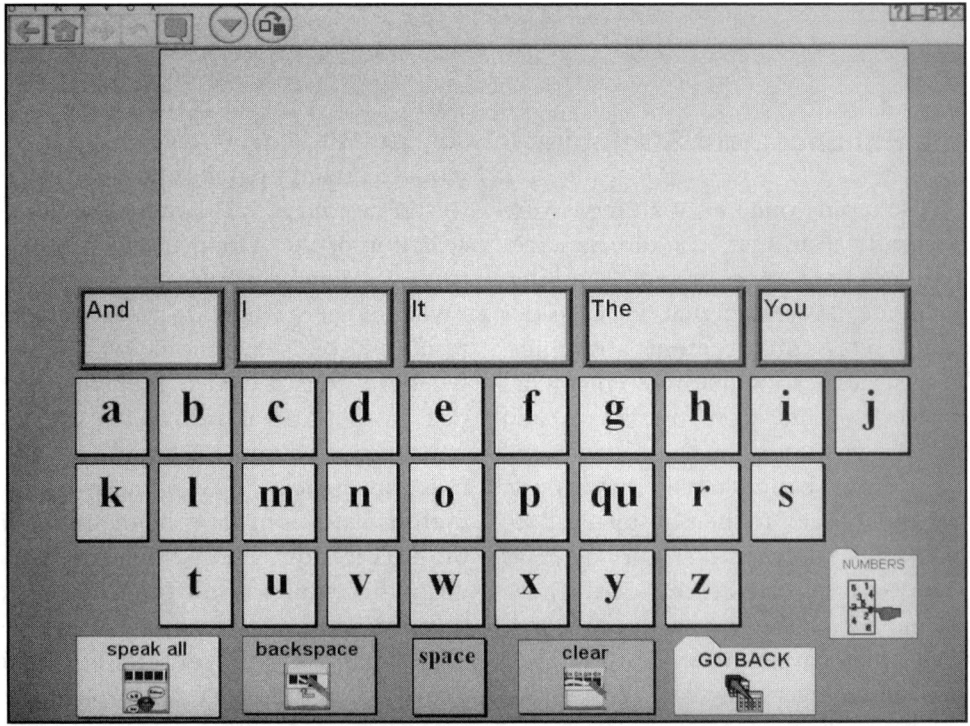

Figure 6–27. IOWA template—Alphabetic keyboard.

As with the QWERTY keyboard, scanning through the alphabet serially or even with a row-column scheme often is too time consuming. So, here too, we have created a version with bailout buttons (Figure 6–28).

Both the QWERTY and alphabetic layouts, although familiar to users, have been considered ill suited for scanning. In their place, AAC system developers have constructed frequency-based layouts (Figure 6–29). In these layouts, the keys are laid out in rows and columns based on their frequency of occurrence in written language. In the case of Jean Dominique Bauby, his clinician provided an auditory scanning of the alphabet using the frequency of occurrence of letters in written French. As with the other layouts, even this frequency-based layout can lead to delays if an inappropriate row is selected. So, even for the frequency-based keyboard layout, we have created a version with bailout buttons (Figure 6–30). Many AAC systems provide a number of additional alternative keyboard layouts for individuals who cannot deal with full keyboard layouts because of limited fine motor skills or who need to access the keyboard utilizing a scan selection method. In these layouts the patient selects a letter in a two-step process. The first button selection picks the group of letters in which the target letter occurs then the screen zooms in to allow the patient two select the particular letter in the group.

For all our alternative keyboard layouts, we include a set of word prediction buttons that engage the AAC system's word prediction algorithm. At this point,

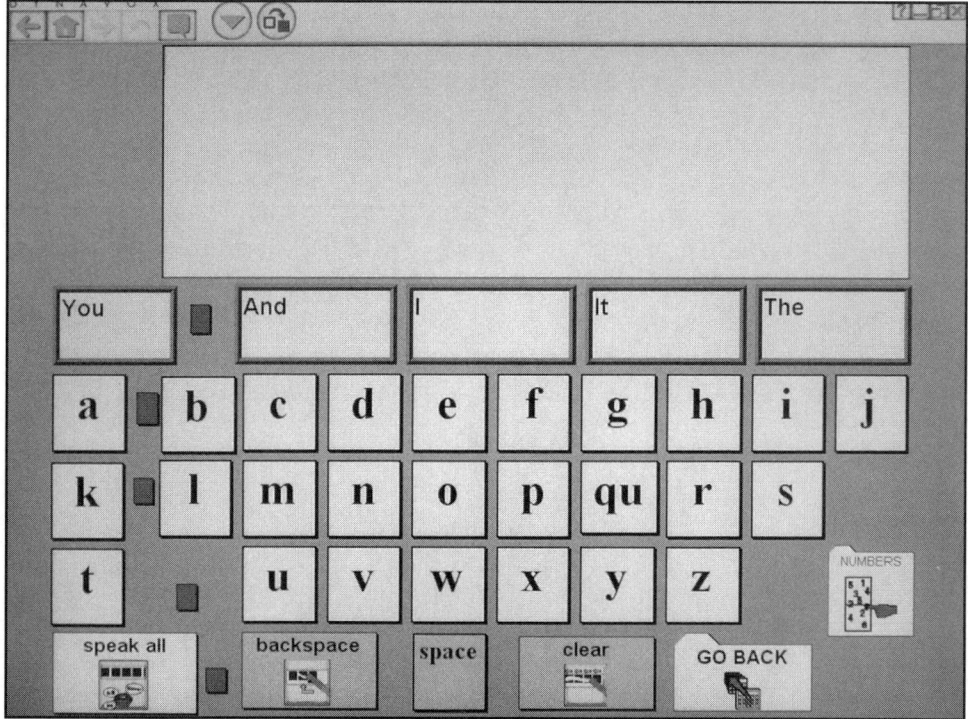

Figure 6–28. IOWA template—Alphabetic keyboard with bailout buttons.

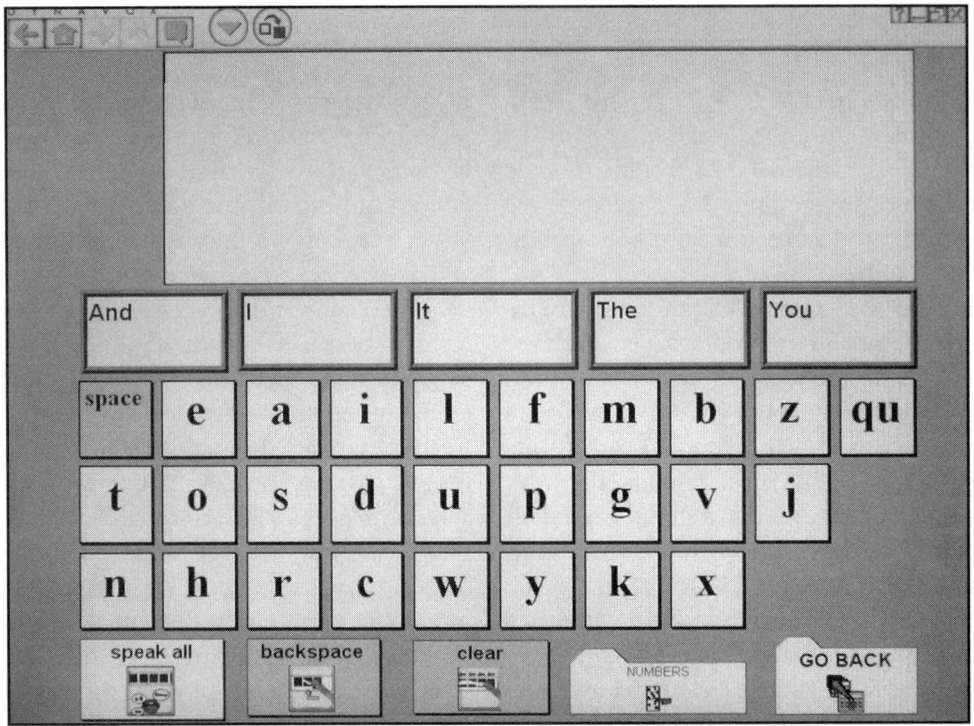

Figure 6–29. IOWA template—Frequency keyboard.

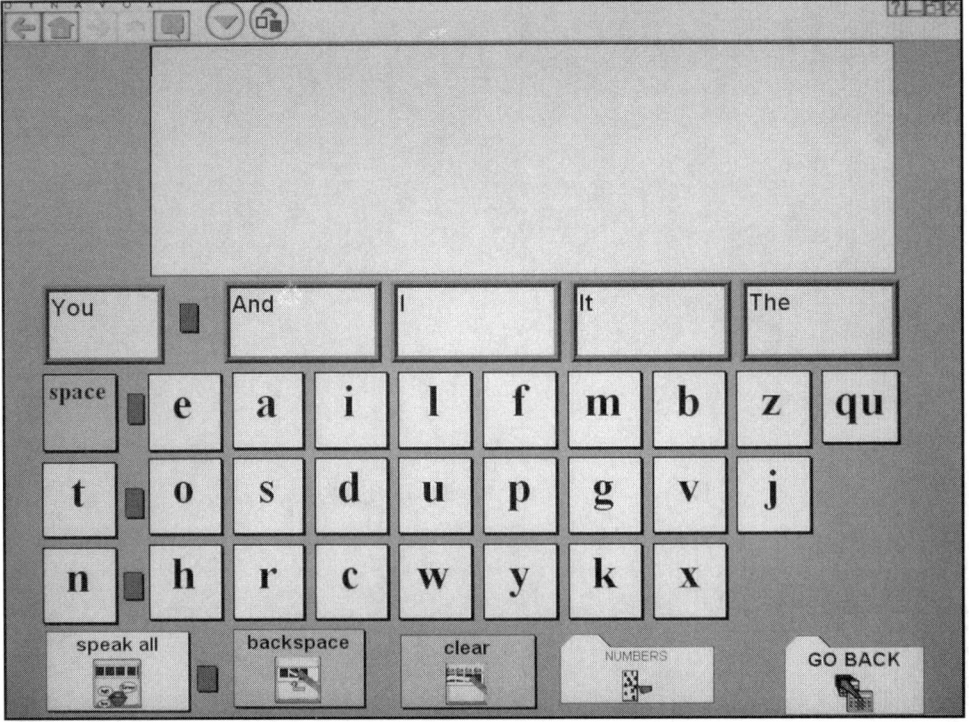

Figure 6–30. IOWA template—Frequency keyboard with bailout buttons.

all high-tech AAC systems provide some form of word or phrase prediction. As the user begins to select individual keys, the set of predictor button above the keyboard and below the message window are updated. If the system has predicted the intended word, then the patient merely needs to select the predictor button displaying the intended word rather than continue spelling out the word. In most systems, one can select the type of prediction to be used. The prediction can be driven by the underlying word frequency values in the default prediction database or by a dynamic database that updates the frequency values based on the usage by the patient. A third alternative involves using a recency representation rather than a frequency representation of the lexical database. Thus, the prediction algorithm produces the most recently used words that share letters with the word currently being typed. Some systems include a syntactic category field in the lexical database and with a grammatical constraint component in the prediction algorithm can use the syntactic context to further restrict the predicted words. Historically, traditional AAC users have not taken advantage of word prediction. Likewise, many of our patients have also ignored the predictor buttons. The reported reason for the rejection of this potentially keystroke saving function is that the content of the predictor buttons is often semantically unrelated to the intended word, so users find the predictor buttons are distracting and cause them to lose their train of thought. In some systems, one can also have the option to use phrase prediction. In this case, potential phrases based on the keys selected are displayed on the predictor buttons. Although this produces choices that are more likely to match the intended message, the problem is that most systems do not dynamically set the font size for the content of the predictor buttons and so the entire phrase is not visible on the predictor button. Not being able to see the end of the word/phrase makes it difficult to be certain that the predicted item is a match for the intended one.

The use of abbreviation expansion has also been used in AAC systems for quite some time. The system stores a two-column table that includes the abbreviation and the expansion (word or phrase). Then, when the user enters the abbreviation, the system produces the expansion of that abbreviation. Some systems automatically perform abbreviation expansion whereas others require the user to enter a designated key (often the key associated with the space bar). The latter option requires an extra keystroke, but avoids the potential code collision that would arise from abbreviations and whole words sharing initial letters (e.g., SUL, which could be the abbreviation for "see you later" or the beginning of a word like "sultry" or "sultan") or from overlap of related abbreviations (e.g., B4 for "before" or B4N for "before now"). Historically, introducing abbreviations was thought to require extensive training to learn and retain the abbreviations and their meanings. As such, introducing abbreviations in acute care short-term AAC usage settings was considered to be impractical. We learned from the case of our ALS patient (described in Chapter 2), who had to use Morse code, that learning many abbreviations may not be a challenge for all patients.

A recent societal change has also made the learning of abbreviations a nonproblem. With the advent of instant messaging (IM), a larger and larger segment of the population is using abbreviations to communicate on a daily basis. Although IM began with kids, almost everyone who uses a cellular phone or E-mail uses a fairly large set of abbreviations on a daily basis. We have taken several hundred of the most commonly used IM abbreviations and added them and their expansions to the abbreviation table in the AAC systems. Thus, the patient merely types in the IM code and the system expands and speaks the intended message. Unlike test-messaging via cellular phone, which requires both sender and receiver to understand the IM code, use of the IM codes in an AAC system does not require the conversational partner to view the message window or know the IM codes' meaning. Many of our patients want to communicate with relatives who may not be able to come to the hospital by phone. With a speakerphone at the bedside, the patient can quickly construct messages using the IM codes and the AAC system produces the voice output associated with the expansion. This ability to communicate with family and friends via phone has been a real boon to intubated and tracheotomized patients, who would otherwise be incommunicado.

Shortly after we had started adding the IM codes to our systems, while we were doing our rounds of patients in the intensive care units who were using our AAC systems, one of the nurses intimated that a female patient in her 60s might not be cognitively intact. We inquired why the nurse had come to that conclusion and were told that the patient appeared not to know how to use the keyboard function and that her spelling was atrocious. When we watched the patient using the system it became obvious that the patient was not typing words but was producing what looked like IM codes. When we asked the patient what she was doing she indicated with full and completely spelled words that she was using IM codes and wished that the system could recognize them. She said that she had been using the IM codes for several years text-messaging her daughter who lived in Australia. We quickly enabled abbreviation expansion for her and consequently she was much more efficient in her use of the AAC system and, as a result, the nurses' perception of her cognitive status changed dramatically.

We typically have a number of high school students working in the lab over the summer and they assisted in compiling the list of the most commonly used IM codes. As one might expect, some of the codes they included had rather colorful expansions. We opted to leave those codes in so that patients would be able to express themselves in whatever manner they wanted to (see also Chapter 11, Case E).

For patients who will need to access the AAC system using head or eye tracking one may need to modify the template layouts. These patients make template selections by directing their gaze to a particular button on the template. The system performs the action associated with the button if the patient holds his or her gaze for a designated time interval (dwell). To avoid unintentional selections the dwell setting can be adjusted so that not all gaze shifts will result in button selections. We have found that some patients find the effort associated with "not looking at a button" can exhaust them. To that end we have modified the template set so that the center of each page can serve as a neutral 'resting space' from which the patients move to make selections. Figure 6–31 provides an exemplar of this alternative layout.

The companion DVD includes multiple versions of the Iowa template in the Dynavox User format. We provide our default template as well as a template modified for use with head and eye tracking which includes the resting space shown in Figure 6–31. We also provide a Spanish version of the Iowa template that can be used in settings where the patient and staff can communicate in Spanish (Figure 6–32). To accommodate the situations in which the nurse and patient do not speak the same language (see Chapter 11, Case A) we include a template that has 'patient' pages that label the button selections in Spanish but speaks English as well as a "nurse" page that labels the button selections in English and speaks Spanish.

The DVD also includes versions of the Iowa template in the Speaking Dynamically Pro™ and Viking user formats. The DVD also includes two sets of template pages developed with the Mayer-Johnson BoardMaker Plus™ software. The first set is in the BoardMaker format and requires the BoardMaker software to view, edit and print the template pages. The second set can be viewed and printed without any proprietary software.

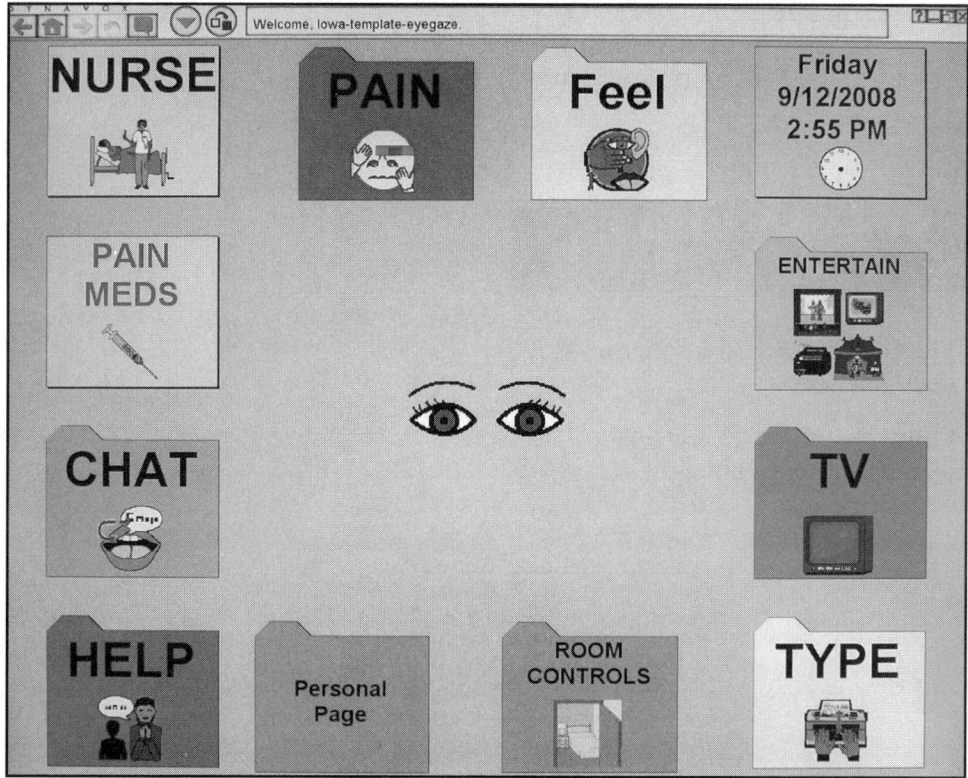

Figure 6–31. IOWA template—Eye/Head tracking layout.

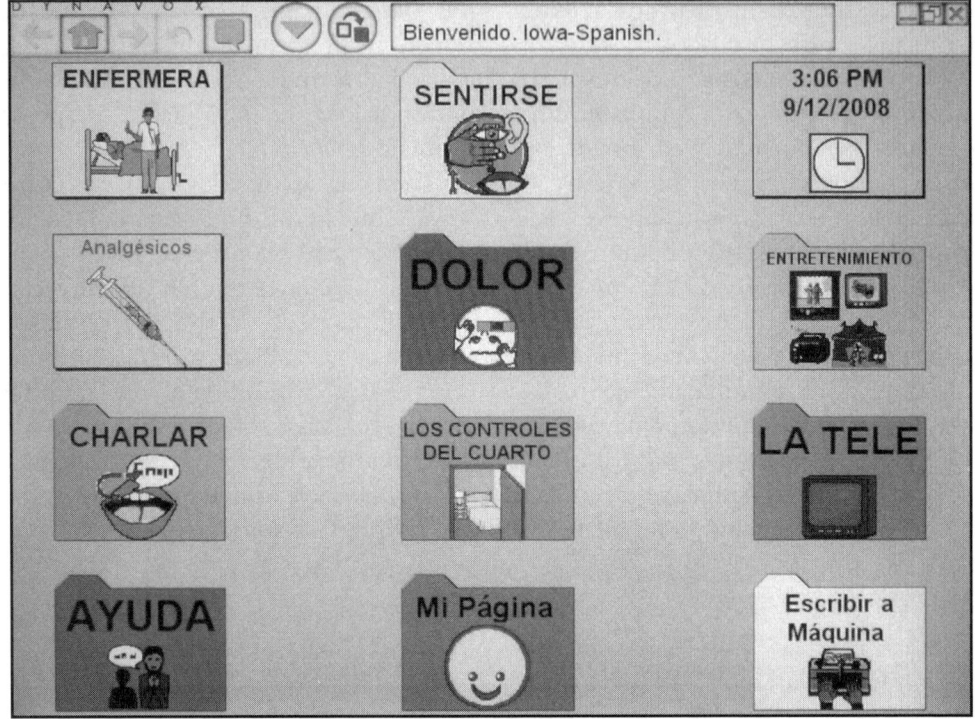

Figure 6–32. IOWA template—Spanish version

VIDEOS ASSOCIATED WITH THIS CHAPTER

Video clip 6–1. Row-column scanning demo.

Video clip 6–2. Pop-up link demo/same as Video clip 4-5.

7 Mounting and Access Issues

Technology allows us to control and travel through our environments when using our arms and legs alone is not sufficient. Before the development of the electric light bulb, we could only control room illumination if we could reach the candles to light them. To reach those high chandeliers in fancy castles and palaces, extra technology was required. In some cases, it was ladders and in other cases it was a pole with a lighting candle and candle snuffer. Today, a light switch allows us to turn a light on the ceiling on and off without having to be able to directly reach it. Although when the bulb burns out and needs to be replaced, we too need the older technology to reach and change the bulb.

The light switch is a great piece of technology that allows us to do something without being in proximity of the actual light being turned on and off. As long as I can reach the switch, the technology allows me to turn the lights on and off. A TV remote allows me to control the TV without having to physically touch the controls on the TV. Some say the technology has a down side in that in contributes to obesity and lack of muscle tone. For the individual who cannot physically get to the TV to turn it on, the remote is essential. But what happens if I cannot reach the light switch or the remote is not where I can reach it? If the technology is not accessible, it is worthless.

The nurse call is a form of technology that allows us to summon the nurse to come to our room when we do not have the ability to get out of bed or the lung power to yell for the nurse. A variety of switches have been used to give patients an effective nurse call (see Chapter 5). Some use fairly simple low-tech solutions and others use more sophisticated high tech-integrated circuit solutions. Regardless of the type of technology used, if the patient cannot reach and activate the nurse call, then the patient is in the same boat as the small child who cannot reach up to flip the light switch. It is not enough to ensure that a switch has been selected that the patient can activate. We have to ensure that the switch is positioned and mounted so that the patient has continuous access to the switch.

Standard nursing protocols require that, prior to leaving a patient's room, the nurse makes sure that the nurse call has been positioned where the patient can access it. Hanging the nurse call pendant behind the bed or lowering the bed rail that has the call button integrated into the rail makes the nurse call inaccessible. Both of these actions might be necessary when performing some bedside care. The problem is that, in the rush of things, the nurse may forget to reposition the switch. This also happens too often when a patient is transferred from the bed to a chair or back to bed again. Nurses are perhaps more vigilant about repositioning the nurse call than others involved in the care of the patient including family members.

Access to a switch is also crucial for patients who receive medication for pain via a PCA pump (patient-controlled analgesia). The literature suggests cognitively intact patients one can achieve good pain management by giving them control over when the analgesic medication is administered. Self-administered medication appears to work well; patients who use a PCA use less medication to manage their pain. Like the nurse call, if the switch linking the patient to the PCA pump is not where the patient can access it, then it is as if the patient is not on a PCA.

For the patient who needs to use an AAC system for communication and environmental control, access to the AAC device is essential if the patient is to benefit from having the AAC system. So if the device is not positioned where the patient can see and activate the options that have been programmed into the device, then the device might as well not be in the room at all. Like the nurse call and the PCA control, care must be taken to ensure that the device is always accessible and that repositioning is essential each time the patient's position changes. Because these AAC systems must be positioned at the bedside, they often are in the way and must be moved in order to perform patient care and mange transferring the patient in and out of bed.

So whether we are talking about the simplest nurse call or the most high-tech AAC technology we have to address the issue of accessibility. That accessibility has two human factors components. The *patient-related factor* requires innovative use of technology including mounting solutions. In some cases, this requires something as simple as a safety pin to keep a switch attached to the patient's gown. In other cases, it may require more complex specialized mounting hardware that needs to be uniquely adapted to the particular physical challenges facing the patient. Some of these solutions will require the assistance of a biomedical engineer, occupational therapist, or physical therapist. The *caregiver-related factor* really requires an educational solution. That solution needs to ensure that the caregivers understand how the technology works and, most importantly, that they must be vigilant that the technology is where the patient can access it.

This chapter addresses the patient-related factors and provides specific examples of how we have handled the physical accessibility issues. The chapter on nurse and allied health training provides some insight on how to address the caregiver-related factors (see Chapter 12).

DEVICE MOUNTING SOLUTIONS

The key to making AAC systems accessible is making sure that they can easily be (re)positioned at the bedside and that, once positioned, allow the patient to easily use the system. This principle applies equally to low- and high-tech systems.

Hand-Held Implementations

In those cases where the caregiver is the AAC system (as in the case of Jean Dominique Bauby, whose clinicians/aides used an oral scanning through the alphabet), it is essential that they position themselves where they can see the patient to note when the patient makes a selection response. In such cases, it is equally important to make sure that the caregiver is positioned so that the patient can see the caregiver and hear the caregiver's voice. Because many intensive care settings are noisy and a flurry of activity, positioning is essential if the patient is to hear the caregiver. The advantage of a direct line of sight positioning is that the caregiver is able to discern changes in subtle facial expressions that might signal critical information. Figures 7-1A and 7-1B illustrate optimal and nonoptimal positioning of the caregiver relative to the patient. In situations where a communication board is used, it is also essential for the caregiver to hold or position the communication board where the patient can see the board. In cases where the patient is using direct selection by pointing to the desired element on the board, it is also critical that the board be positioned where the patient can reach it. Figure 7-2 illustrates the situation where the caregiver holds the board. Note that the caregiver should be standing in such a way that he or she not only makes the board accessible but can clearly discern what selections the patient is making. If the communication board is an ETRAN in which the patient uses eye gaze to make the selections, it is essential that the board be held up where the patient can comfortably make gaze shifts to indicate the selections. Figure 7-3 illustrates an effective positioning of an ETRAN. Care should be taken to position the board so that the patient is able to make gaze shifts from primary gaze. To minimize strain, the board should be positioned so that the patient does not need to maintain an extreme eccentric gaze. Care should be taken not only to position the board appropriately in terms of horizontal gaze but also appropriately in terms of vertical gaze. It is sometimes difficult from the caregiver's perspective to gauge what an optimal position might be for a bedridden patient. As the patient's position in bed may change periodically and where the caregiver can stand may vary given all the equipment surrounding the bed, it is essential to establish a protocol for board positioning prior to each communicative interaction with the patient. So everyone who will interact with the patient using the communication board should start each interaction with some questions about whether the board is positioned properly for the patient. This protocol should include ascertaining whether the patient's glasses (if the patient uses glasses) are on. Video clip 7-1 demonstrates how such a positioning protocol can be implemented.

Bed Tray Implementations

In situations where a bed tray can be positioned by the bed, communication boards can be placed on the bed tray. As with hand-held implementations, care must be taken that the board is visible and accessible. A flat placement of the board on the tray would be very difficult for a patient who must lie flat and would not be able to see or reach the surface of the bed tray.

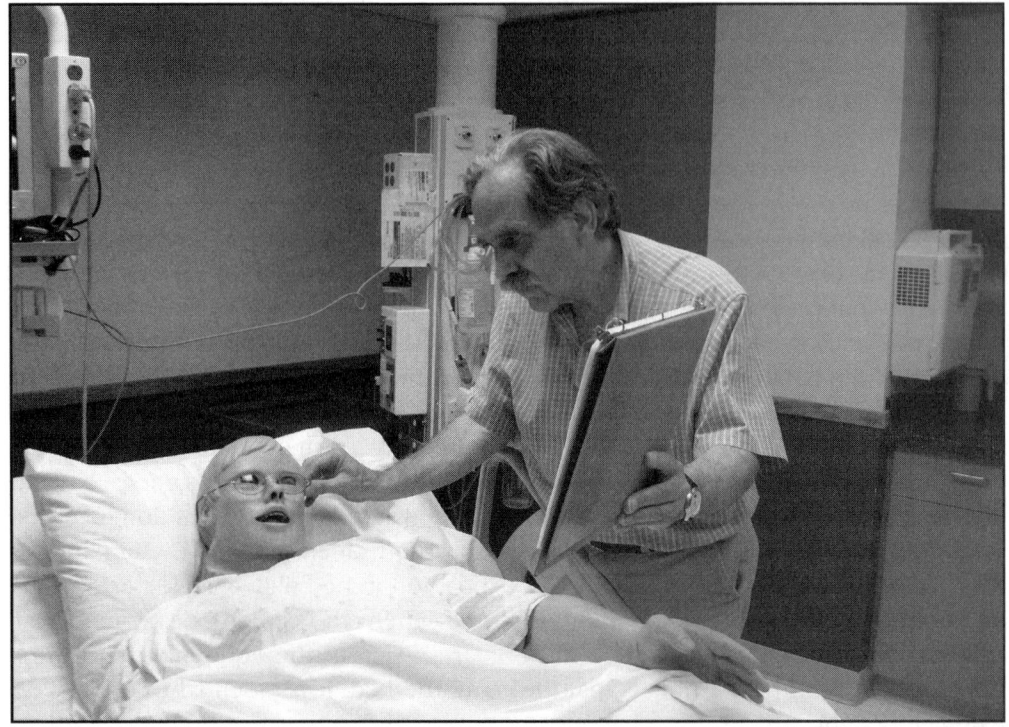

A

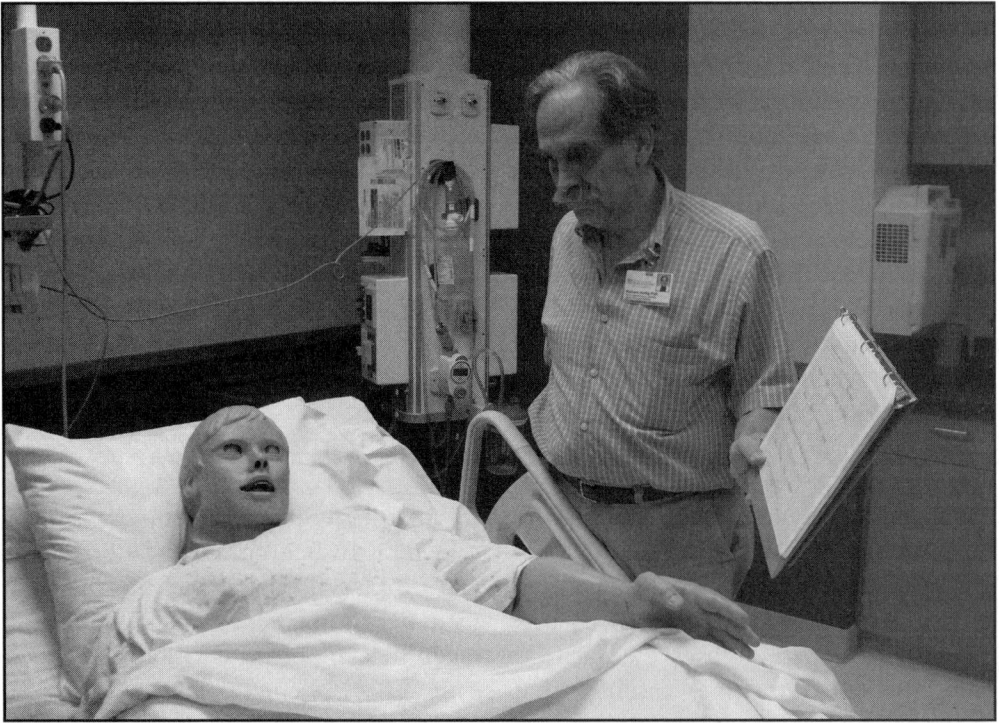

B

Figure 7–1. **A**. Optimal position for hand-held communication board. **B**. Nonoptimal position for handheld communication board.

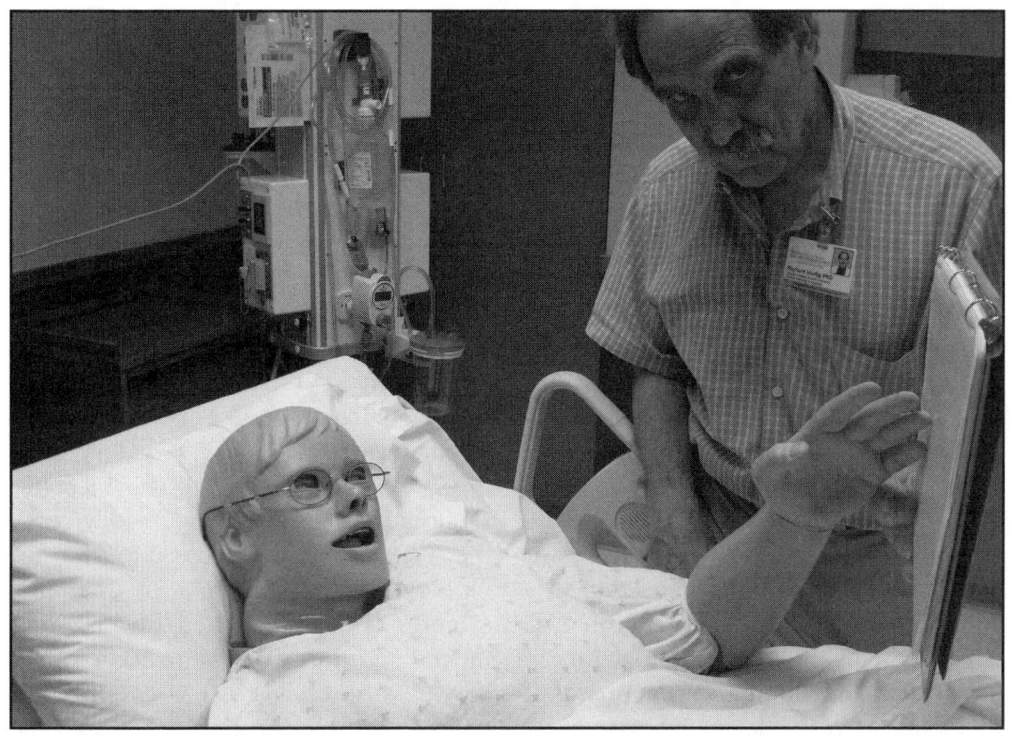

Figure 7–2. Optimal position for handheld communication board-direct selection.

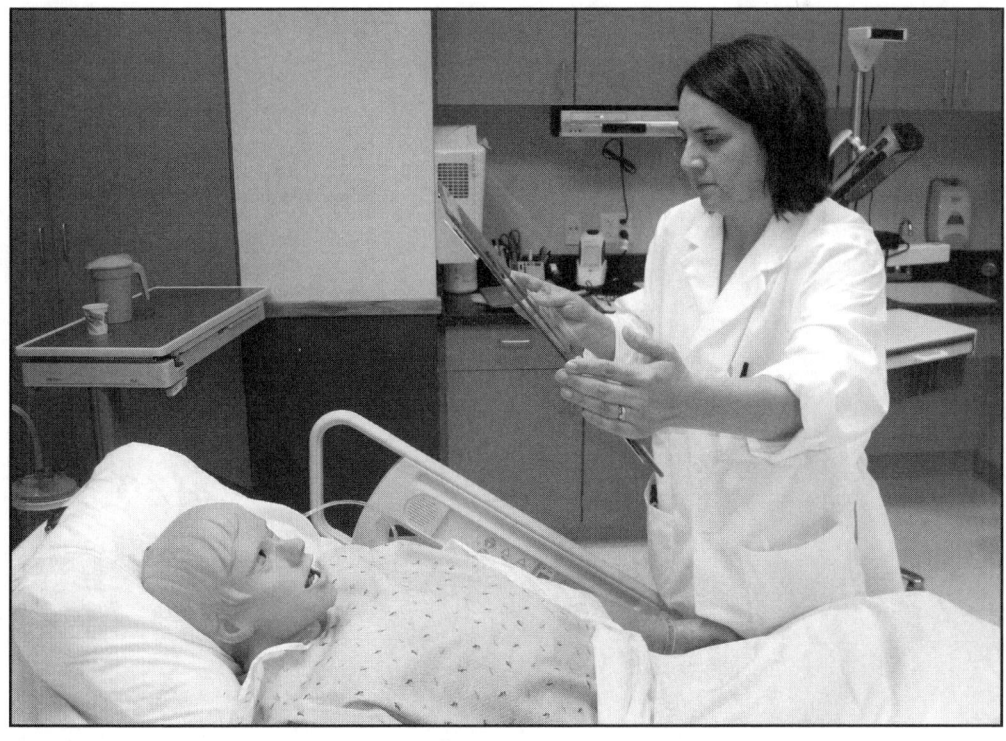

Figure 7–3. Optimal position for ETRAN board.

If the patient can sit up, then a flat placement might be appropriate (Figure 7-4). Care should be taken to secure the board so that, as the patient makes a pointing gesture he or she does not accidentally push the board off the bed tray. The board can be held in place by using tape, Velcro, or Dycem (a nonslip product that can easily be put on and removed). Alternatively, the bed tray can be used with an easel that can allow positioning of the communication board at an angle that makes it visible and accessible (Figure 7-5).

The bed tray also can be used in situations where a mid- or a high- tech AAC device is being implemented. As with the use of low-tech communication boards, it is essential that the device be positioned so that the patient can see and access the device. Care needs to be taken that the device not be able to slip off the bed tray to fall either on the patient or on the floor. Depending on the weight of the device, either a material like Dycem can be used to keep the device from slipping or the device can be clamped to the bed tray. Many devices come with mounting plates that allow for their use with tabletop or wheelchair mounts. The mounts can be securely attached to the bed tray (Figure 7-6). These systems allow for greater flexibility in positioning of a device so that it is visible and accessible even for patients who must remain totally supine (Figure 7-7). As the bed tray is often moved and the patient's position in bed may also be changed it is essential for caregivers to periodically assess that the device positioning is appropriate.

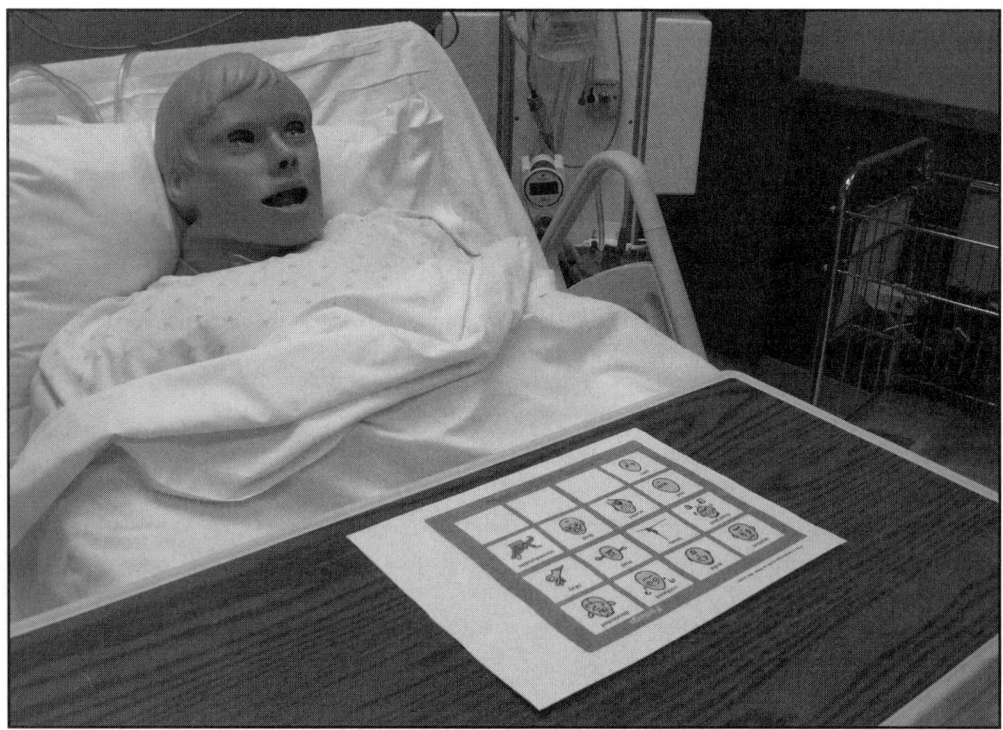

Figure 7-4. Communication board on bed tray: flat position.

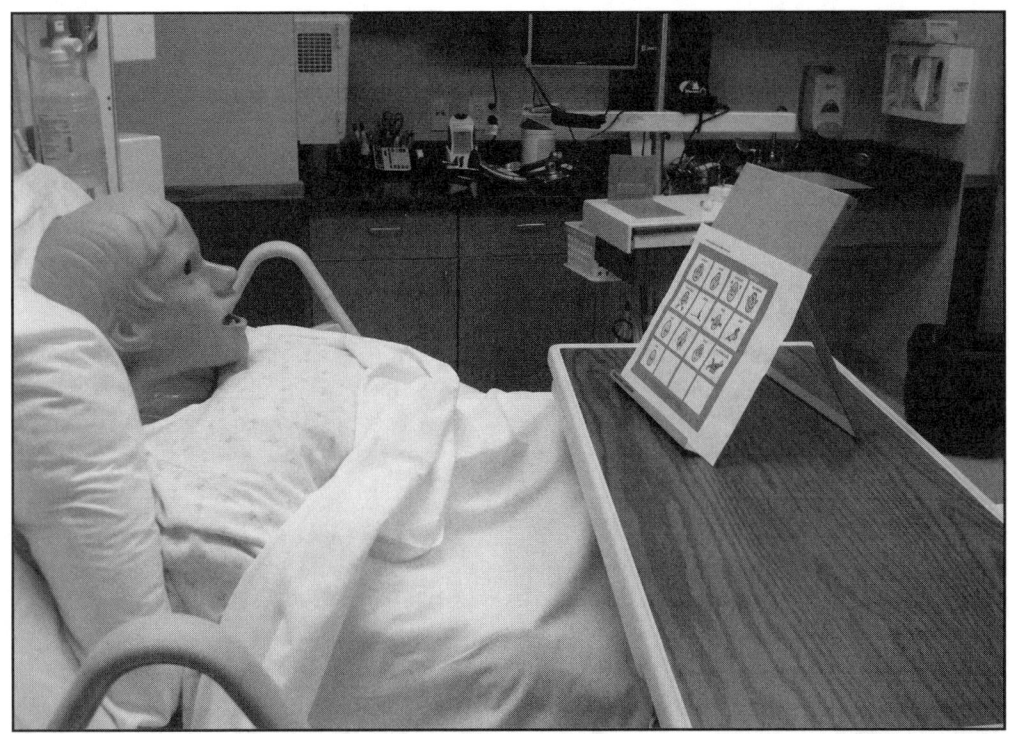

Figure 7–5. Communication board on bed tray: angled on typing stand.

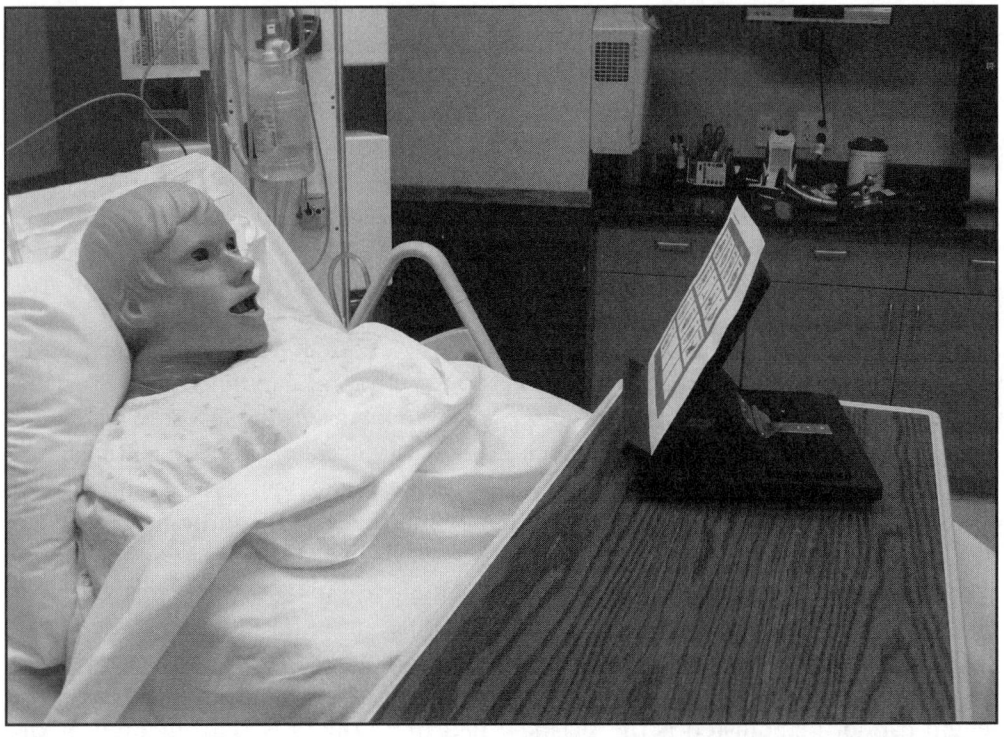

Figure 7–6. Communication board on bed tray: angled suction mount.

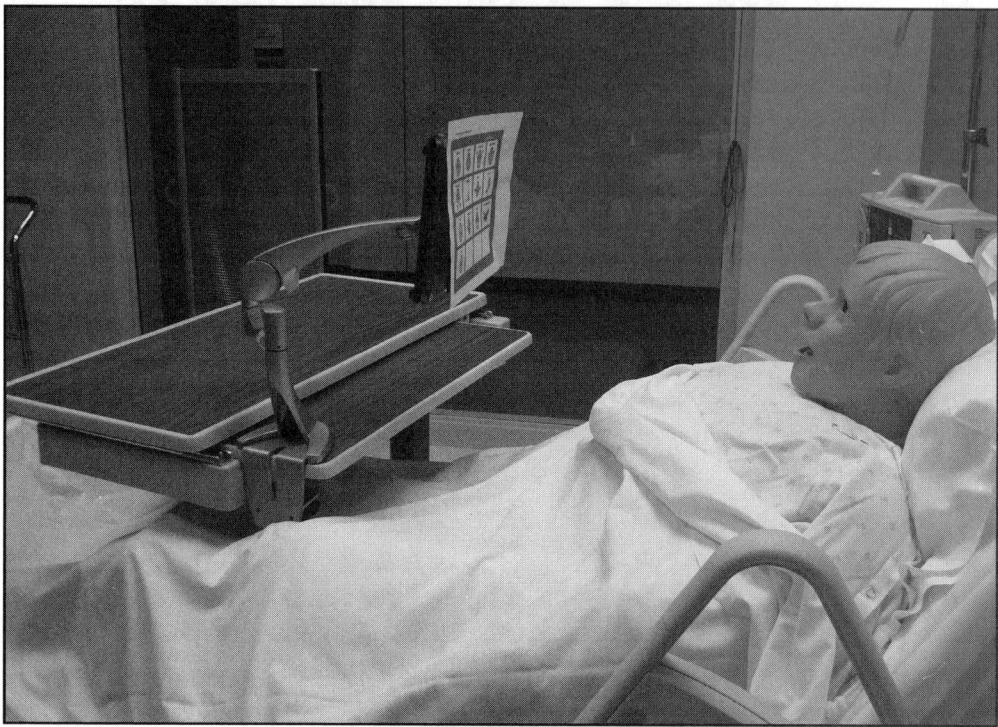

Figure 7–7. Communication board on bed tray mounted on Ergatron Neoflex Monitor Arm.

Bed Rail Implementations

In many intensive care settings, it is not possible to use a bed tray. In some cases, the special beds used will not accommodate a bed tray; in other cases, the sheer volume of other bedside equipment (i.e., IV poles, mechanical ventilators, hemodialysis machines, and cardiac monitors) precludes the use of a bed tray. One alternative that can be used with low-tech systems and smaller high-tech devices is to use some form of mounting arm that can be attached to the bed rail. For lightweight communication boards, one can use a simple gooseneck like the ones used with podium microphones (Figure 7-8). An alternative to the gooseneck whose length cannot be adjusted is the plastic Loc-Line tubing (Figure 7-9). For heavier AAC devices, one can use a flexible arm that can be clamped to the bedrail (Figure 7-10). These flexible arms originally were designed for positioning photographic equipment and have the advantage that they allow many degrees of freedom in positioning.

The use of bed rail mounting must be done with some caution. Because bed rails need to be raised and lowered with some regularity in intensive care settings, care must be taken that the mounting does not interfere with the bed rail mechanics. Devices are also more vulnerable is such situations and care must be taken that the mounts and the devices will not be damaged by bed rail movements. A common problem encountered with bed rail mounts is the pinching or disconnection of switch and power cords.

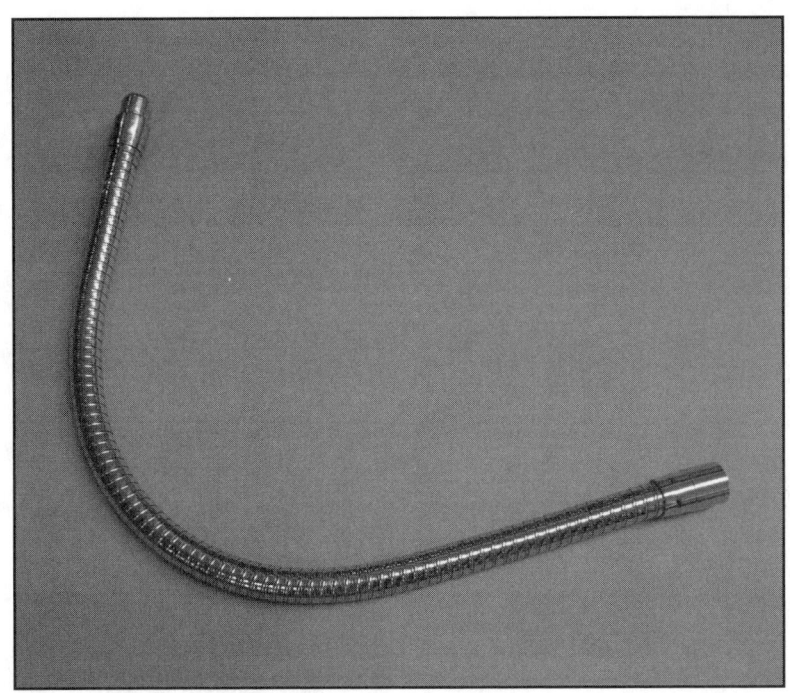

Figure 7–8. Flexible gooseneck.

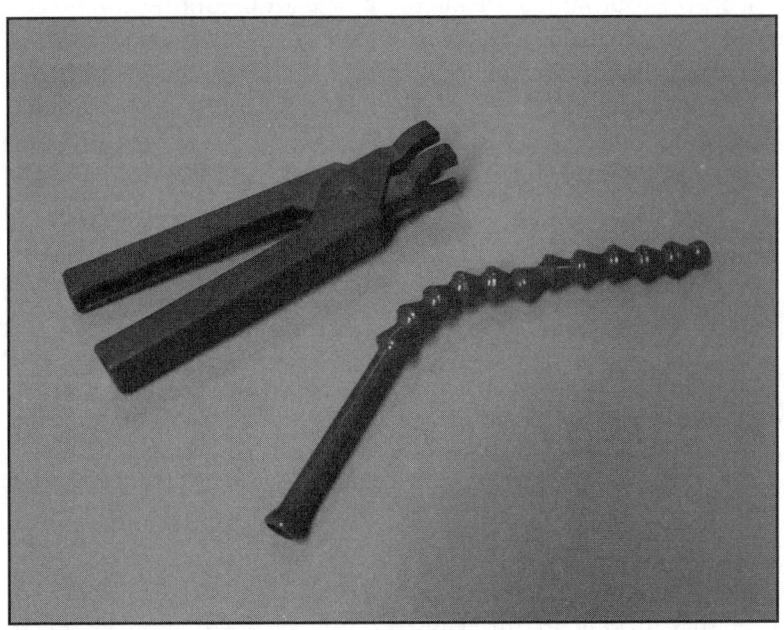

Figure 7–9. Loc-Line tubing.

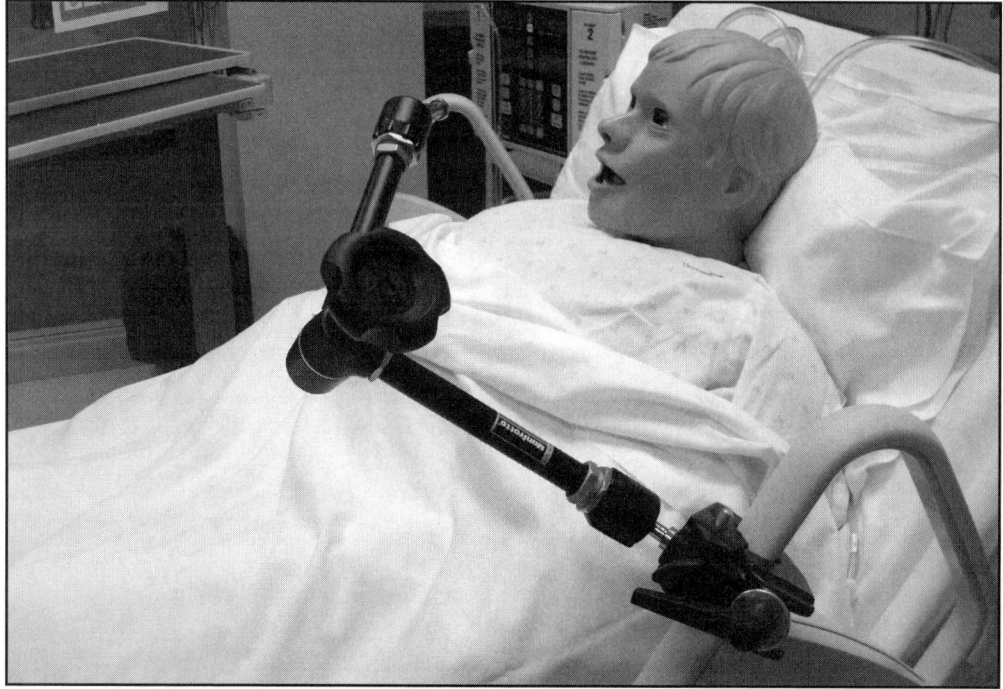

Figure 7–10. Bogen magic arm clamped to bed rail.

As with bed tray implementations, one needs to establish a routine that ensures that the patient can see and access the AAC system each time the patient is moved in the bed or when the bed rail position is changed.

IV Pole Implementations

For patients who are more acutely ill, bed tray and bed rail solutions are often inadequate for a number of reasons. First, the limitations on flexibility of positioning may make it difficult for the patient to see and easily access the device. Second, because of the space limitations, it may not be feasible to use a bed tray. And, finally, the frequency with which the bed rail is adjusted may make it an unreliably placed platform for an AAC system.

The IV pole provides a flexible alternative for mounting and positioning AAC systems. The smaller footprint of the IV pole by comparison with the bed tray makes it easier to use in the crowded space at the bedside. Unlike the bed tray, which must slide underneath the bed, the IV pole can be used in conjunction with a wide range of hospital beds, including those with limited clearance. It is typical to see multiple devices attached to a single IV pole so adding a flexible arm and attaching a device to one of the IV poles being used at the bedside is an option that may be considered (Figure 7–11).

When considering such a mounting solution, it will be necessary to coordinate with the appropriate nursing staff to ensure that movement of the pole to optimize positioning of the IV pole for the patient will not interfere with the IV

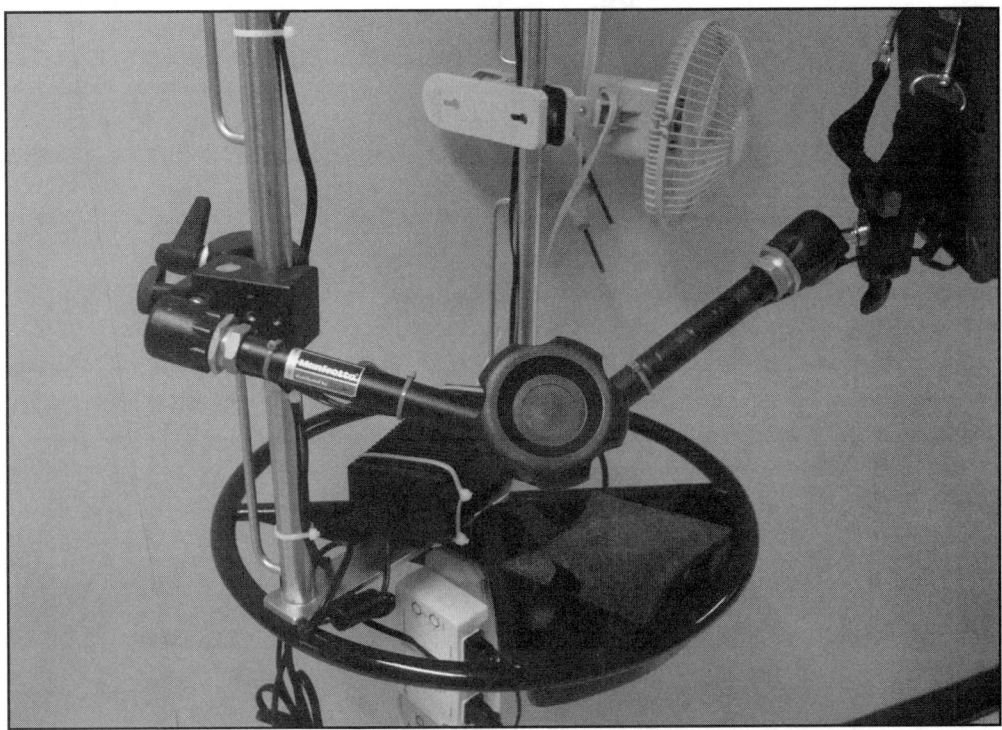

Figure 7–11. Bogen magic arm clamped to IV pole.

lines. In addition, this option should be considered for only low-weight AAC systems as care must be taken that a device extending from the pole not raise the risk of the IV pole tipping over.

As the high-tech AAC systems often also include providing access to environmental control units, it is necessary to be able to mount those units in proximity to the AAC device. To that end, having an integrated AAC delivery system and keeping track of all system components on one freestanding IV pole is preferable to adding components to other IV poles being used for medical care. There are a number of advantages to this approach.

First, it provides a platform that does not need to be shared with other bedside functions and as such can be positioned to optimize the communication of the patient. The other advantage of everything mounted on a single pole is that the system can easily be moved to accommodate the need to perform medical procedures and cares. Second, it clearly identifies the AAC system and its components as an integrated entity. We have been using independent IV poles at UIHC with a fair amount of success because the entire system is preset on an IV pole, can be quickly brought to a patient, and requires minimal setup at the bedside. Figure 7–12 illustrates the IV pole system we have developed. It has a 50-pound weight on its base to allow use of heavier devices that can be positioned well out from the base of the pole. The pole has a set of large lockable casters that make moving the pole easy and also allow it to be locked into place. The

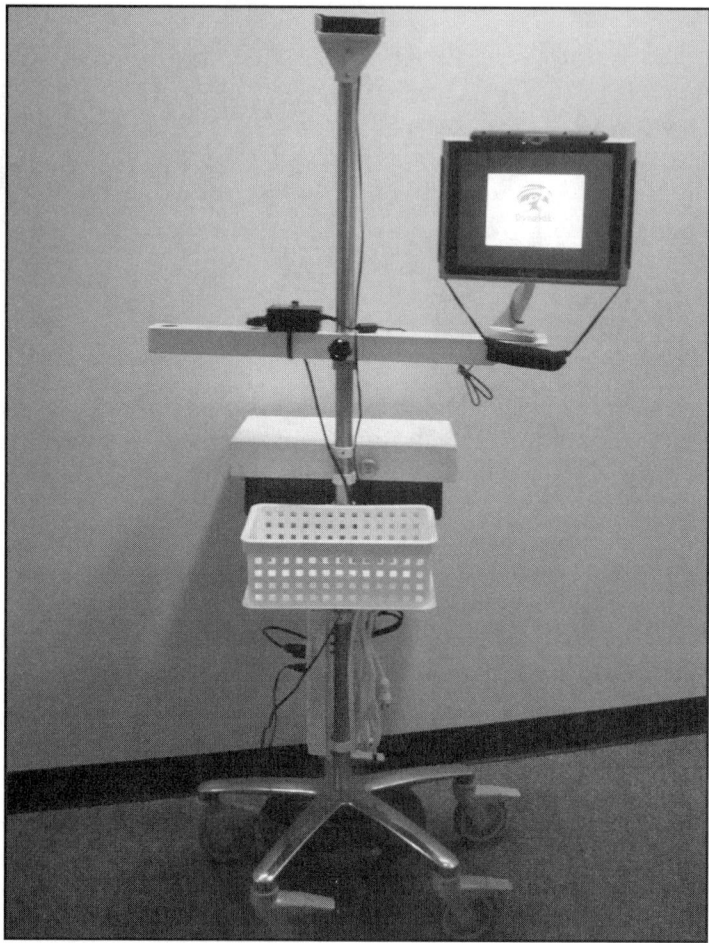

Figure 7–12. Iowa AAC pole.

pole has a hospital-grade power strip that allows all the components of the AAC system to be attached and plugged into a single AC circuit. This is essential for use of X-10 systems for pain management and ECU (see Chapters 8 and 9). The pole has a height adjustable bar with a flexible Ergatron Arm mounted at the end. This allows us to raise and lower the device as well as to rotate and tilt it to the optimal position. The design of the adjustable bar allows us to either position the pole at the side of the bed and extend across the bed (Figure 7-13) or to position the pole behind the bed and come up over the patient's head (Figure 7-14). The pole has a mounting bracket at the top for an X-10 IR receiver (Figure 7-15) to optimize use of the AAC devices' IR environmental control functions. Finally, to keep ancillary equipment such as specialty switches, pointers, and a keyboard and mouse together with the system, the pole is equipped with a lockable storage drawer (see Figure 7-12). Video clip 7-2 illustrates the manner in which an AAC device mounted on an Iowa IV pole can be positioned for optimal access.

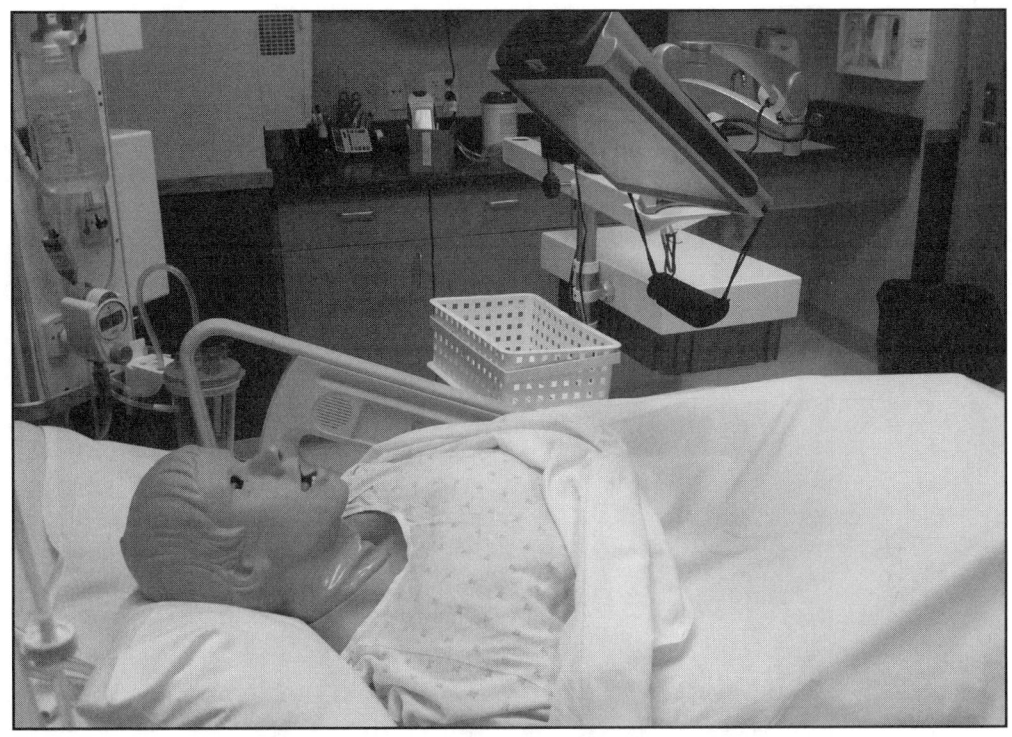

Figure 7–13. Iowa AAC pole from side of bed access.

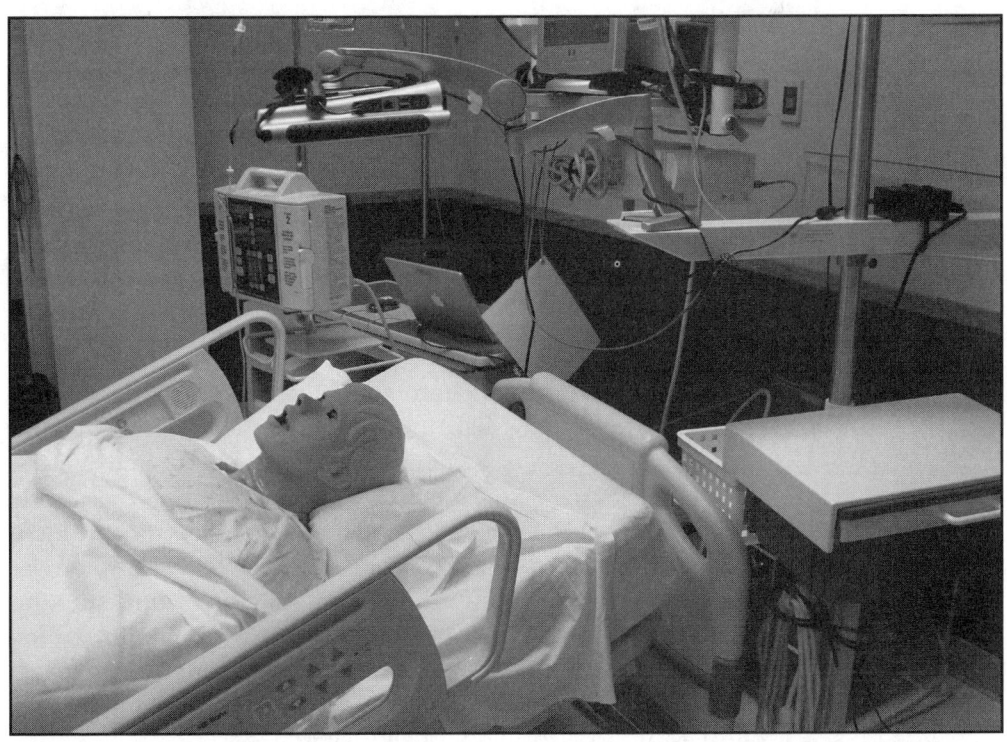

Figure 7–14. Iowa AAC pole from behind the bed access.

101

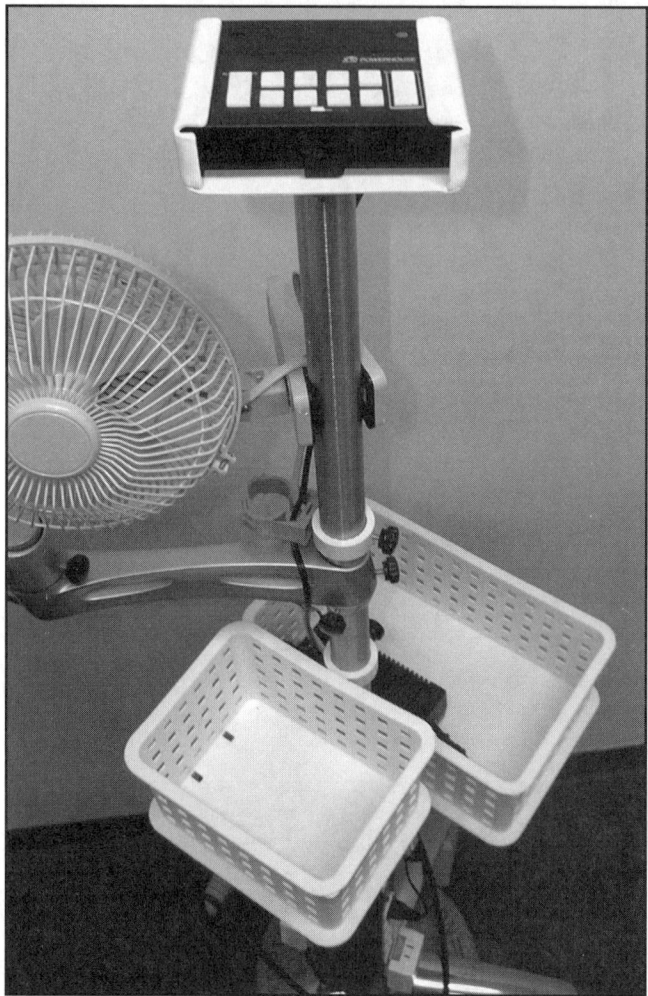

Figure 7–15. Iowa AAC pole IR (infrared) receiver.

SWITCH ADAPTATION AND MOUNTING SOLUTIONS

For many patients in acute care, positioning a switch to make it continually accessible requires a careful assessment of the patients' ability to activate the selected switch and an assessment of the ability, independent of positioning, to access the switch. Even if one has an array of switch technologies with which to evaluate a patient, there will be cases where patients will not be able to activate the standard switches. In those cases, one needs to decide whether the problem stems from inherent limitations of the switch or from limitations in the mounting/positioning of the switch. In the following sections, we address approaches to switch adaptations and to mounting options for switches.

Adapting Switches

Wherever possible, one should use the most commonly available switches. In many cases, a simple adaptation can make a switch accessible to the patient. Often these adaptations can be made with materials readily available at the bedside. To illustrate how this can be done, consider making a conventional nurse call pendant accessible to patients who cannot isolate a digit to touch the nurse call button or who cannot generate sufficient force with a single finger to directly activate the call light. Using a gauze pad, a tongue depressor, and some tape (Figure 7-16), a lever can be made that can both increase the 'target zone' and reduce the force necessary to activate the switch. Figures 7-17A and 7-17B provide two views of an adapted nurse call. In cases where the patient cannot see the switch, one can use tape, soft Velcro or Dycem to provide a textured surface that will provide tactile feedback to let the patient know they are positioned over the switch (Figure 7-18).

Mounting Strategies

For both standard and adapted switches, the ultimate determinant of successful use by a patient is the mounting or positioning of the switch to ensure consistent access to the switch. For patients with some limitation of mobility, who can use the conventional nurse call pendant, it is essential that nurses and caregivers make sure that the pendant is within reach each time they leave the patient's bedside.

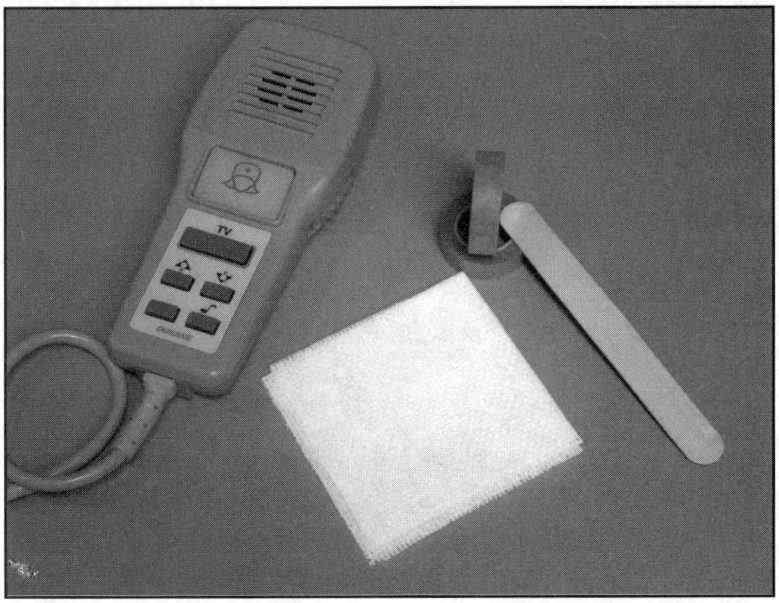

Figure 7–16. Simple materials (tongue depressor, gauze pad, tape) to adapt nurse call pendant.

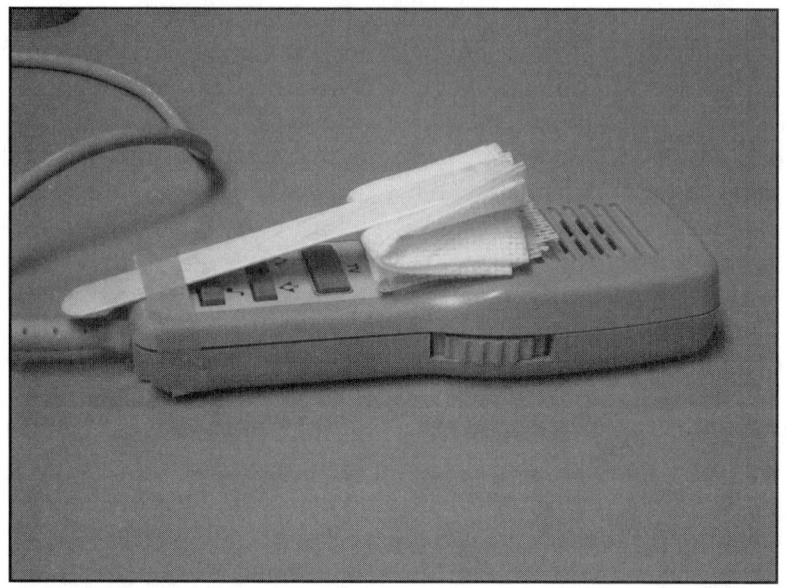

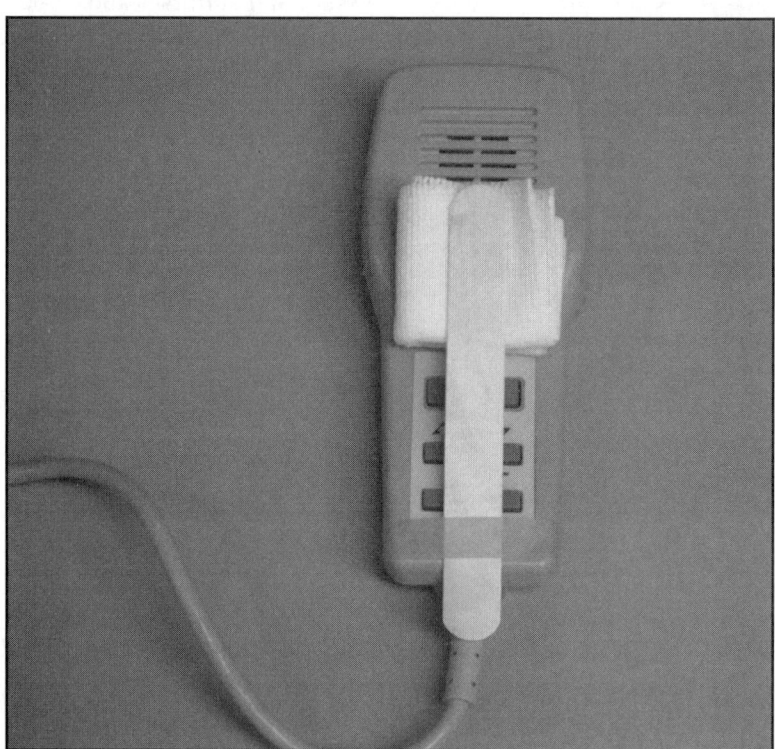

Figure 7–17. A. Adapted nurse call pendant—view 1. **B.** Adapted nurse call pendant—view 2.

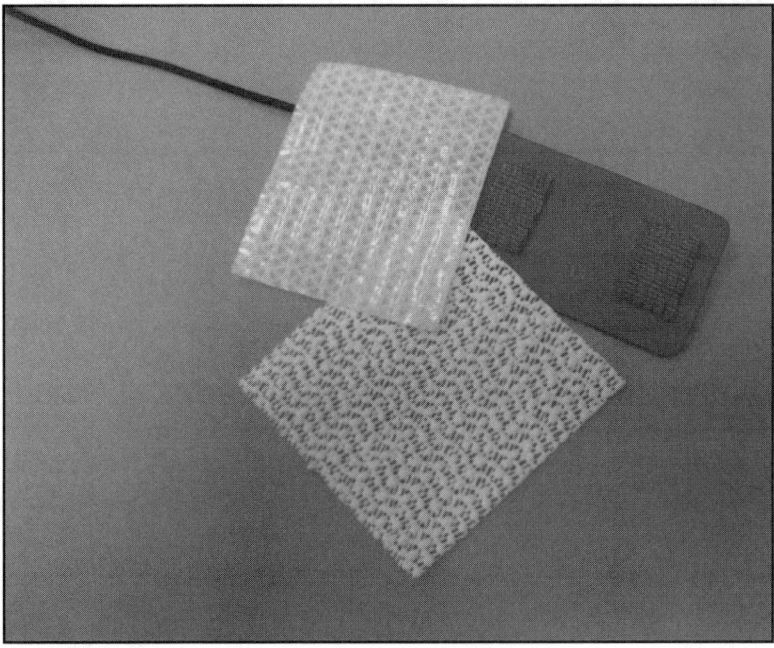

Figure 7–18. Texture materials/Dycem, Velcro.

To ensure that the pendant does not fall out of reach, it is typical for it to be clipped or pinned to either the patient's nightgown (Figure 7-19), a sheet (Figure 7-20), a pillow (Figure 7-21), a towel roll (Figure 7-22), or strapped to the bedrail (Figure 7-23). In many cases, this is sufficient; however, one solution may not be equally good across different patient positions. For example, for a patient whose arm only has a functional biceps, pinning a flat pressure plate switch to the patient's gown works well only when the patient is sitting somewhat upright. In this situation, the patient can adduct the arm and make contact with the switch and gravity takes the arm off the switch when the patient relaxes the biceps. But, when the patient is supine, once the patient has adducted to make contact with the switch, the inability to abduct leaves the patient unable to reactivate the switch. Therefore, it is essential that a switch and positioning solution be determined for each position that the patient will be put in. Although not optimal, this may require not only a different switch mounting for each position (sitting vs. supine) but also perhaps a different type of switch. Care must be taken in such cases to ensure that the patient understands what switch is being used at any particular time.

One problem with using the patient's gown or soft bedding surfaces is that they offer little resistance and, therefore, the patient's gesture may displace the switch rather than activate the switch. This is particularly true when using some form of pneumatic pressure switch.

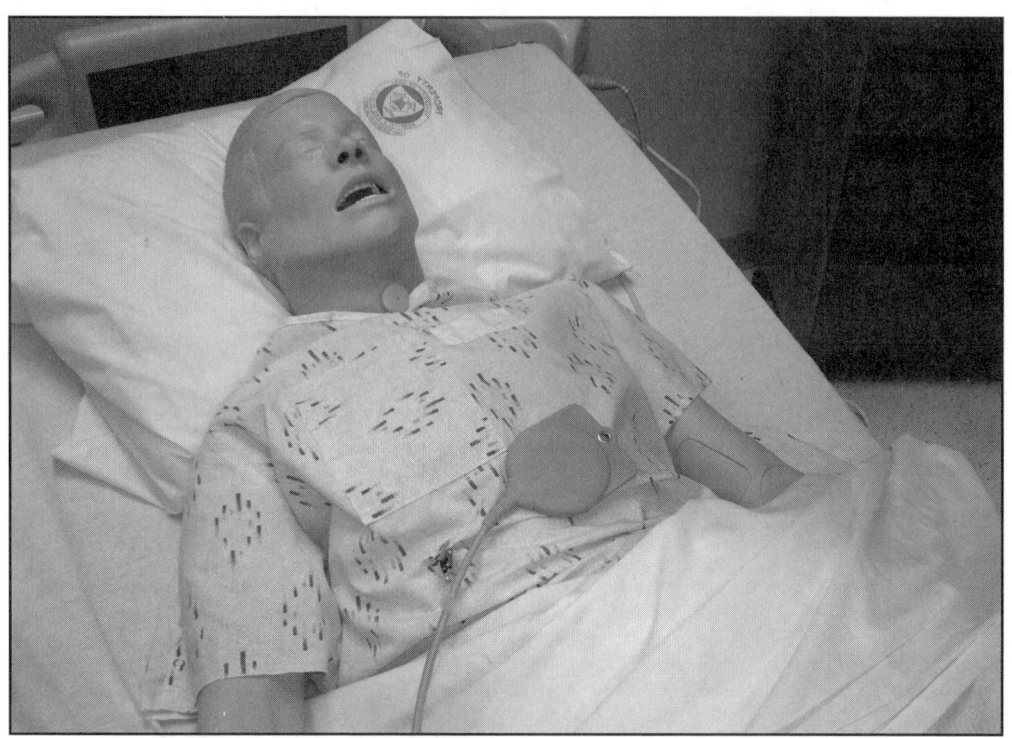

Figure 7–19. Switch pinned to gown.

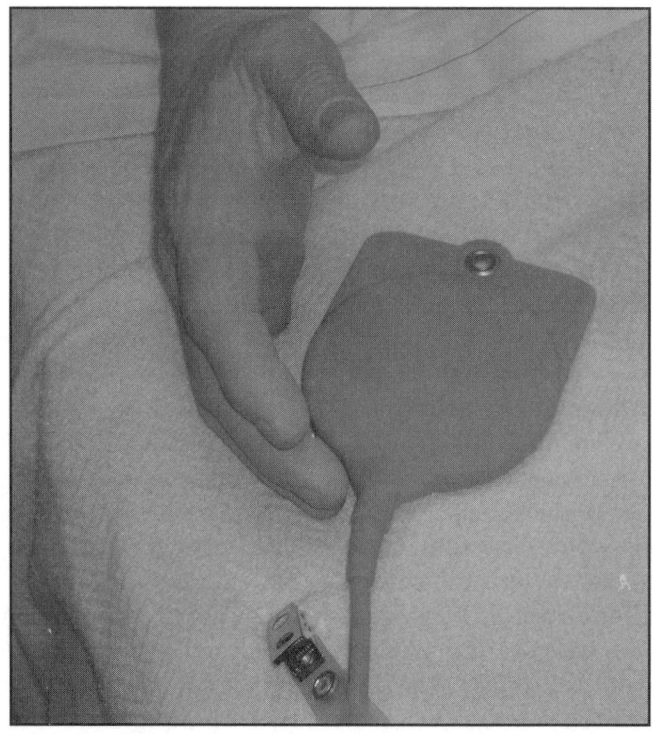

Figure 7–20. Switch pinned to sheet.

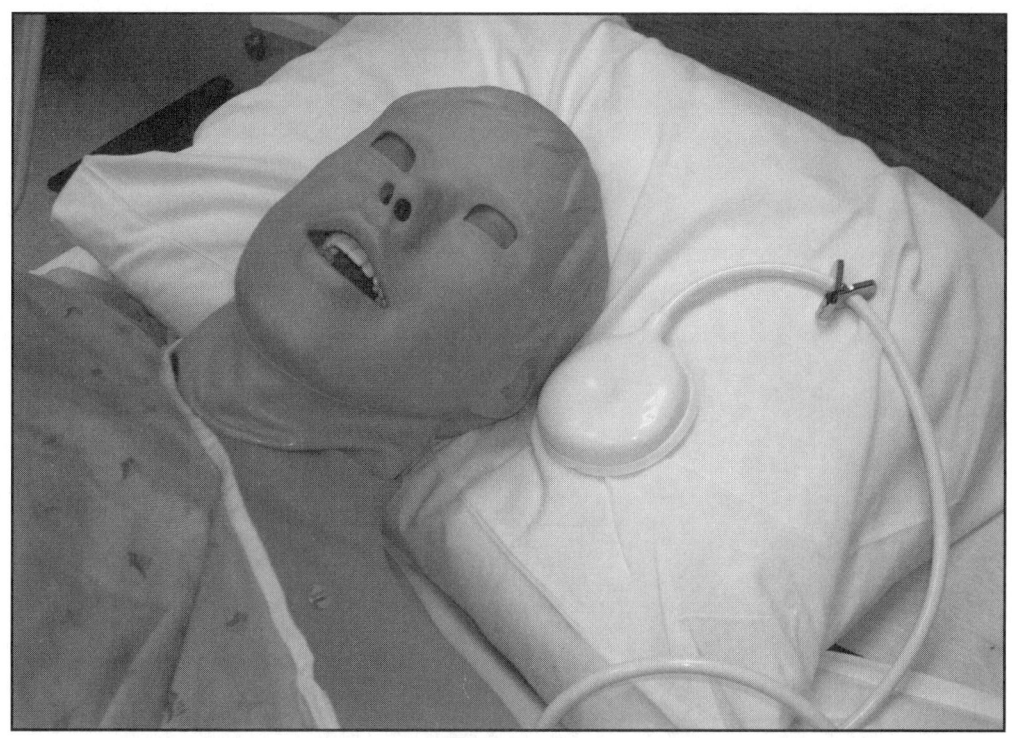

Figure 7–21. Switch pinned to pillow.

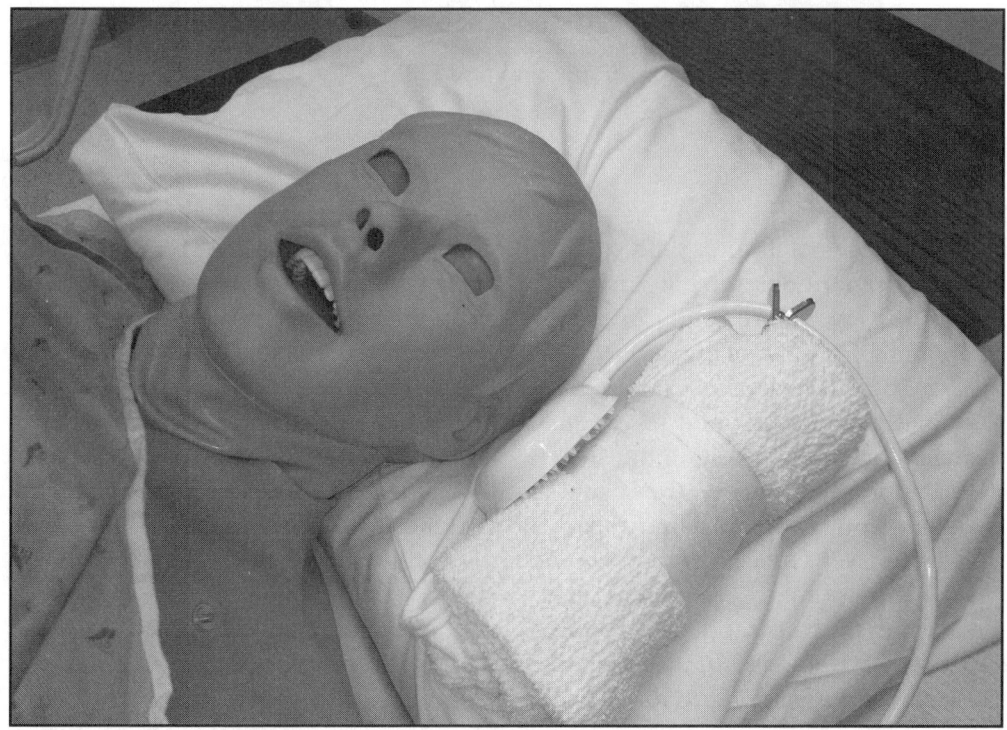

Figure 7–22. Switch pinned to towel roll.

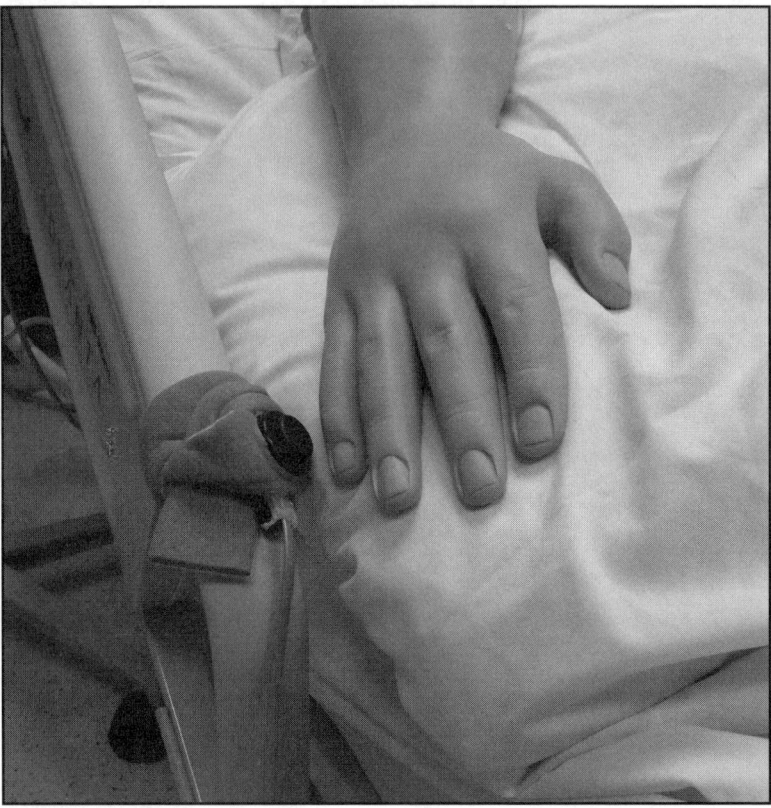

Figure 7–23. Switch strapped to bed rail.

This problem can be addressed by mounting the switch on a rigid surface. A square of thermoplast (splint material; Figure 7-24) works well and can usually be obtained from the occupational therapy service. We have also used thermoplast that has been shaped to produce an angled bracket to position the switch at the appropriate angle. This material is easy to work with and can be shaped with a hairdryer. One can cut slots in the thermoplast to attach straps that allow the mount to be strapped or pinned down. We have also used thicker material like lexan and plexiglass, to make angle brackets. The switches are then attached to these brackets with Velcro. This allows easy modification of position of the switch on the mounting plate. This approach to switch mounting allows using head rotation (Figure 7-25), a shoulder shrug (Figure 7-26), lateral hand/arm movements (Figure 7-27), lateral leg movements (Figure 7-28), or foot movements (Figure 7-29). This type of mounting system allows for the use of a wide range of switches to accommodate the force and displacement that the patient can generate. As with the use of the nurse call pendant, care must be taken each time the patient is repositioned to ensure that the mounting plate and switch are properly placed. This is especially critical when the patient is severely limited in generat-

MOUNTING AND ACCESS ISSUES 109

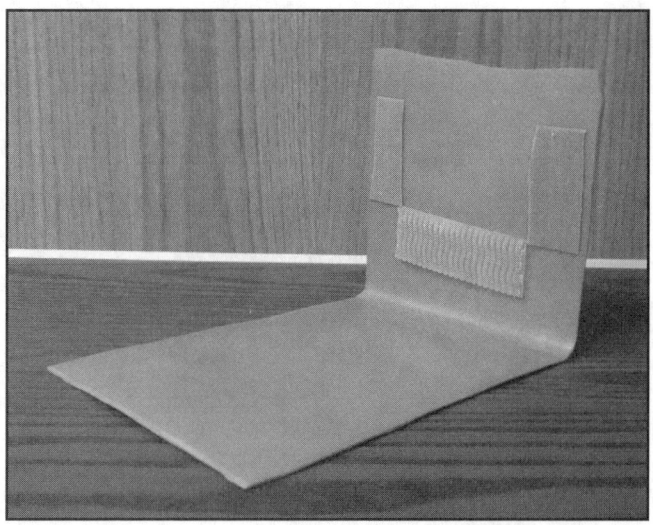

Figure 7–24. Thermoplast—splint material.

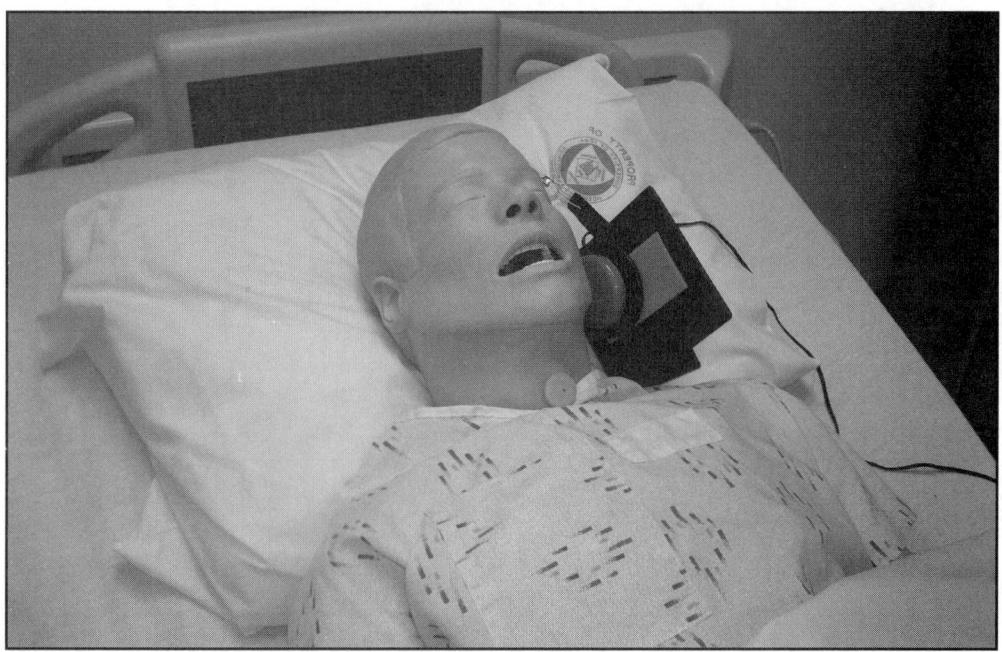

Figure 7–25. Angle bracket—head position.

ing a voluntary gesture. In addition to clipping the plates, one can also stabilize them by using small bean bags (filled with heavy beads), which form a better platform for the uneven surfaces of the bedding and pillows (Figure-7-30).

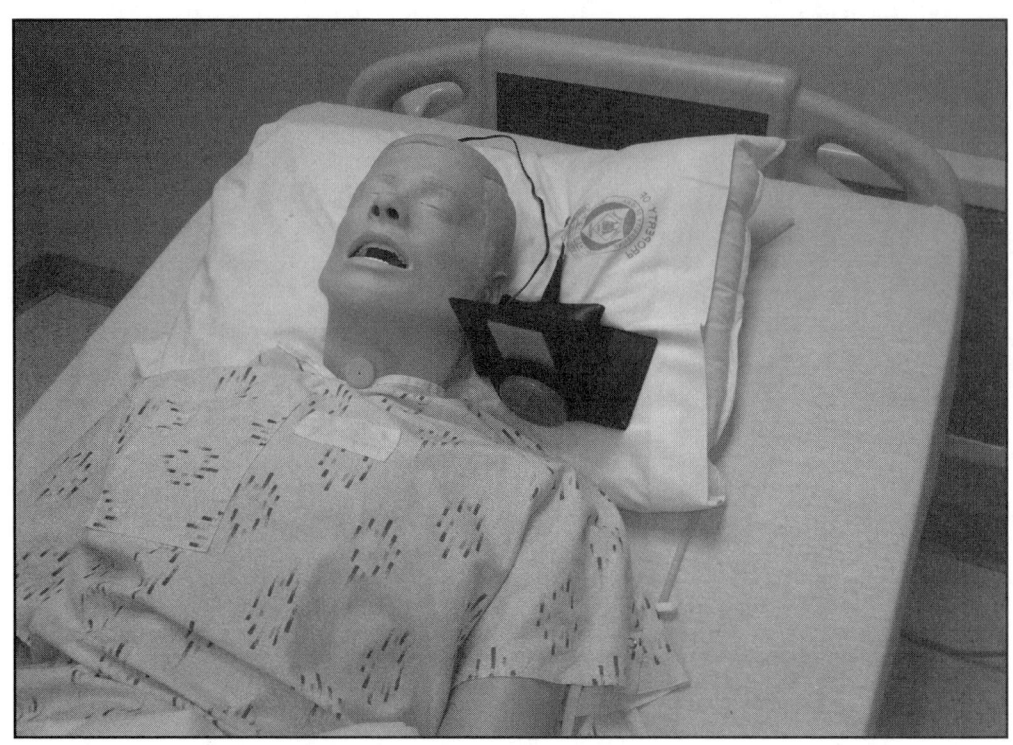

Figure 7–26. Angle bracket—shoulder position.

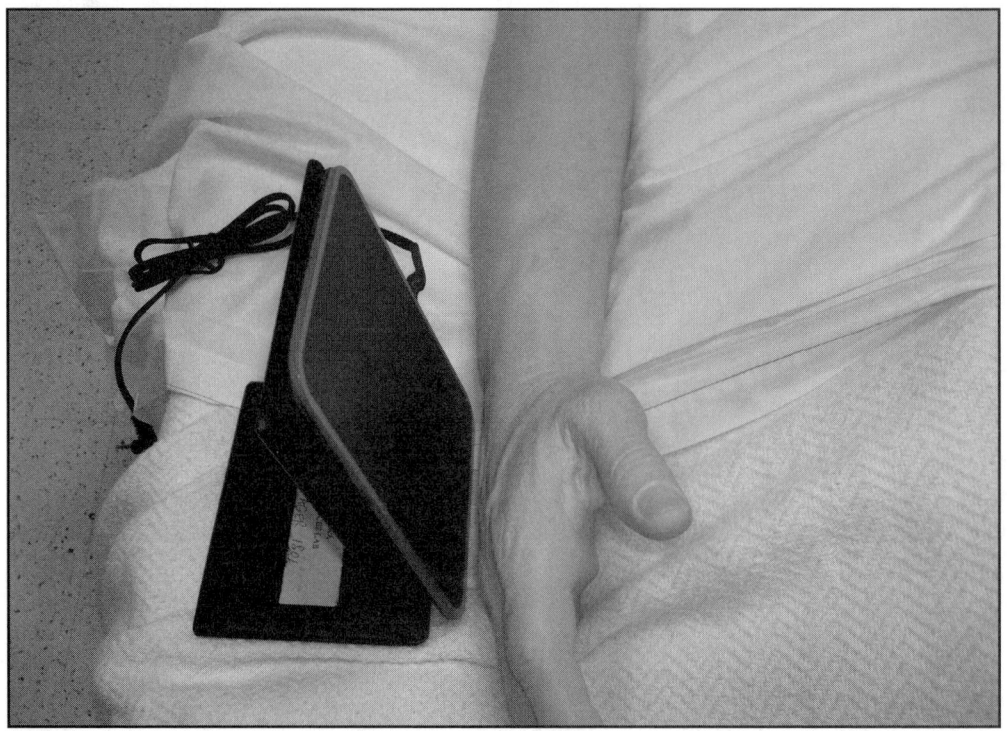

Figure 7–27. Angle bracket—arm/hand position.

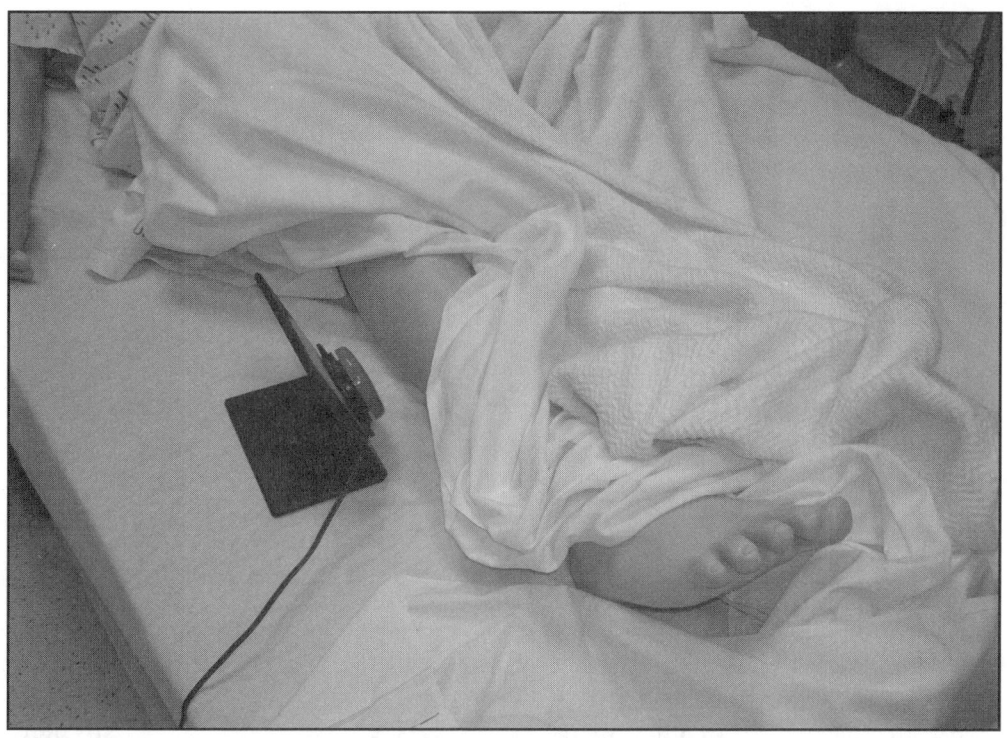

Figure 7–28. Angle bracket—leg position.

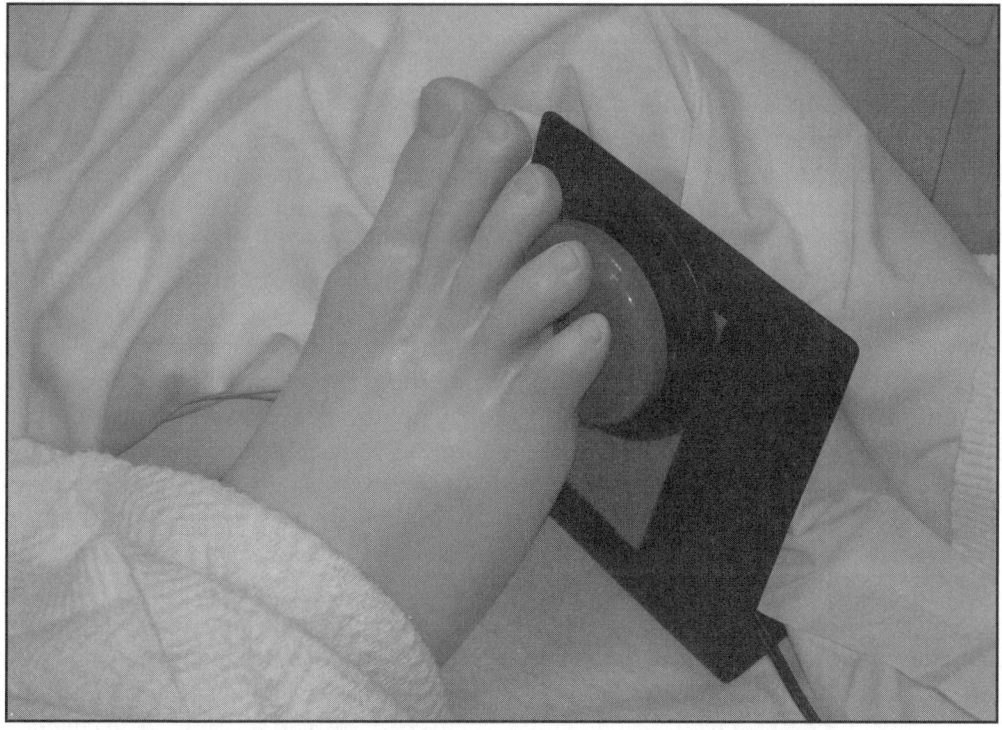

Figure 7–29. Angle bracket—foot position.

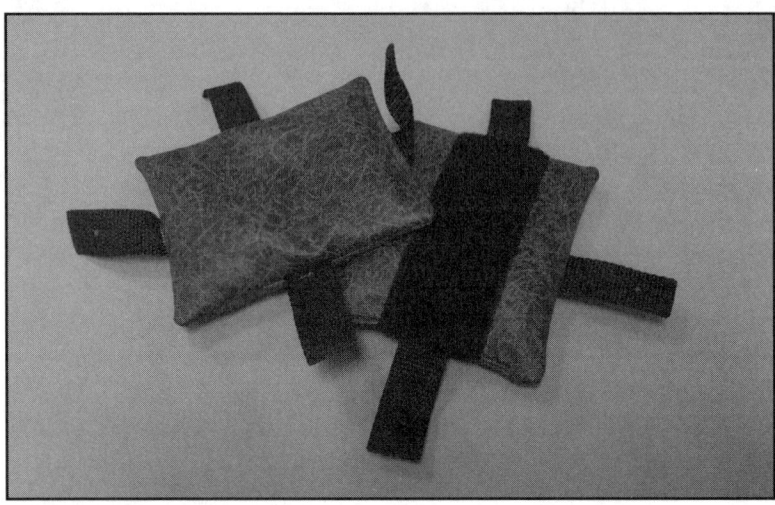

Figure 7–30. Bean bag for mounting switches.

An alternative approach utilizes a flexible switch mounting platform. One approach utilizes clamping a goose neck (Figure 7-31) or Bogen arm (Figure 7-32) to the bed or to an IV pole. The switch can then be attached with Velcro to a small plate attached to the gooseneck or Bogen arm. Both allow adjusting the position of the switch in all three dimensions. If the patient can generate only small displacements with minimal force, both of these solutions work well as the patient's gesture will not push the switch out of reach. For patients who cannot control the force of their gestures, the Bogen arm is a better solution because, once tightened, the orientation of its components will not be altered by the patient's gesture. One drawback of the gooseneck is that its length cannot be adjusted, making large changes in position difficult to accommodate. The Bogen arm is better suited for this, but its drawback is that it is bulkier and may interfere with access to the patient by medical staff.

We have recently started using some flexible plastic segmented tubing (Loc-Line; Figure 7-33). This is extremely lightweight tubing that can be shaped to allow positioning of the switch from any angle. Another advantage of this approach is that we can easily shorten or lengthen the tubing; like children's snap beads, the individual Loc-Line segments can be added or removed with a simple tool that can be purchased along with the Loc-Line tubing, which comes in small segments, longer straight segments, and angle segments. Because the Loc-Line tubing is hollow, it is possible to pass switch cables and pressure bulb tubing through the Loc-Line, thereby reducing the possibility of something getting hooked on the cable or pinching the pressure bulb tubing. Like the gooseneck and Bogen arm, one can mount the Loc-Line to the bed rail or to plates similar to those illustrated in Figures 7-25 through Figure 7-29. Because repositioning the Loc-Line is very simple and easier to use than the Bogen arm or gooseneck, it is more likely that staff will take the time to make the small adjustments necessary to accommodate changes in the patient's position.

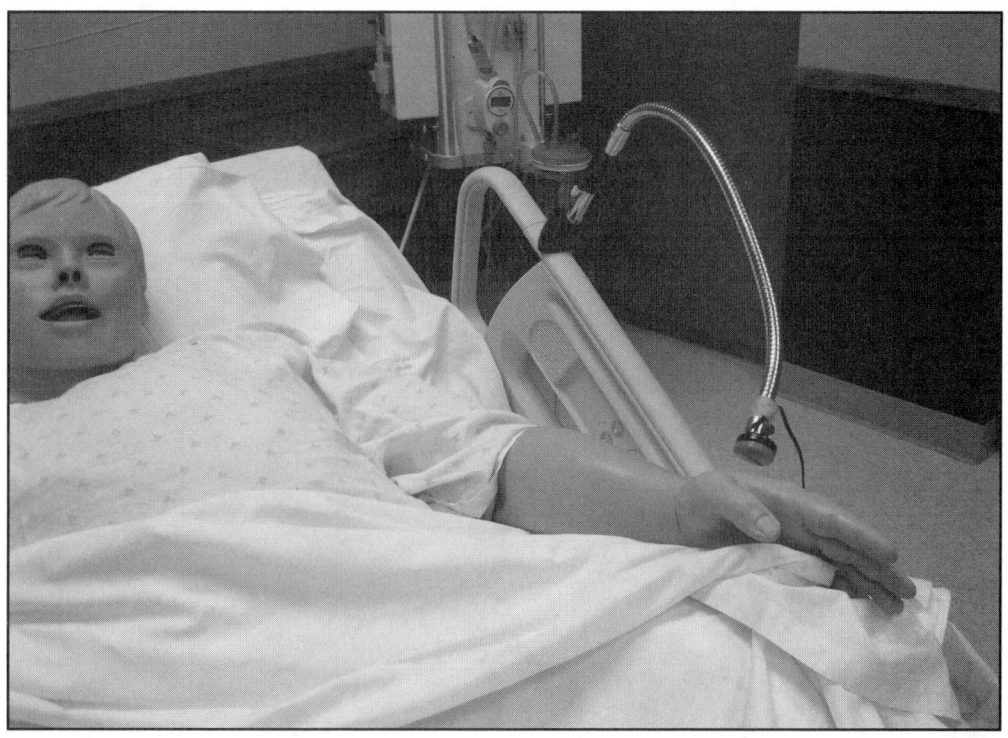

Figure 7–31. Gooseneck.

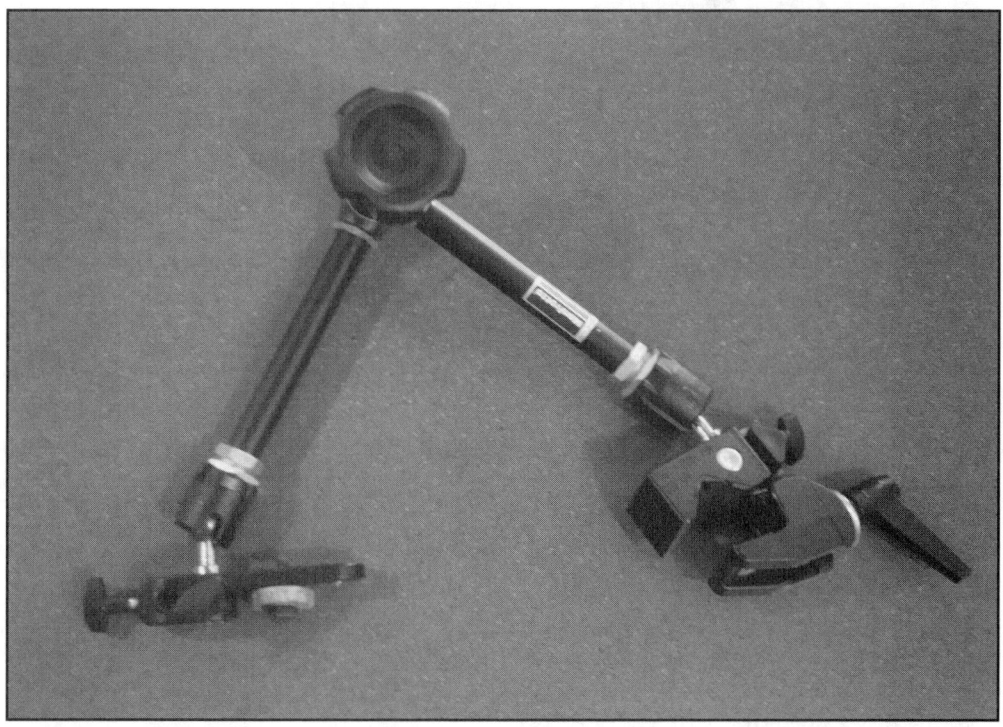

Figure 7–32. Bogen magic arm.

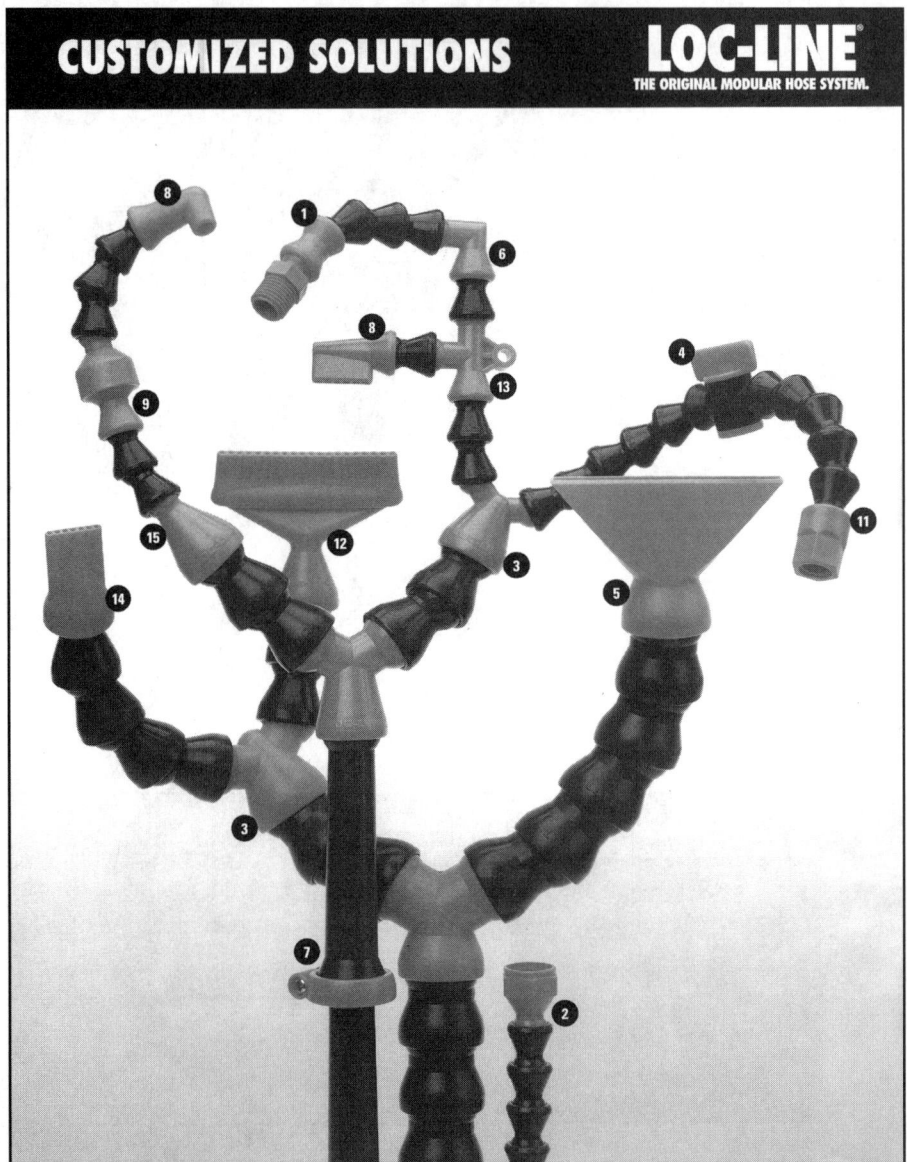

Figure 7–33. Loc-Line flexible tubing.

The best way to accommodate for changes in the patient's position, which result from repositioning by the staff or from the voluntary and involuntary positional changes initiated by the patient, is to find a way to use the patient's body or a medical device fixed to the body as the platform for the switch. Such a mounting strategy would ensure that the switch is properly positioned regardless of the patient's position.

Patient's Body as Platform

Using straps or tape, switches can be attached directly to the patient's head, limbs, or body. The most common solution involves attaching a switch to the hand with an elastic strap (Figure 7-34) or to a hand splint (Figure 7-35). This works well with patients who can squeeze a pneumatic bulb or use thumb or fingers

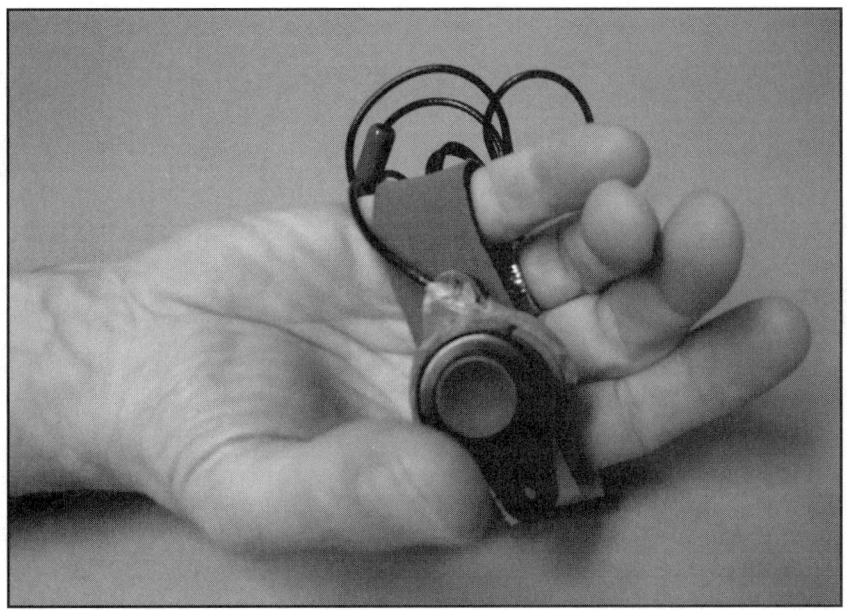

Figure 7–34. Elastic strap on hand.

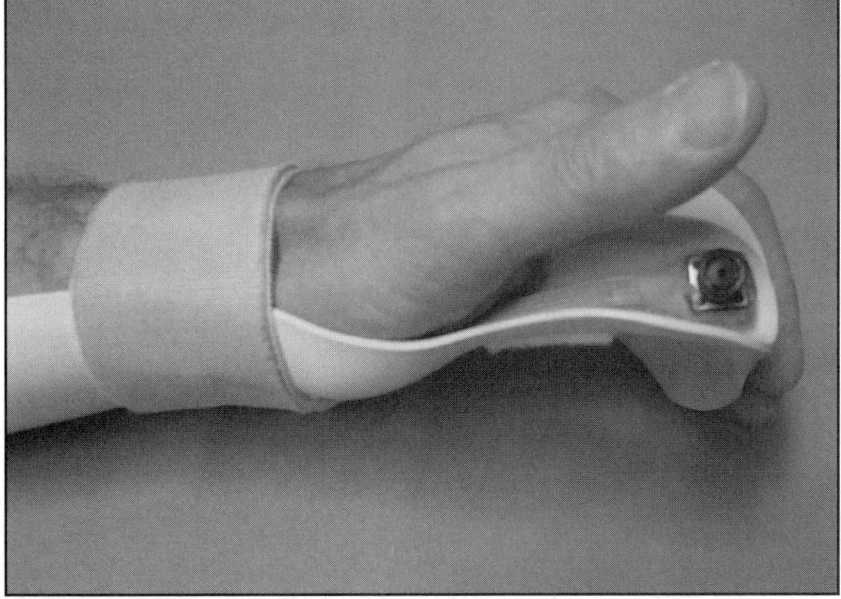

Figure 7–35. Hand splint.

to depress a small switch. We have also used this with patients who can extend their arms out to the bed rail but, because of positional changes, may not be able to hit a particular target zone on the bed rail to which the switch is attached (Figure 7-36). This can also work with a patient who can extend the leg or depress the foot (Figure 7-37). By attaching the switch to the patient, all the

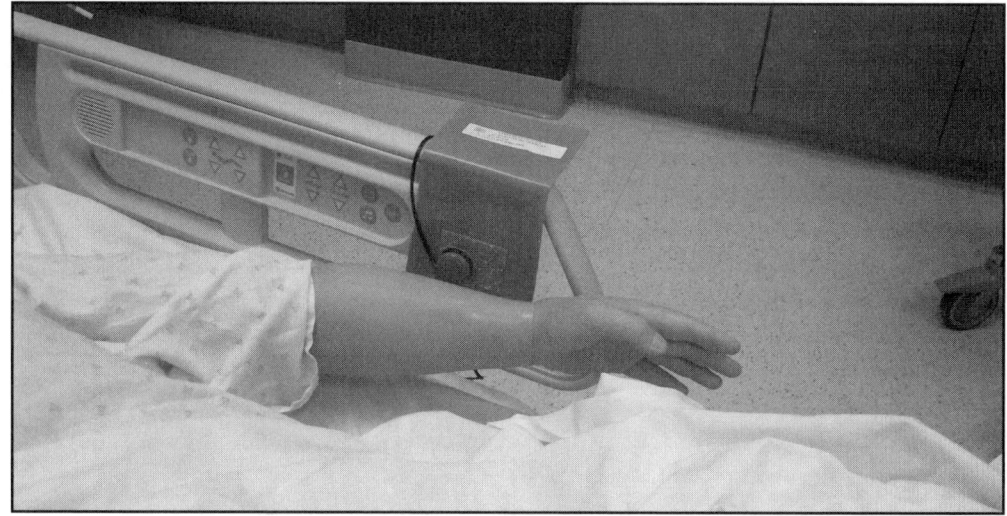

Figure 7–36. Hand movement to a switch mounted on the bed rail.

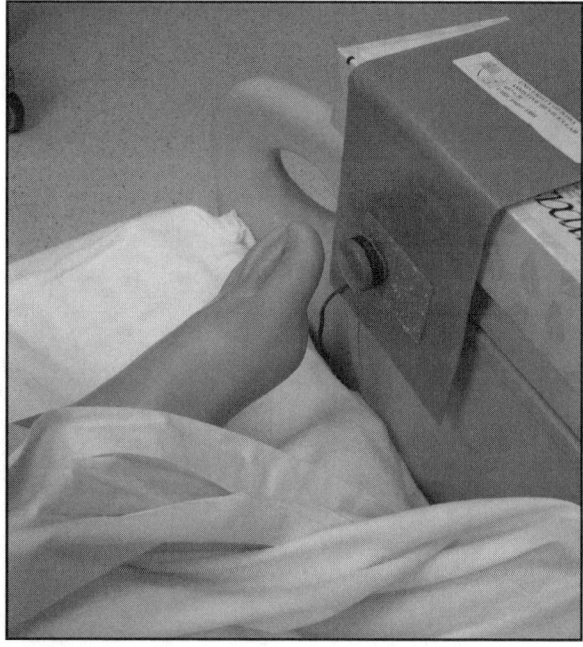

Figure 7–37. Foot movement to a bed-mounted switch.

patient must do is contact the bedrail which then causes the switch mounted on the patient's body to be activated. In a couple of cases where the only gesture the patient could generate involved bringing the knees together, we attached the switch to one knee with an elastic strap so that when the patient brought her knees together the switch was activated.

In cases where the patient uses a sip-and-puff switch or a small pressure bulb switch, the straw or bulb can be held in position with a flexible wire hung over the ear and/or taped to the cheek (Figure 7–38). This allows the patient to reach for the switch with movements of the lips and or tongue.

Medical Device as Platform

For patients who have been fitted with a halo brace for treatment of a cervical spine trauma or as a follow-up to spinal surgery, the brace can be used as a platform for a Loc-Line mounted switch. Figure 7–39 illustrates how the loc-line tubing can be used with a ball clamp. Figure 7–40 illustrates how the Loc-Line and clamp are attached to the halo brace to position a pressure bulb within reach of the patient's mouth. We have also used this configuration with charge transfer proximity switches for patients who can push out their cheeks with their tongues. In this case, the switch is positioned about one centimeter from the cheek (Figure 7–41). For patients who can lower their jaw slightly, the switch can be positioned just below the chin. In cases where a patient is transitioned from a halo brace to a cervical collar or started off with a cervical collar, the Loc-Line tubing can be attached to the collar using a mounting block (Figure 7–42) that can be fastened to the collar with a cable clamp or with Velcro (Figure 7–43).

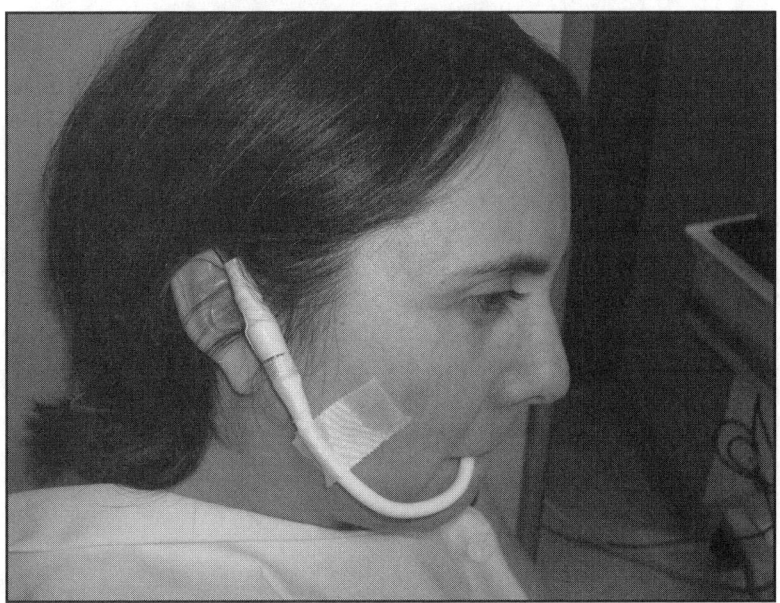

Figure 7–38. Sip-and puff switch mounted over the ear and taped to cheek.

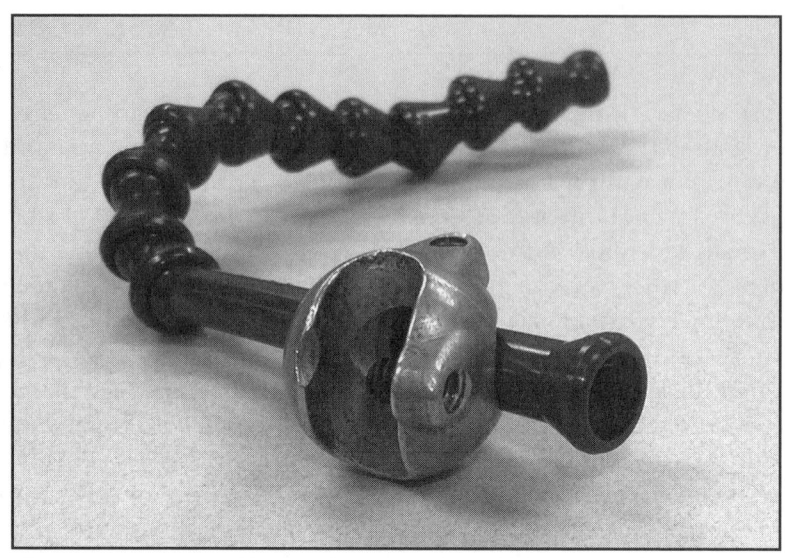

Figure 7–39. Loc-Line with ball clamp.

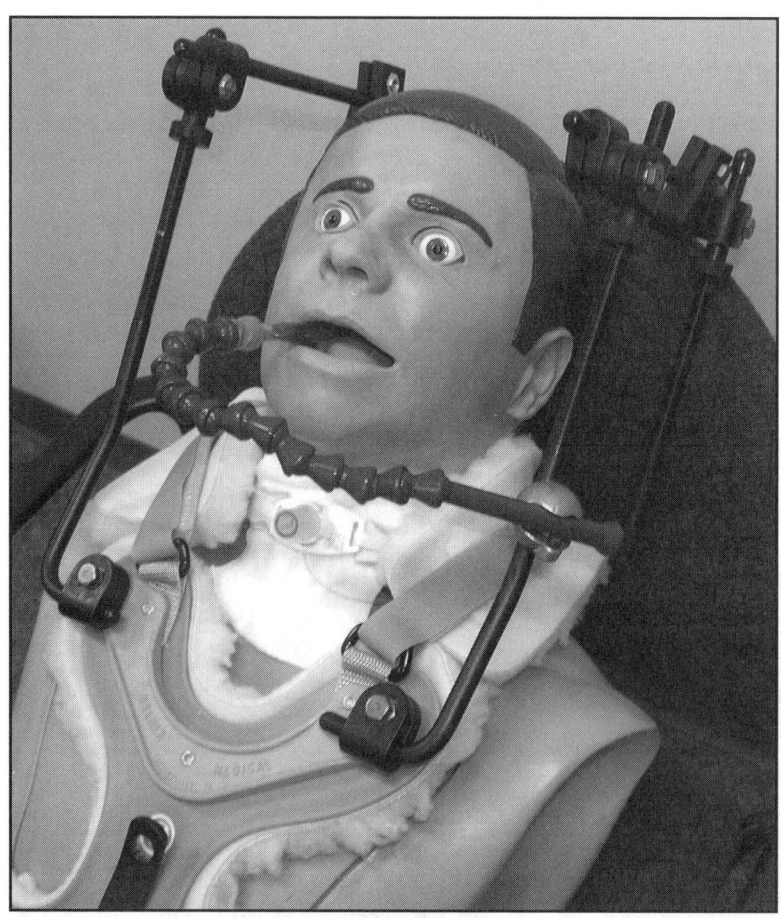

Figure 7–40. Loc-Line mounted to halo brace.

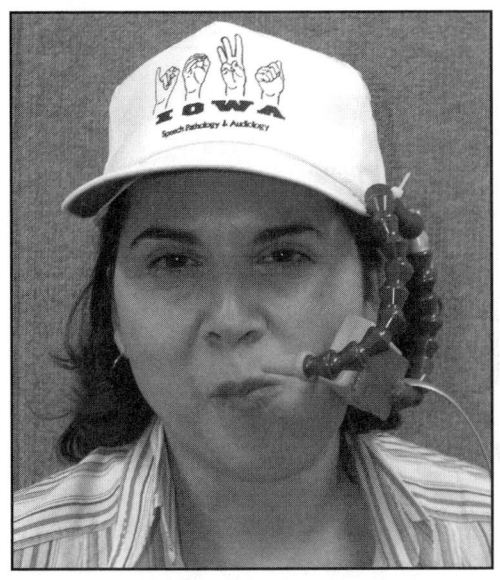

Figure 7–41. Loc-Line mounting to allow tongue in cheek to activate proximity switch.

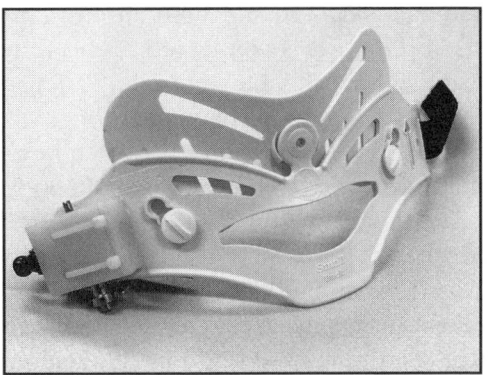

Figure 7–42. Loc-Line mounting block (locally made).

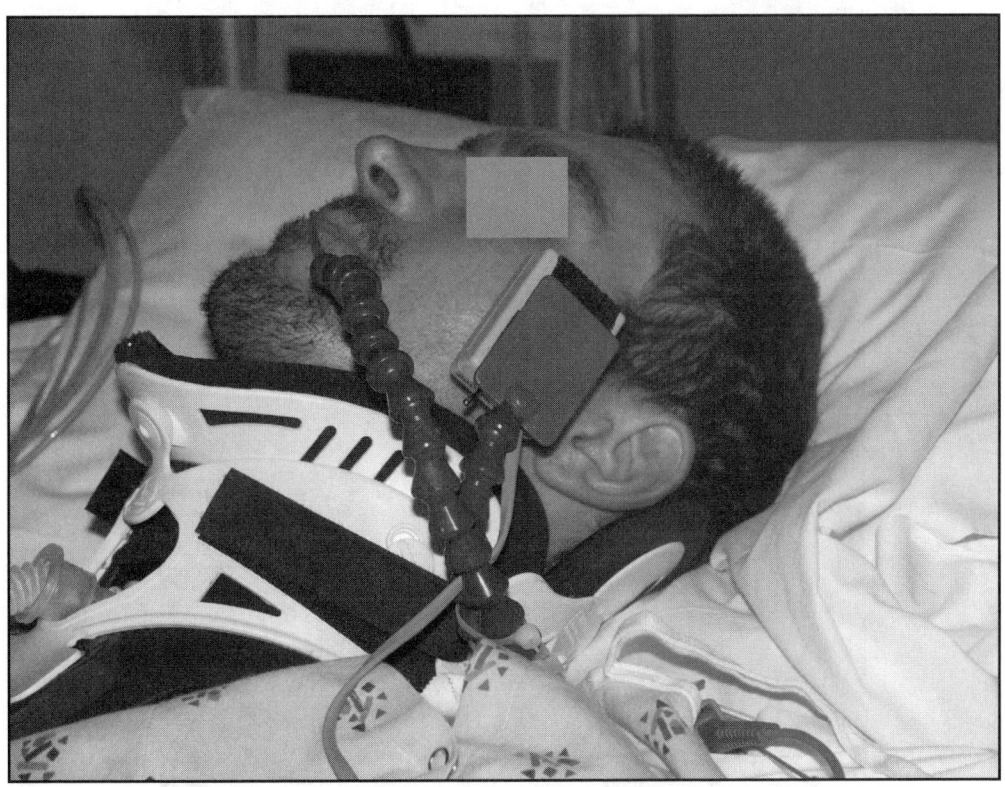

Figure 7–43. Loc-Line mounted to cervical collar brace.

Many critical care patients experience a period of ventilatory support. Acute trauma patients and some postsurgical patients are intubated with an endotracheal tube that is connected to the ventilator with a flexible vent line. Patients requiring longer term ventilation may have a tracheostomy and the trach tube is then connected to the ventilator. In both cases, the connecter at the patient's end of the vent line can be used as a base for a Loc-Line mounted switch. We have developed a light nylon adapter (Figure 7-44) that can fit over the vent line connector. The Loc-Line can then be snapped on this adapter and allow the positioning of the switch at or near the mouth (Figure 7-45).

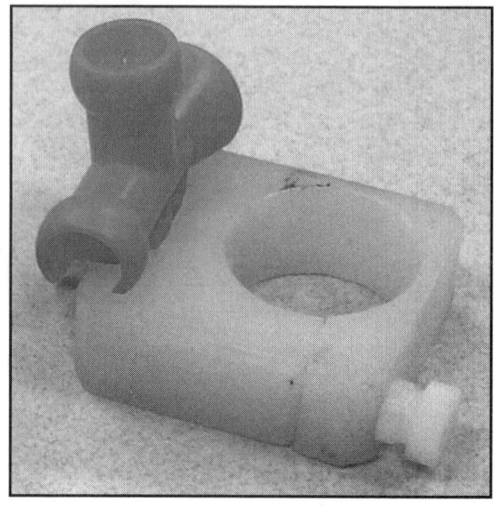

Figure 7-44. Vent line adapter for Loc-Line tubing (locally made).

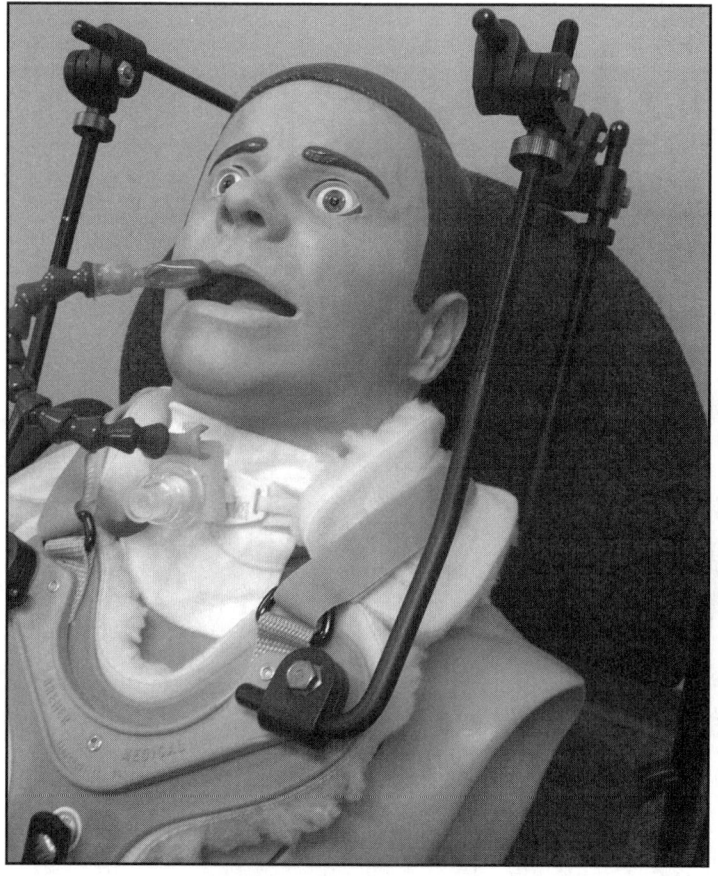

Figure 7-45. Vent line mounting with Loc-Line adapter.

This proximity makes it easy for patients to quickly access their switches. Many of these intubated patients cannot produce the oral pressures that are required by conventional sip-and-puff switches. For that reason we have used a small silastic pressure bulb (Figure 7–46). Some older patients (with either an endotracheal tube or a tracheostomy) have preferred keeping the small pressure bulb switch between their lips rather than extending or puckering their lips to reach the bulb when they wanted to activate the switch and control their AAC system (Figure 7–47). This led some of the ICU nurses to rename our switch the adult pacifier. The Iowa Smart Switch or any switch that can be programmed to distinguish small pressure changes from the higher amplitude pressure changes associated with the voluntary squeeze of the bulb allows the patient to keep the pressure bulb in the mouth at all times. What the halo brace, the cervical collar, and the vent line have in common is that they keep the switch accessible to the patient, regardless of the patient's positioning in the bed.

Eyeglasses as Platform

For patients who can wear glasses, the frame can also be used as a viable platform

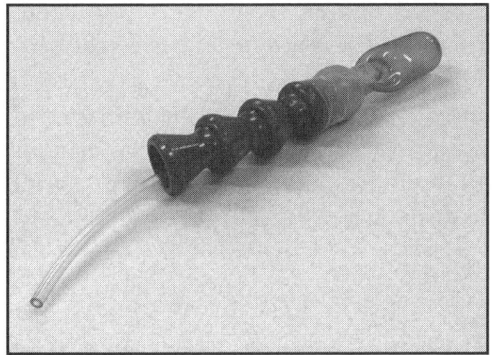

Figure 7–46. Silastic pressure bulb for pressure switch.

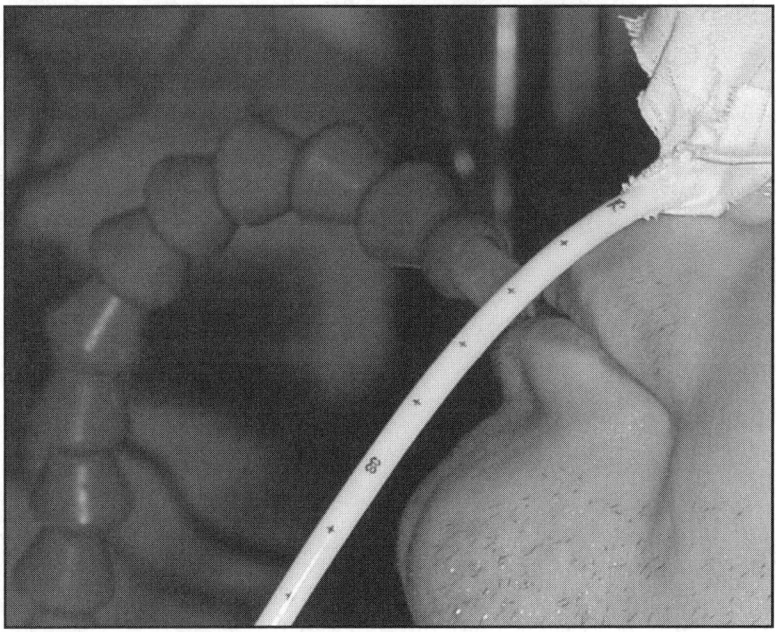

Figure 7–47. Pressure bulb in mouth.

for mounting a switch. Like the medical device platforms, the glasses can maintain a fixed positioning of the switch regardless of the patient's positioning in a bed or chair. Figure 7–48 illustrates how a small flexible wire attached to a stem of the eyeglasses' frame can allow positioning a switch. This is most commonly used with a blink/wink switch, which uses reflected infrared light to discern eyelid movements. To be effective, the switch circuitry must be programmable to distinguish the high-velocity natural blink from the lower velocity associated with the voluntary blink/wink. In some cases, we have also used this mounting approach to suspend a pressure bulb down to the corner of the mouth.

Baseball Cap/Visor as Platform

In some cases where we began with a halo-mounted switch, we typically would switch to a collar-mounted switch as the patient progressed. As we are an acute care facility, patients are often discharged before they can function without a collar. Because of a variety of medical and social services reasons, some of our patients remain hospitalized after their cervical spines have been stabilized. Although the patient and medical staff see the "loss" of the collar as a "good thing," we are left with the problem of finding an alternative stable platform for the switches that these patients with quadriplegia need in order to access AAC

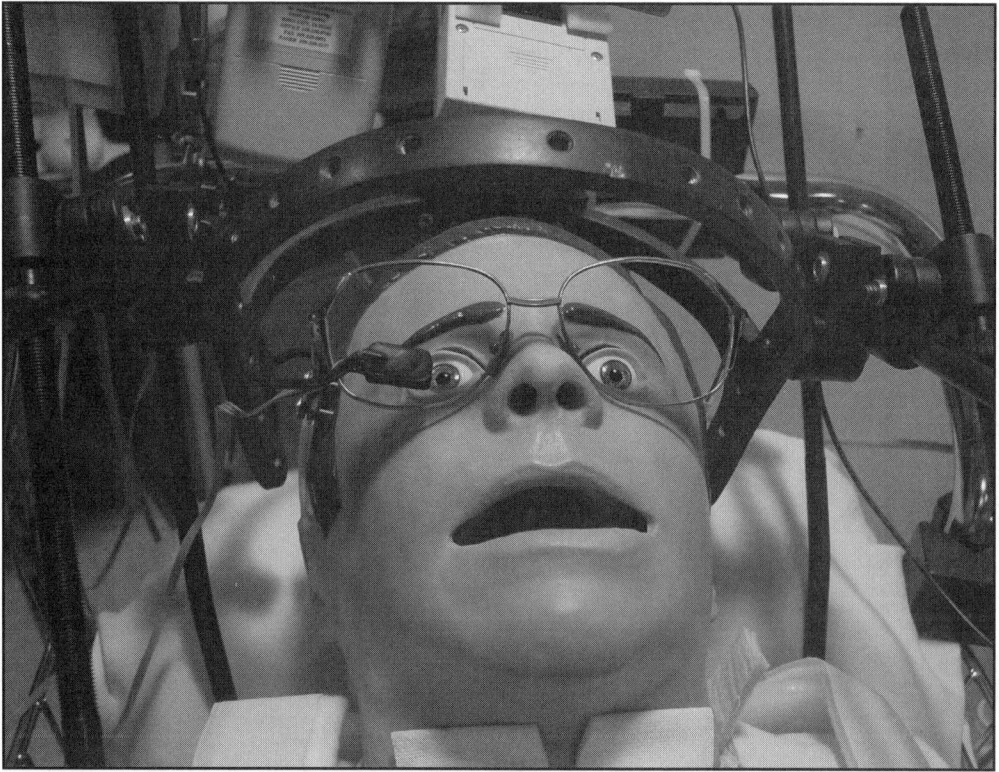

Figure 7–48. Eyeglasses as switch mounting platform.

and ECU systems. One of our patients was fond of wearing baseball caps and his family gave him one to wear as soon as his halo brace came off. No matter when we came to see him, he always had a baseball cap on, so when the cervical collar ceased to be an option for mounting a switch, we utilized a Loc-Line manifold (Figure 7-49) as a mounting plate that we could attach to the side of the cap. The Loc-Line tubing could then be extended down to the cheek or mouth to provide access to a switch (Figure 7-50).

Special Mounting Case: Auto-Suction

For many intubated and trached patients managing oral secretions is a problem and patients find themselves having to

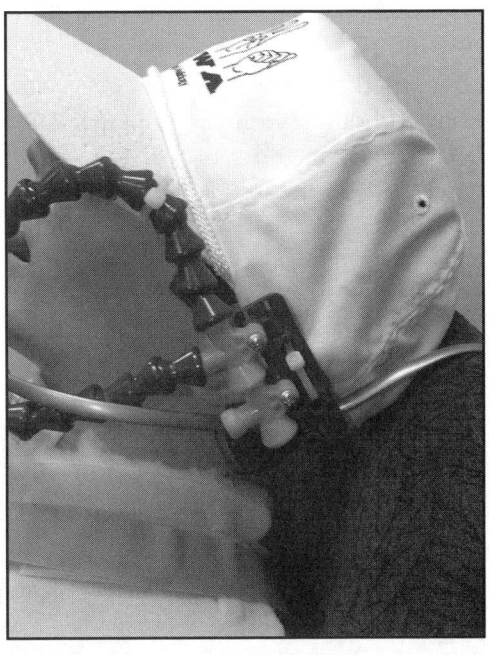

Figure 7-49. Loc-Line manifold.

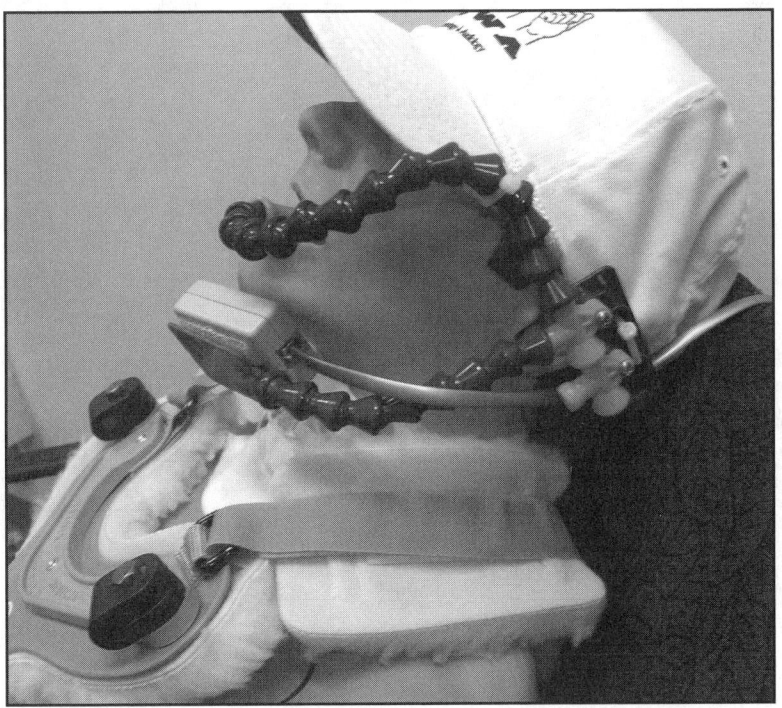

Figure 7-50. Cap-mounted Loc-Line tubing with switch.

ask for suctioning with great frequency. Patients often feel very dependent and concerned about respiratory complications. Although our AAC templates make it easier for patients to ask for mouth cares and suctioning, some patients remain leery of constantly asking for care. So, when we developed the baseball cap mounting system, we had the option of suspending a second Loc-Line tube from the cap. We threaded a catheter that was connected to the vacuum line through the Loc-Line tubing so that it was positioned where the patient could reach it by pursing his lips (Figure 7–51) and thereby could suction his mouth without assistance.

VIDEOS ASSOCIATED WITH THIS CHAPTER

Video clip 7–1. Board positioning check (checking for patient's glasses).

Video clip 7–2. Iowa AAC pole-positioning protocol.

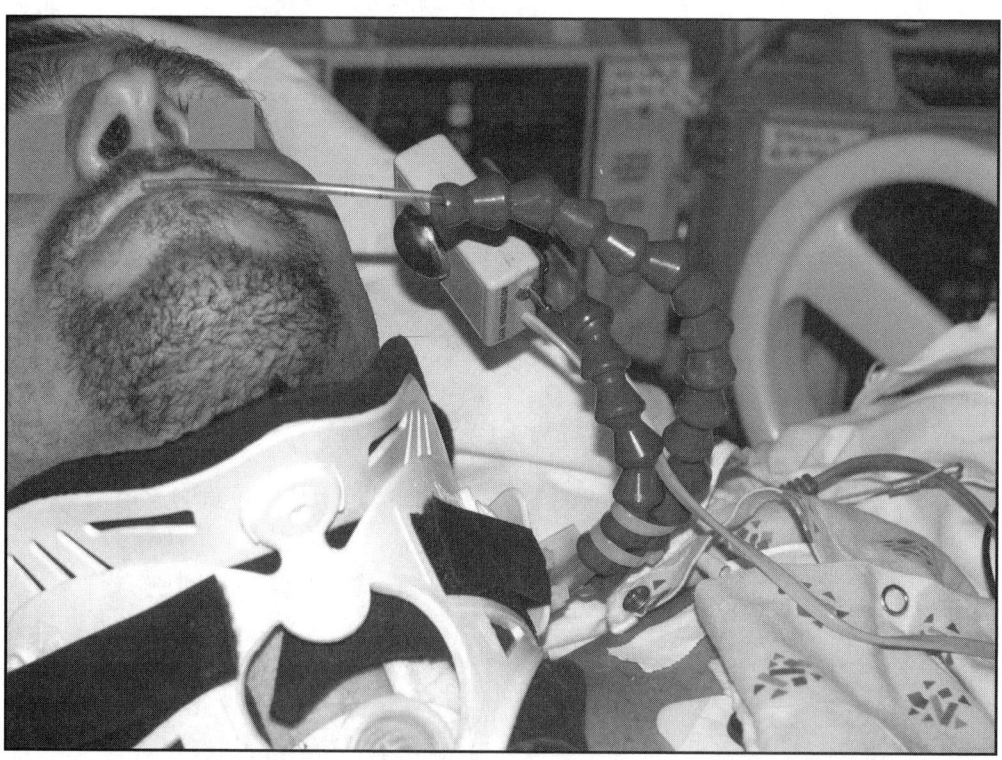

Figure 7–51. Auto suction setup using Loc-Line tubing.

8 Pain Management

One of the most consistently reported needs of critically ill patients is effective management of pain. It is generally accepted that magnitude and duration of pain have a direct impact on a patient's state of mind and, consequently, on the trajectory to recovery. Managing pain is essential to the well-being of the patient. JC now requires health organizations to have effective pain management programs in place (Weissman, 2003). Effective pain management also influences patients' perceptions of how much their doctor cares about them (Weissman, 2003) and probably their willingness to be active participants in their care plan. Interfacing assistive technology in acute care settings to allow the verbally or motorically impaired patients to request analgesics for pain or to provide the patients with the ability to activate patient-controlled analgesia (PCA) pumps would greatly facilitate pain management and the patient's state of mind. Such use of AT for pain management has been experimentally implemented at the University of Iowa Hospitals and Clinics (Hurtig & Downey, 2006). PCA pumps allow the patient to self-administer a predetermined intravenous amount of the prescribed medication. PCA pumps often are used during the recovery phase to relieve postoperative pain, although they are also used for patients with chronic pain. The PCA allows the patient to control pain medication by pressing a control button whenever he or she experiences pain. These devices are programmed by the nurses to allow only a limited dose per interval of time so the patient cannot receive an overdose. Use of PCA devices is common in intensive care settings. The value of the PCA is that it allows the patient to stay ahead of the pain and potentially require less medication while providing more comfort for the patient and, most importantly, some sense of control. This "sense of control" can be critical in allowing the patient to feel less anxious and reducing potential frustrations that the patient may experience. It also allows the patient to be a participant in his or her care on the path to recovery. The advantages of the PCA pump include:

- Patients feel less apprehensive about pain following surgery because they know they have control in their hand—by simply pushing a button.
- The physician determines the amount (dosage) based on the patient's weight to prevent an overdose.
- Narcotic addiction can be avoided because the drug is taken on a short-term controlled basis.
- Pain relief is available around the clock—no need to wait for a nurse to deliver pain medication.

- Medication does not need to be swallowed or injected with each dose.
- The PCA unit is "programmed" to control the dosage. The unit "locks out" if the dosing frequency is exceeded.
- Patients are assured they are receiving the correct medication and dose prescribed by their physician.
- Doses are smaller and available more frequently, which helps prevent sleepiness and weakness.
- Pain is more consistently controlled.
- Dosing at regular intervals reduces the overall amount of medication needed to control pain.
- Prior to expected activity (e.g., physical therapy, getting out of bed), the patient can self-dose to control pain during movement.
- Most cognitively intact adults and children can use PCA.

Although the use of PCAs is common and appropriate for most patients, it is not uncommon that their use has been limited with patients in intensive care settings, who experienced extensive trauma that precludes their ability to vocalize the need for pain medications, or who need to be immobilized for a variety of reasons (e.g., to prevent accidental self-extubation).

The inability to vocalize is often inappropriately taken as a sign that the patient's cognitive state cannot be assessed and therefore one cannot determine if a patient could be a candidate for a PCA. Similarly, for the patient who is immobilized, the inability to access the standard PCA switch also is often taken as an exclusionary criterion. Patients who cannot generate the force necessary to activate the push button of the standard PCA cord are also often excluded from PCA use. Note that, when such exclusion occurs, the patient faces an access barrier that could easily be overcome by interfacing AT with the PCA pump. Adapting a PCA pump is an appropriate and ethical alternative when traditional PCA use is rendered nonfunctional due to the physical status of the patient. The AT equipment needed to make such an adaptation may be minimal. The solution often comes in identifying the voluntary gesture that the patient can consistently produce and finding a switch that can transducer that gesture. Because the PCA is activated with a simple push-button switch, substituting an alternative switch should be fairly simple and may require an adapter cable. For more detail, see Chapters 5 and 7 which address selecting alternative switches and how to mount them. In situations where a patient has both communication and pain management needs and only can control a single switch, one can use an AAC device that provides both speech output and environmental control (ECU). One can then utilize an X-10 relay module to function as the alternative input to the PCA. It is important to note that this in no way interferes with the programming of the PCA that ensures that the patient can not administer more than the prescribed dose. The ability to provide an assistive technology solution to provide patients access to PCAs will depend on the specific PCAs available and on locally determined bio-safety regulations that might preclude using the X-10 relay modules with medical devices. The next chapter provides greater detail on how ECUs can be used.

9 Environmental Control Units (ECUs)

Controlling one's environment is a key element to a sense of autonomy. When a short-term or long-term condition limits that autonomy there can be a significant negative impact on an individual's psychological and physical well-being. An inability to get up and turn the lights on as it gets dark can not only raise anxiety but also raise the possibility of physical risk if one attempts to engage in activities in the dark. Being dependent on others raises the burden on caretakers and also raises the risk of depression as one feels helpless in one's environment. Recall Jean-Dominique Bauby's eloquent description of his feelings when an aide turned off the television during a soccer match and left him in the room alone and unable to access the TV controls or call for assistance. Current technology, allows a wide range of remote control of electronic devices in the hospital and the home environment.

Most individuals have, from the comfort of a couch or an easy chair, turned on their TV and been able to cruise through the available channels. The earliest remotes could do little more than turn the TV on and off, adjust the volume up or down, and step through the channels in a linear fashion. These remotes had a limited set of keys. Pressing a key resulted in the remote putting out a coded IR (infrared) or RF (radio frequency) signal that the TV or other device could sense and then perform the desired response (e.g., power on). Given the limited set of options, each key had a unique function and learning those functions posed little if no burden on the average user.

The contemporary remote control can control not only the TV but also a whole array of home entertainment equipment as well as home automation systems (Figure 9-1). With the additional functions came a proliferation of keys on the remote and the need to produce a sequence of key strokes to accomplish certain functions. The modern remote poses a challenge to many users, because of the vast number of programming options. One result of this complexity is an underutilization of all but the most common functions. Some high-end remotes incorporate visual displays and access to built-in help functions to aid the user deal with the complexity and take advantage of the added functions.

A few remotes have eliminated the need to remember the particular keystrokes needed to accomplish a particular function by incorporating speech-recognition technology (Figure 9-2). The

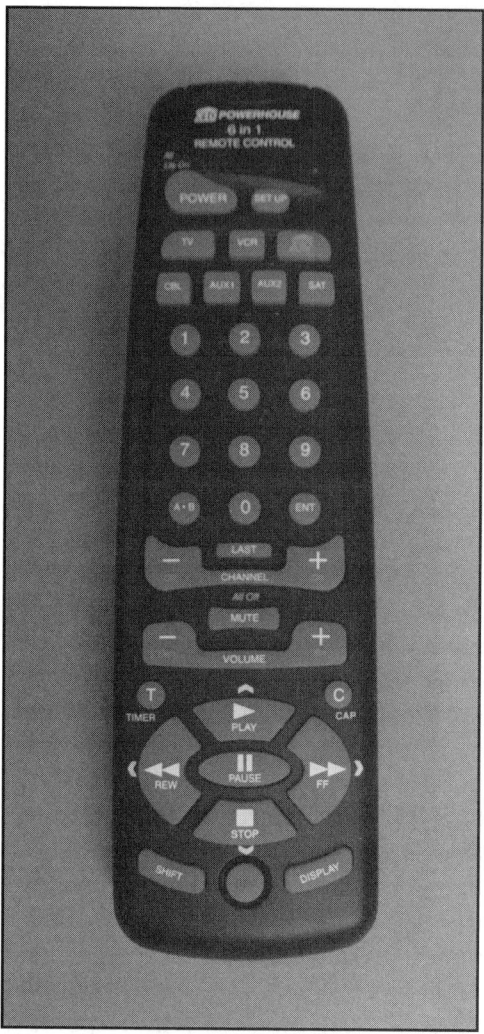

Figure 9–1. Universal remote control.

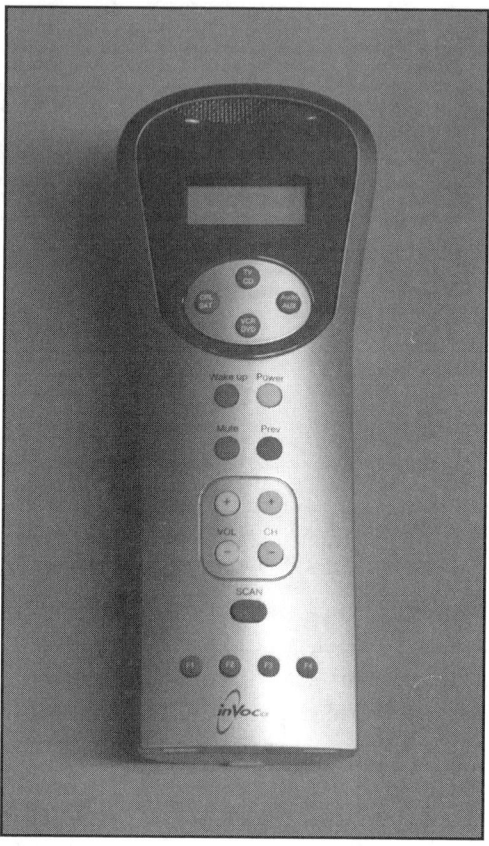

Figure 9–2. Voice-activated universal remote.

user trains the remote to recognize a particular oral command and associate it with a particular keystroke or sequence of keystrokes. Thus, all the user needs to do is produce the target phrase and the remote executes the required keystrokes. The user no longer has to remember what a particular channels numerical code is. All that he or she must do is utter the unique name for the channel. For example, if the user wants to select the Food Channel, all that he or she needs to do is utter the phrase "food channel." For the patient who is unable to physically activate a multiple key remote but who has stable speech, the remote controls that utilize speech recognition provide a reasonable alternative.

In addition to controlling home entertainment, remote control has been used to permit home automation. Again from the comfort of the couch, one can turn lights on and off, turn appliances on or off, control heating and cooling systems, control electronic drapes, and remotely lock and unlock doors. As with the TV remotes, the controller emits an IR or RF signal that identifies a particular device and the state that the user wants the device to be in. Unlike the TVs or VCRs which have a built-in receiver for the IR or RF signal, home automation systems require additional devices to achieve their desired outcomes. The systems typically include a receiver unit (Figure 9-3 [IR] and Figure 9-4 [RF]) that is plugged into an AC wall plug. The receiver translates the signal it receives into a stream of pulses which are placed on the 60 cycle AC line. This pulse stream is carried throughout the house via the AC wiring. Custom wall switches (Figure 9-5) and relay modules (Figure 9-6) are assigned particular address codes corresponding to the pulse streams. When a unit encounters a pulse stream with its address code, it changes its state as a function of that pulse stream (Figure 9-7, detail of X-10 module address settings).

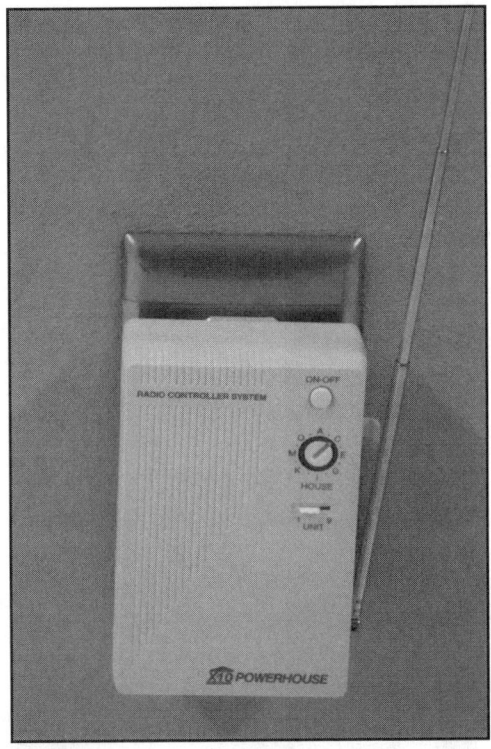

Figure 9–4. RF (radio frequency) receiver X-10.

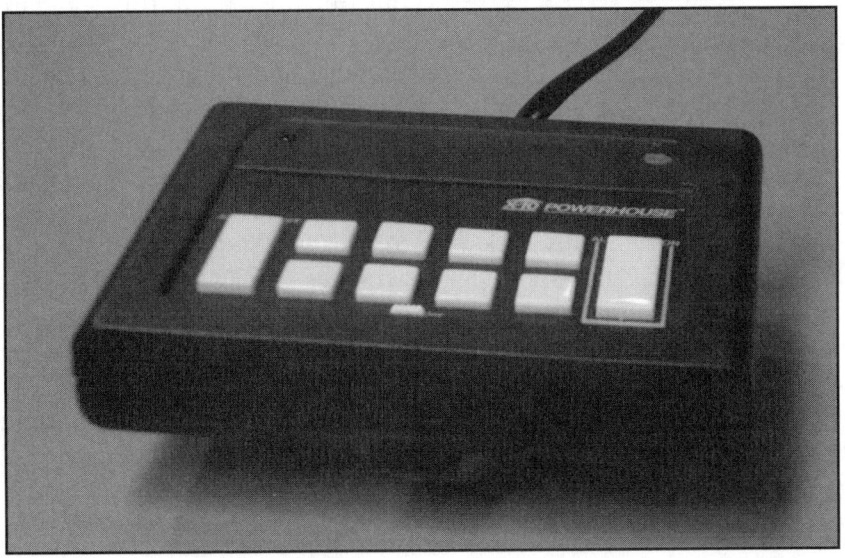

Figure 9–3. IR (infrared) receiver X-10.

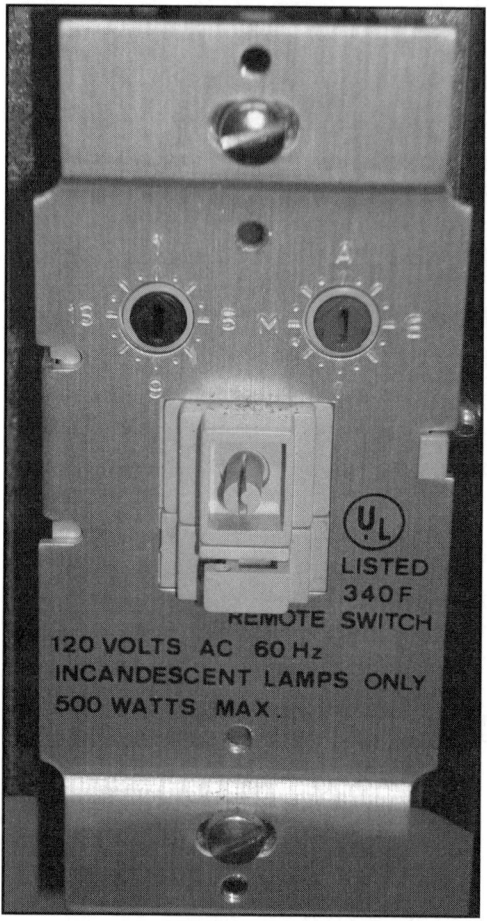

Figure 9–5. Custom wall switch for X-10.

As we indicated in Chapter 3, for a hospitalized bedridden patient, control of the environment (e.g., lights, TV, fans) may be severely limited. This lack of control can have significant psychological impact on the patient. Major trauma patients are extremely susceptible to a fairly rapid onset of depression as they realize that their lives as they knew them will forever be different and that they may well be dependent on others for everything from feeding, bathing, as well as positioning and mobility. The ability to provide electronic ECU to even those most impaired patients not only has the potential of reducing the post-trauma depression but also creates the hook by which one can convince patients to utilize the same switch access that gives them ECU for other functions, communication in particular.

In the previous chapter, we suggested that the ECU function that is part of high-tech AAC systems can be utilized to control PCA pumps and allow patients access to pain medications. In the Iowa Template (see Chapter 6), we provide patients not only with messages to indicate the locus of the pain and that they need medications for pain but also a button that sends an IR signal to an X-10 receiver that is coded to correspond to the X-10 code sequence associated with an X-10 relay module that is set on "momentary" and whose relay contacts are wired to replace the standard switch button closure of the standard PCA switch. Thus, even a patient who can produce only the smallest, low-force voluntary gesture can access the PCA. This typically is accomplished by having the AAC system operate in scanning mode. When the template button corresponding to the PCA is highlighted, the patient activates the switch which causes the AAC device to emit the coded IR signal that the X-10 IR receiver mounted at the top of the IV pole detects and converts to the pulse stream that will trigger the X-10 module connected to the PCA.

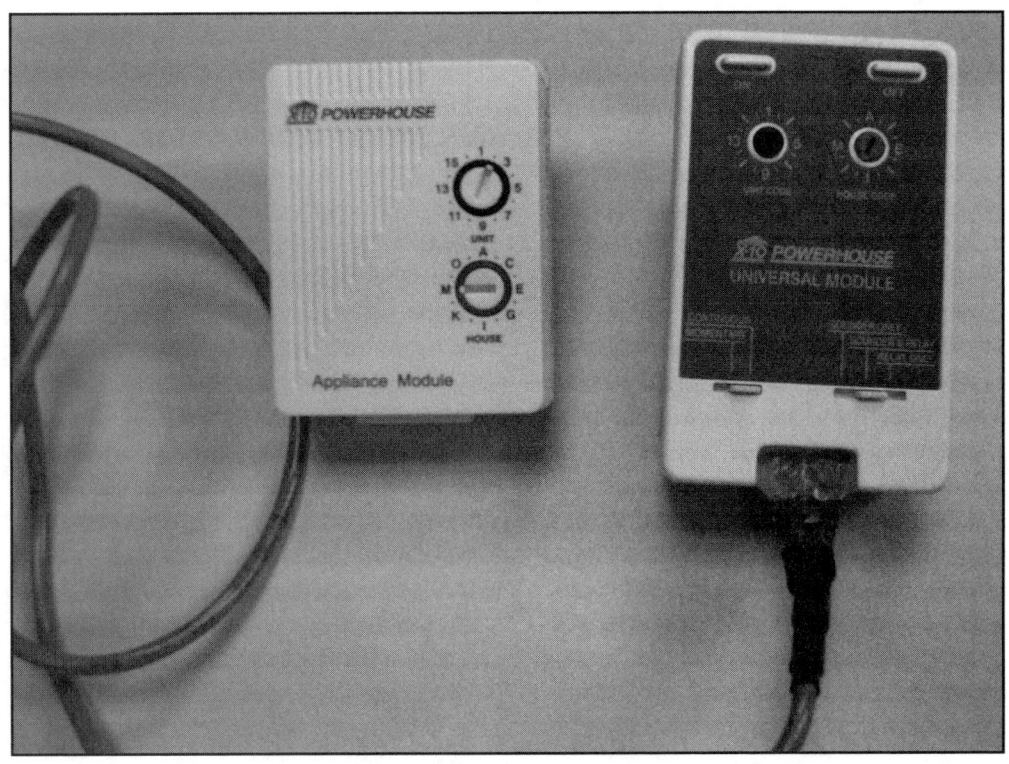

Figure 9–6. X-10 relay modules for appliances and devices requiring switch closure.

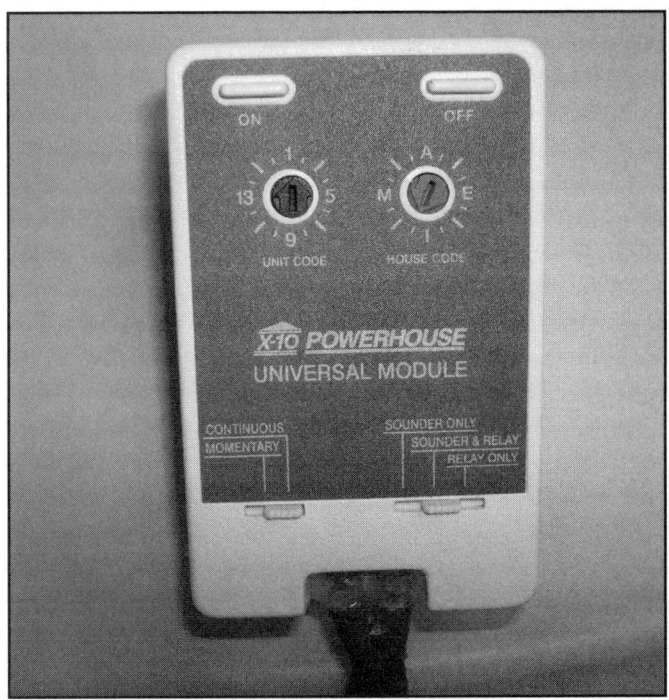

Figure 9–7. X-10 house and unit address code selection.

10 Bad News—Communication Issues

Sophocles gives us one of the earliest (442 BC) literary references to the problems of delivering *bad news*. Being blamed or worse, being killed, for being the messenger who gives bad news has been a recurring theme in eastern and western literature. Shakespeare makes reference to such unwelcome messengers in a number of his works (*Henry V*, Pt. 2 and *Antony and Cleopatra*). It is not just the potential of physical harm that messengers fear; it is also dealing with the psychological consequences of the message on those who receive it. The messenger becomes the "bad news" and so has to be the target to the reaction to the news.

Fear of a negative reaction often leads one to avoid talking about the possibility of a negative outcome. When there is no way to avoid talking, one is nevertheless torn about what to say and how to say it. We fear broaching the topic as well as how to respond when the topic is inescapable. Physicians, nurses, and family members are uncomfortable and patients often do not talk or raise questions for fear of having to confront the answers they will get. Everyone seeks the "right" or "good" way to deal with the *bad news*. Unfortunately, avoidance merely postpones the inevitable and delaying the news may do nothing to diminish its potentially devastating impact.

If one could, one would prefer to say "you will recover" or "you will live" but for many patients in acute care, the reality is that they may not leave the hospital with all their physical and mental functions intact. Life as they have known it has ceased. They may never walk on their own, breathe without the help of a respirator, or be able to talk and carry on the daily activities that defined their lives and identities. Unfortunately for some, even such a drastically altered life is not in the cards. For them, life will be measured in hours or days.

Conversations about dying are not easy, even when the patient is able to speak. All participants in such conversations weigh their choices of content and form and proceed with extreme caution. Each side is concerned about the feelings and reactions of the other. Often, once the topic of impending death has been broached, conversations move with greater ease.

For the patient who is incapable of speaking or writing without some form of assistive technology, the situation of dealing with "bad news" is all the worse. They have no way to indicate they understand what they are being told and no way to ask questions or express their feelings and wishes. AAC solutions can provide patients with an opportunity to participate in such end-of-life conversations.

The problem is: how does one program an AAC system to allow for such conversations? Thus, we are burdened not only with how to tell the patient about his or her impending death but also with the challenge of what options to provide the patient so that he or she can play an active and interactive role in the subsequent conversations. The problem we face is that, just as there is no one perfect way to deliver bad news, there may be no single set of responsive options to provide in an AAC system.

In so many respects, the problem with the "bad news" scenario is no different from any of the other scenarios that we need to address in building AAC systems. The approach to building systems to deal with such scenarios needs to be based on an understanding of what a patient might want to know and talk about as well as how to give the patient a means of expressing his or her personal voice. Ethical and legal issues must also enter into how the systems are built and structured.

Let us start with these latter issues, as they necessarily influence how we will deal with the content and voice issues. The first and fundamental question deals with "who tells what to whom" (Fitch, 1994). In the typical American hospital, if there is such a thing, a member of the medical staff will meet with family members to deliver the bad news to them prior to delivering the message to the patient. Whether for fear of the "shoot the messenger" reaction or out of direct concern for helping people cope with the information, the task of being the messenger is left to the member of the care team who would have the most natural rapport with the family members. In some settings, more than one member of the medical team participates in such meetings (Curtis, 2000, 2004; Curtis et al., 2001; Curtis et al., 2002). One may deliver the unwanted news while the others provide the hand holding and the shoulders to cry on. There is no question that there is wide range of how such meetings transpire. The range of empathy and an understanding of how the information in the message will be processed by the family members play a critical role.

A good outcome is not just a consequence of having empathy and being informative. We know it is painful to hear a loved one will die or be permanently disabled and we presume to know enough about the patient's condition to explain the patient's condition. Knowing the right message and the right way to deliver it often are more a function of who we have to tell than a function of the specifics of the patient's condition. One of the most poignant examples of this can be found in the disastrous failure documented in Anne Fadiman's chronicle of the miscommunication between doctors and a Hmong family in her book, *The Spirit Catches You and You Fall Down* (1997). Although the case Fadiman describes involves a collision of cultures, it points out that the assumptions that underlie doing the right thing need to be carefully thought through. In this case, a failure to understand who the medical team was talking to and how the messages they were providing were being understood led to a cascade of tragedies. All too often, the message is provided to whomever is available in the waiting room and does not take into consideration individual family and cultural traditions about medical decision-making (Waters, 1999).

In the situation where the communication must involve patients in acute care, who because of their medical condition may not be able to speak or write, the success of that earlier conversation with family members is all the more critical.

In the case of children or adults who are deemed incompetent, there is a tendency on the part of many to take the position that they need not get the whole bad news. This is often a joint decision taken by family members and the medical team. With infants and toddlers, the bad news message is never delivered. With young children, there is great reticence to deliver the message, and with adolescents and teenagers, there is trepidation about the reaction to the message. The decision about whether or not to deliver the message is based on feelings that the child might either not grasp the import of the message or that the child would not have the means to psychologically deal with the import of the message. The risk of not having the bad news conversation is that given the nature of acute care and the patient's condition there is a likelihood that the news will slip out in unintended ways at inopportune moments when the patient's family and primary care team may not be available to cushion the blow. A lot of individuals come in contact with patients, many of whom may not be part of the primary care team or immediate family. These individuals may or may not be aware of what the patient knows. Statements they may make directly to the patient or in conversations they may have with others that may be overheard by the patient can "spill the beans" with all the negative consequences. In one case, while the parents and medical team were discussing a teenager's prognosis and how to tell her about her condition and the treatment options, a surgical resident entered the patient's room to do a prebiopsy examination and proceeded to discuss the procedure and the possible outcomes of finding evidence of lymphoma. The patient's reaction and screams could be heard by the horrified parents and medical team in a conference room way at the other end of unit. This patient had the means to communicate her reaction to the *bad news* and had the means to participate in the subsequent discussions about the treatment protocol and its potential outcomes. What would have happened if she had no means to communicate? This case exemplifies the need to make sure that everyone is aware of what a patient has and has not been told.

In the case of competent adults, the tendency is to provide them with information about their state as soon as it is available. Prior discussion with family members often occurs and delivering the news is often done in their presence. The desire to not be the lone messenger delivering the bad news often postpones the message until family members can be present. The problem that often arises is that the patient's care is ongoing and everyone on the unit may know of the patient's condition with the exception of the patient. So, as in the case of the child with lymphoma, some trauma patients in acute care settings discover that they may have a life-threatening condition or that they will be permanently disabled from interactions with medical staff who are unaware of what the patient has or has not been told. In both the accounts of Julia Tavalaro (1997) and Jean-Dominique Bauby (1997), there are instances in which they recount their reactions to such indirect ways in which they learned of what people thought of their conditions. In their cases, their inability to speak or write left them helpless and unable to either solicit corroboration of the information or to engage in a conversation in which they could express their feelings or engage in an active way in their treatment.

In Bauby's case, individuals would tell him things but not solicit any response or acknowledgment of comprehension from him. In a scene in the film based on Bauby's book a physician entered his room and in a cavalier manner said that he would have to suture one of Bauby's eyes shut; the doctor then proceeded to do it with no thought of Bauby's reactions or desires. To make things worse, the doctor talked about coming back from a great vacation skiing. Remember Bauby is a locked-in syndrome patient who cannot move anything but his now single open eye.

In our society and dominant culture, patient autonomy is considered highly important. Except for young children and incompetent adults, in the end, it is the patient who should decide what treatments to accept or reject. Thus, we accept that the patient plays a significant role in decisions about whether they should be resuscitated in the case of cardiopulmonary failure or whether they should receive transfusions. Where this construct of autonomy faces the most challenges is in cases where decisions involve the withdrawal of life support. Here, moral and ethical beliefs of patients, family members, and medical staff often collide and the belief in patient autonomy may not trump these other beliefs (Waters, 1999). Who decides whether a ventilator-dependent patient does or does not continue to be kept on the ventilator? There are many who might want to keep the 'truth' from the patient. This can place staff and family members in an ethical dilemma (Fowler, 2004).

Assuming that a patient can neither speak nor write, the challenge facing the person designing the AAC system for the patient is how to provide an easy way for the patient to actively participate in what may be "end-of-life" or "end-of-life as you have know it" conversations. To meet this challenge, it may be useful for the communicative needs of such conversations to be broken down into expressions of comprehension, expressions of reaction, and expressions of desires.

Expressions of comprehension are those that allow patients to affirm not only that they have understood what they have been told about their condition and what the prognosis is, but also allow the patients to ask questions to gain a further understanding of the situation. For example, a patient who has been told that he has sustained a spinal cord injury that has resulted in his being placed on ventilatory support may, in order to truly understand his situation, want to ask whether he will have to stay on the ventilator. Expressions of reaction are those that allow patients to let people know how they feel about the news they have received. Understanding how a patient is psychologically responding to the situation may play a critical role in the approach to treatment; including, among other things, management of depression and anger. Finally, and perhaps most importantly, expressions of desires allow the patient to become an active participant in critical decision-making about treatment goals.

For the patient who is limited to providing a gaze shift response to indicate yes and no, the approach to giving the patient the ability to provide these three different types of expressions will be limited to how well the conversational partners are able to construct their questions so that the patient's communicative needs are addressed. The following is an example of an interaction with the patient and how such questions may be structured.

Staff: Hello Mr. Jones, we have some things we would like to tell you about your condition. So that we are sure you understand what we are saying and so we can know what you want, I will be asking you some questions. I want you to respond using your yes/no response of looking up for yes and down for no.

Patient: (looks up)

Staff: We have reviewed the x-rays of your spine and it looks like you have sustained some significant damage. The reason you are on the breathing machine is that the nerves that control your breathing have been damaged. Do you understand what I am saying?

Patient: (looks down)

Staff: You sustained damage to the control of the breathing system, so the machine is doing the breathing for you. Do you understand?

Patient: (looks up)

Staff: Right now we don't know if you will be able to breathe on your own. Do you understand?

Patient: (looks down)

Staff: Is there a question you want to ask me about that?

Patient: (looks up)

Staff: I will try to guess what question you want to ask. Okay?

Patient: (looks up)

Staff: Are you asking if you will need to stay on the ventilator?

Patient: (looks up)

Staff: We don't know at this point if you will be able to breathe on your own. I know this must be upsetting.

Patient: (looks up)

Staff: Do you have any questions you want me to address?

Patient: (looks down)

Staff: Is there anything else you want me to explain?

Patient: (looks down)

Staff: We'll let you rest now. Okay?

Patient: (looks up)

This first conversation allowed the bad news to be presented and afforded the patient an opportunity to indicate a level of understanding, a reaction, and some control. However, one should not assume that the patient has a full understanding of the gravity of the situation or of the consequences of maintaining or withdrawing ventilatory support. Any decisions about maintaining or withdrawing treatment require repeated conversations that should be witnessed by a number of individuals including family members so that there is a consensus on how the patient responded. Just as with advanced medical directives, in these situations one should always attempt to verify the patient's choice prior to taking action.

One of the questions that is very difficult to ask is: "Do you want to have life support withdrawn?" It is a difficult question for all involved and unfortunately is one that ends up needing to be asked in situations where there is disagreement among family members about the wishes of the patient with regard to end-of-life decisions. In one case, that we refer to as the "dueling siblings" case, a retired gentleman fell and sustained severe spinal cord injuries. He was effectively rendered a quadriplegic and could not breathe on his own. The two daughters differed radically in what they thought their father would want. One said that her father had been a vigorous and active man who would not want a vegetative existence. The other said that her father was a fighter and that he would never want to give up no matter what his circumstances. Each daughter wanted to be the decision-maker and each could not accept the decision of the other. The nursing staff, on the basis of their interactions with the patient, was confident that the patient was sufficiently aware of his situation and needed to be part of the conversation. It was apparent to the impartial observer that he was tracking the situation and that he was distressed by the siblings' conflict. The Assistive Technology Service established a communication system that allowed the patient to demonstrate a level of competency that would indicate that he could participate in these end-of-life decisions. The outcome was as good as one might hope. The patient indicated that it was his wish to be withdrawn from life support. By itself, that was comforting to one sibling and accepted by the other. However, giving this intubated patient a means of communicating allowed him not only to play a significant role in this most difficult situation but it also enabled him to indicate what he wanted each family member to do after his death. In the end, it was the ability to have those final wishes made explicit that left the patient, family, and staff able to accept the outcome of withdrawing life support. In this case, perhaps because all parties respected the patient's right to autonomy, everything worked. However, there are many cases where the outcome may not be so well accepted.

When everyone genuinely accepts the patient's right to participate in the decision, then posing the question of withdrawal of life support can take the form of asking the question and verification that the patient understands the consequences. In situations where one party or the other questions the patient's ability to rationally decide, the form and content of the alternatives presented to the patient become controversial. Some might argue that the patient can only be asked if he or she wants to live and that, by asking a question about withdrawing life support, we are unduly directing a patient or putting words in the patient's mouth.

In a similar vein, some might argue that, no matter how alert and competent the patient may appear, there is no way they can give truly informed consent to have life support turned off. However, it is unclear that family members under stress are in any better position to do so. For most people, patients, and family members, this is a novel and most likely unplanned for situation. They do not know what questions to ask or really understand what all the alternatives are. Typically, hospital staff, from their experiential base, lay out the possible scenarios for the family members.

So why is laying out the options on a communication board for the patient any different? The key is that everything should be contextualized for the patient. Just as hospital menus are tailored to the dietary needs/restriction of patients, communication boards also need to be tailored to a patient's particular medical status. One would not want a patient to first encounter the possibility that they are dying by reading across the set of utterances on a communication board and seeing the phrase "Am I going to die?" On the other hand, it is a legitimate question that many patients want to ask. So how and when does one give a particular patient access to such a question? A good rule of thumb in making decisions about the content of an AAC system is to determine that the patient understands how an AAC system works and that the selection options are to give the patient the widest range of options given the knowledge of what other patients in comparable situations have asked and wanted to talk about. What that means is that if one makes the phrases "I want to be taken off life support" and "I want to be kept on life support" available, then one should provide an explanation of why they are included and that they are there so that patient can indicate what he or she wants.

If a patient is limited to asking yes/no questions, then one has to consider how to ask the question. For many patients unfamiliar with physiologic systems, their answers to the question "Do you want to live?" may not be the same as answers to "Do you want us to keep you on the ventilator?" So it may be prudent to approach the end-of-life decisions from a range of questions rather than a single one focused on the withdrawal of a medical intervention. Likewise, for patients who can use an AAC system, it is essential that they have the multiple response options available to them. So, as painful as it may be for family members to see some of those phrases in the AAC system, it needs to be presented as a means to provide an opportunity of expression that a patient with the ability to speak would normally have. Absent a technology that can read the patient's mind, alternative message options are the only way to ensure that a patient can make his or her wishes known. A set of options for a communication page for potential end-of-life conversations may, among other things, include:

Questions:

How bad is my situation?

Will I be able to breathe on my own?

Will I be able to move my arms and legs?

Will I be able to eat regular food?

Statements:

I want to live.

I want to live no matter what.

I want to stay on life support for now.

I want you to do whatever is necessary to stay alive.

I don't want to stay on life support for long.

Take me off life support if . . .

Take me off life support, I want to die.

It is probably unwise and insensitive to generate a one-size-fits-all template to use with all patients facing an end-of-life decision. How these options are actually phrased and organized, as well as how the context for the end-of-life conversations is presented, all need to be informed by the physical and cognitive state of the patient and the family members as well as their cultural background and its approach to death and dying. The only way to avoid the pitfalls exemplified in the case of the Hmong child with epilepsy (Fadiman, 1997) is to ask questions and be attentive to the responses of the patient and family members when confronted with elements of the bad news. Most importantly, one needs to think twice before proceeding with an approach if responses do not seem to fit with our expectations.

Although we accept that we often have no way of knowing enough about any individual patient or family to anticipate every issue that might come into play in the *bad news* scenario, many clinicians have never systematically considered how a bad news scenario would play out in their own family. It may not seem natural to think about how you might tell your child, parent, or other family member that they are dying or that they will be permanently disabled. Thinking about how you would approach such a situation not only gives you a sense of what your patient's family members may be experiencing but also lets you make explicit what you might consider your options to be. To get a patient's perspective, think about how you would want to get the bad news if you were the patient and consider what kinds of follow-up questions and discussions you might want to be able to participate in. Considering these scenarios in the abstract may provide only a loose approximation to the real cases one would encounter in clinical practice. We should not succumb to the societal reticence to talk about death and dying. We need to consider how we would talk with our patients and their families and how we would construct an AAC system for a patient. If we do not do this, we are likely to stumble at a time when there may be no time for a second chance. Our patients and their families may not be prepared for the bad news conversation, but we cannot afford not to be.

11 Cases

The following cases are provided to highlight some of the lessons learned in our attempts to implement AAC with patients in acute care settings. We present them in part to highlight the diversity of what may be confronted in these settings and to illustrate instances of success as well as failure. To protect patient confidentiality and privacy, all the names and initials we use in this chapter are pseudonyms.

A. SOLVING THE LANGUAGE BARRIER

Imagine walking into a doctor's office for a procedure that can carry the risk of complete paralysis or even the possibility of death. Can you image how nervous or scared you might feel? Now imagine that you are walking into a doctor's office in a foreign country and engaging in a dialogue regarding your symptoms and possible risks but a communication barrier exists because the patient and the doctor do not speak the same language. How can you be assured that the doctor understands your comments and how do you alert the doctor that you do not understand what he is saying? Certainly, having to contend with a language barrier during any medical procedure or hospital stay can be a challenge. Language barriers are problematic for both the patient and the medical staff who are faced with the task of caring for the patient. If the patient cannot identify feelings of discomfort or pain successfully, the entire admission may be a frustrating and painful experience for all. Imagine not knowing what is going on with your health and being uncertain about the events that are going to happen next. Having a nurse to reassure that you are doing okay is no longer a given. This can be a very scary and uncomfortable situation. This scenario plays itself out in hospitals across the United States. At the University of Iowa Hospitals and Clinics (UIHC), Iowa's only comprehensive academic medical center, we are finding that changes in the demographics of the Iowa population as well as the fact that some individuals come from all over the world to receive state-of-the art care and to benefit from innovative surgical procedures developed by faculty members. For example, many individuals with some form of pathology of the cervical spine come to UIHC to undergo a transoral surgical procedure pioneered by Dr. Arnold Menezes. As a consequence of the trans-oral approach to the cervical spine, there is considerable swelling of the tongue and pharynx that requires that patients be intubated postoperatively for a period of 2 to 5 days.

For such patients, Dr. Menezes requests that the Assistive Technology Laboratory staff meet the patients preoperatively in order to set up a temporary communication system that the patients will use postoperatively.

Recently, a 45-year-old man traveled from a small village in India to be treated by Dr. Menezes. The gentleman, whom we will call MM, was accompanied by his brother, a physician practicing in the United States. MM had been diagnosed with a Chiari malformation Type 1 resulting in neurologic impairment. In particular, MM reported, that for the past 12 years he had experienced numbness and weakness in his right arm and then in both lower extremities that had progressed to a gait disturbance and then weakness in his left arm.

Following our protocol, we arranged to meet with the patient prior to his admission. When we arrived at the clinic to see the patient, we found him sitting quietly in corner of the room with his head down, arms and legs crossed, and appearing most removed from the situation. It was clear that MM demonstrated difficulty in comprehending English. He often requested that his brother translate for him. MM's native language was reported to be Gujarati. It was explained to MM, through translations offered by his brother, that we had several devices that might assist him in communicating with nurses, physicians, and family members during his hospital admission and that we were here today to ask him if he would like us to set up a communication system for him. We also asked him if he would feel more comfortable if common nursing instructions were presented to him in his native language. He raised his head and flashed us the first smile we had seen. His answer was a clear "yes!" One of the few English words MM knew. We explained that we would be using a device that allowed for voice output messages in English and Gujarati.

At the time of this presurgical consult we learned that MM would be admitted for halo crown traction. If the ventral compression of the cervicomedullary junction was reduced, then MM would undergo dorsal decompression and fusion. However, if the compression would not be reduced, then MM would require transoral decompression of his odontoid as well as dorsal fusion. The need to place MM in halo crown traction meant he would be able to talk but it also meant that he would have to be hospitalized prior to surgery for several days. We instructed the patient that we would meet him in his room on the initial day of his admission with a working device. Such a time window of intact verbal abilities is an excellent time to help the patient become familiar with the use of an AAC device and provides the clinician with feedback from the patient as the content is being developed for the patient.

From the first interaction in the neurosurgery clinic, it was apparent how concerned the patient was about being able to communicate with the nurses and the medical staff. At the same time, we were sensitive to how uneasy MM was about being in such a high-tech environment. It was clear to us that we did not want to overwhelm MM and we knew the importance of making sure he had success with his first attempts at communicating with the device. We wanted to ensure that the device selected would be one that would be easy for MM to use and be flexible enough to allow for quick changes at the bedside. Because of the need to have voice output in a language not available in standard text-to-speech systems we needed to select a mid-level device that provided us with the ability to use digitized recordings of words and phrases in the patient's language. We did not need to be concerned about the patient's ability to recognize AAC symbols as MM was literate, a common characteristic of our acute care patients. But we knew we would have to find someone familiar with Gujarati to assist us. At the time of our initial consultation, it escaped us that MM's family could have easily been our "experts." Instead, we looked to a doctoral candidate in our department familiar with Gujarati to assist us and to generate any necessary graphic symbols. Again, because of the need to keep this system as simple as possible, we selected a system that allowed us to use a laminated paper overlay and a dry erase marker. This feature of an easily modifiable overlay along with the capability of digitizing speech led us to select the Tech/Speak communication aid. The Tech/Speak is a simple 32-location overlay that offers 2.2 seconds of digitized (recorded voice) per location. The Tech/Speak provides its user with up to six levels of stored recordings/overlays. Although we did not use more than one overlay/level, the 32 message layout allowed us to provide MM with some core phrases during his hospitalization.

Based on our meeting with the patient and his brother, the following messages were selected for MM's use during his hospitalization:

1. I am hungry.
2. I am thirsty.
3. Wipe my face.
4. I need to go to the bathroom.
5. I want to take a shower.
6. Give me medicine.
7. I need to be suctioned.
8. My lips are dry.
9. Change my sheets.
10. I want to sleep.
11. I want a pillow.
12. It's hot.
13. It/s cold.
14. I am constipated
15. I am having trouble breathing.
16. I am tired.
17. I have a headache.
18. I feel weak.
19. I feel uneasy.

Each message had a key word written in Gujarati with the voice output spoken in English so that the nurse could clearly understand MM. Having the key word written in the Gujarati script allowed MM to be assured he was communicating the correct message to the nurse. In turn, keywords written in English were generated for the nurse to select during his or her communication with MM. The voice output that we associated with the nurse's messages was recorded in MM's native language of Gujarati. To ensure that we had selected the appropriate nursing messages, we interviewed primary care nurses on the units that MM would be on during his admission. The nursing staff suggested the following messages be included on the device:

1. How are you doing?
2. Do you have any discomfort/pain?
3. I need to take your blood pressure and temperature?
4. I need to do a heart exam.
5. I am going to give you some medication.
6. I am going to get your family.

As we worked on selection of specific wording of the nursing messages, we took advantage of our doctoral student's ability to help us understand possible cultural differences. For example, she suggested that a straightforward translation of the phrase "I need to check your vital signs" might not be understood and suggested we select phrases that would be more specific such as "I need to take your temperature."

Figures 11–1A and 11–1B illustrate how the template for the TechTalk was laid out. The template was arranged with MM's messages (Gujarati words/English voice output) written in black on the top three rows of the template. The nursing messages (English words/Gujarati voice output) were written in blue on the bottom row of the template.

One week after our initial meeting in the clinic, MM was admitted to the Neuroscience Inpatient unit and was placed in crown halo traction. Prior to meeting with MM, we asked to meet with one of his family members to review our list of intended messages and to ask them to record the selected messages in Gujarati. MM's nephew volunteered to record the selected phrases. The recording of all 19 messages took less than 5 minutes. We intentionally left five slots on the template open to allow for later additions to the template. We then met with MM that afternoon and introduced the device to him. MM's face immediately lit up and he eagerly participated in the training with the device. MM instinctively knew to select the options on the template grid and he went directly to those with the Gujarati script and used the device to speak with his brother in Gujarati. His brother told us that MM was surprised to see text written in Gujarati. Later, as he experimented selecting the nurse's messages and heard the Gujarati recordings, his eyes widened and he began to sigh and exhaled with some element of notable relief. "Yes, yes, Gujarati," he said. Using his brother as interpreter, he informed us that this was the best machine he had ever seen and wanted to know how expensive it was!

For the next 2 days, MM continued to use the device without difficulty. It was simply placed on his over-the-bed table or positioned on his lap. Family members also were observed holding the device up for MM to access it when it was difficult for him due to the immobilization caused by the halo-crown traction.

After 2 days of traction MM underwent an MRI of the C-spine while he was in traction that revealed persistence of the ventral compression of the cervicomedullary junction. It was then decided that MM would undergo both ventral decompression and dorsal fusion the next day. MM underwent transoral decompression of his odontoid as well as a dorsal fusion.

Postoperatively, MM was transferred to the Surgical Intensive Care Unit where he remained intubated but had access to the Tech/Speak communication device. MM used the device with family members and nursing staff throughout this intubation period. Staff nurses and family raved about the device and indicated it made all parties feel more at ease. MM's brother, the physician, wanted to know how much the device cost and where he could get one for the hospital where he works. Additionally, MM and his family showed our staff the few additions they had added to allow MM to indicate that he wanted to watch TV or listen to the radio. MM also indicted that the print was too small on some of the buttons so family members simply wiped the words off and rewrote them using a large print. Seven days later, MM was extubated and

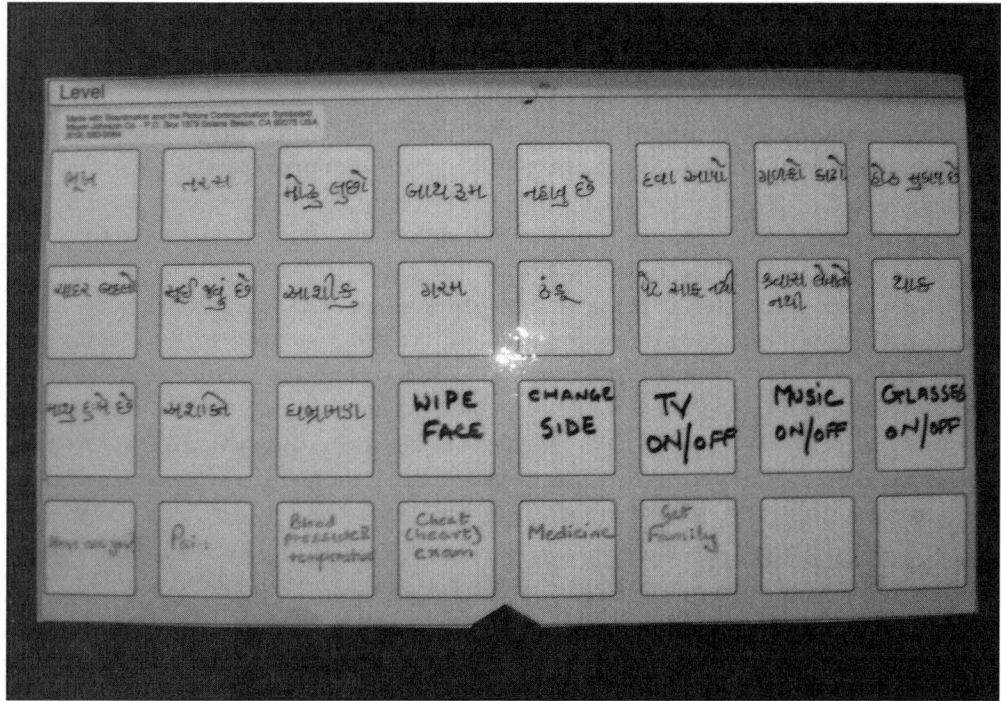

A

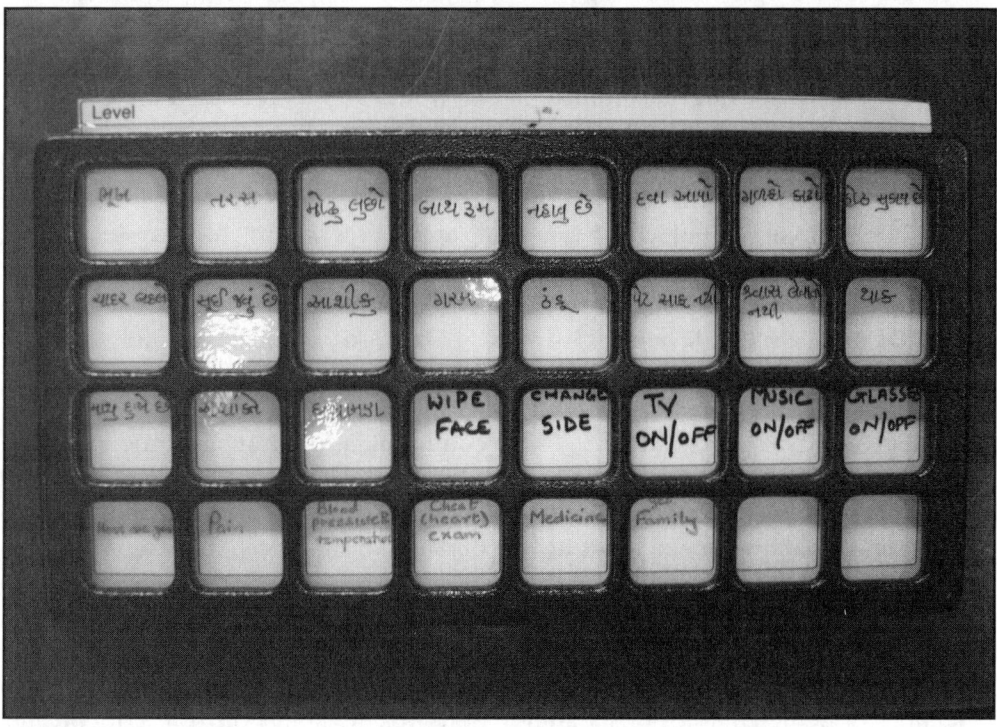

B

Figure 11–1. A. Bilingual set up of mid-tech AAC device. **B.** Bilingual template for mid-tech AAC device.

was transferred back to the neuroscience unit able to use his voice. He continued to use the device in order to more effectively communicate with the staff. He was discharged 11 days later.

Prior to discharge, we interviewed MM about his experiences with the device. His brother served as our interpreter for the interview. The following is a list of our questions and his responses:

- Did the device allow you to communicate your needs? *Response:* "Yes, I was very pleased with the device."
- Was there anything you could not communicate using the device? *Response:* the message "I feel uneasy" was too vague and I had my brother record over this message with the statement, "It's hard to breathe."
- Did you use the device to communicate pain or discomfort? *Response:* "Yes, I used the device often to alert the nurse when I was in pain."
- Do you think you would have been able to communicate about your pain or discomfort as efficiently if you did not have the device? *Response:* "No, it would have been difficult to say I was in pain without the use of the device."
- Was the device positioned in such a way that you could see it? *Response:* "No, but my family helped me if it was hard for me to see and lifted the device up so that I could see it."
- Do you think that the device allowed you to cope with possible feelings of being afraid or upset after the surgery and during your hospital stay? *Response:* "Yes, it was so very helpful."
- Did you use the device to control your environment (i.e., to control the TV or nurse call)? *Response:* "Yes, because I had my brother added messages that asked to have the TV or radio turned off or on." *It should be noted that the Tech/Speak does not provide its user with environmental control options.*
- Who did you communicate with while using the device? *Response:* "I used the device with my family, the nurse, and the doctor and you."
- Was there anything that you would like to change? *Response:* I wish it was positioned in a way that I would not have needed my family to hold it up for me. Any other changes that I wanted we went ahead and just made them. For example, the small print was hard to see so we wrote the words over in a larger print."
- Would you recommend the device to others whose ability to communicate is impaired during acute hospitalization? *Response*: "Yes, without a doubt!" "This system was like a lifeline for my heart!"

This case exemplifies not only the need to provide temporarily nonoral patients with an effective alternative mode of communication but also the need to address the language barrier issue for patients who speak a language that the nursing and medical staff to not understand. Live interpreters for many languages may not be available and, if they are available, cannot be at the bedside for extended periods of time. AAC solutions that enable both the patient and the caregivers to effectively communicate regardless of language barriers significantly enhance care and the patients' emotional state. Our patient's final statement in the exit interview says it all . . . "This system was like a lifeline for my heart!"

B. MAINTAINING A PERSONAL VOICE— ADDING HUMOR

One of the possible reasons that individuals do not accept AAC is that they feel that their own personality and unique voice are lost when using AAC systems. With standard low-tech options used in hospitals, like the preprinted basic communication boards (Figure 11-2), none of the patient's individual communication style can be transmitted. The ability to vary formality as a function of whom the patient is communicating with is lost. The unwillingness to use such communication board, especially by older patients, may in part be due to the potentially inappropriate symbols on the board. For example, the choice of symbol for a urinal may appear inappropriate given the gender of the patient. The presence of a symbol for spouse would be inappropriate for an unmarried patient and might be distressing to a patient whose spouse was deceased. Likewise, a board for pediatric patients that includes symbols for mother, father, and grandparents

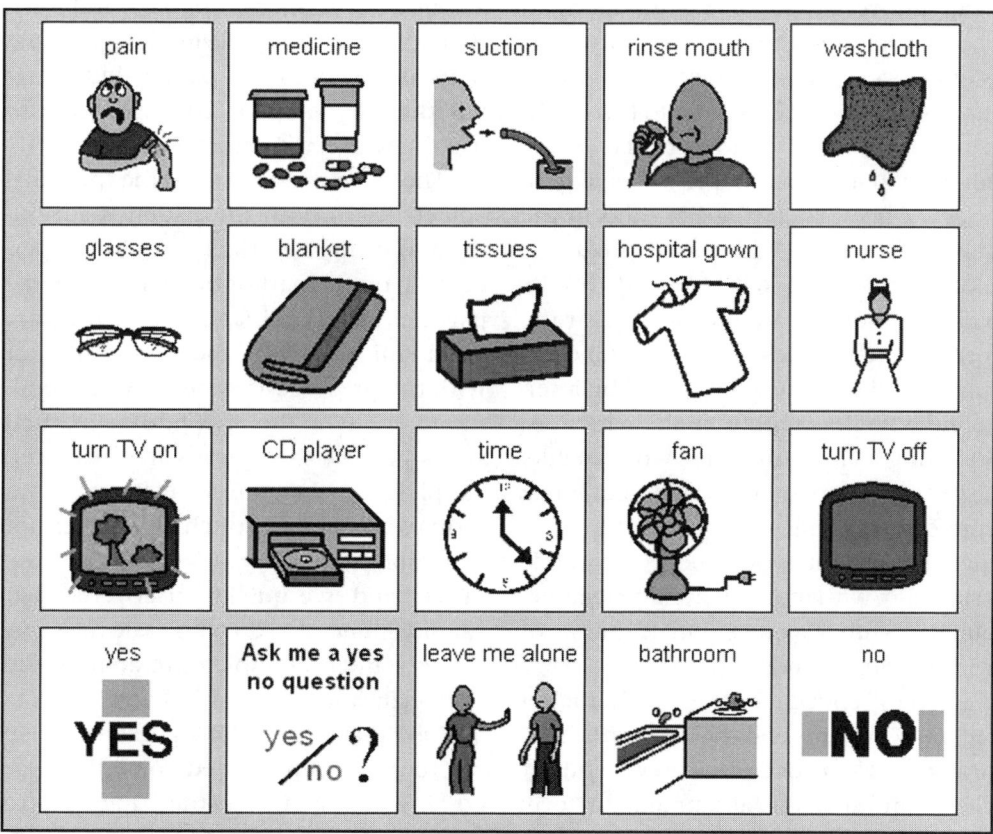

Figure 11–2. Generic communication card.

might be equally inappropriate if the child does not have such relations. Providing the nursing staff with the option to customize the communication board should alleviate some of these problems.

If the boards include more than symbols, then the issue of the appropriateness of the selected words and phrases also needs to be addressed if one wants to achieve acceptance. For patients, particularly those in more intensive care settings, personal privacy and dignity are often compromised. Some bodily functions such as bowel movements and voiding need to become shared activities with individuals who are strangers, of differing genders, and of differing generations. If the communication boards are not customized to the patient's preferred form for requests for assistance with bodily functions, the loss of dignity issue is only exacerbated. "I need to go potty" may be appropriate for a child but might be demeaning for an adult to use. Some adults would feel too prissy having to select "I need to have a BM" and in the context of talking with friends might be more comfortable with "I need to take a crap." A complicating factor is that the form of such requests is perhaps more a function of who the patient will be interacting with than with who the patient is. So asking a family member what an adolescent male patient would feel most comfortable using might generate a form that the patient would be comfortable using only with intimate family members but not with a young female nurse or with visiting friends.

Adding speech output with higher tech AAC systems does not alleviate these problems, as the decisions on vocabulary choice and syntactic and pragmatic form must still be made. With speech output, the fit, or lack thereof with the patient's preferences is all the more critical, as the output will be audible to a wider range of individuals in the patient's vicinity. As a consequence, clinicians will often select/program more formal or neutral utterances that fail to capture the individual speech style of the patient. In cases where the patient is able to participate more actively in the construction of the AAC system, many of these personal voice problems can be averted. This is easiest for individuals who can be seen preoperatively and can meet with the clinician and make selections in terms of both content and form. Obviously, for cases where the patient is already intubated or physically unable to produce audible speech, the process of utterance selection becomes a more complex issue requiring a considerable amount of back and forth with the clinician offering suggestions/options and with the patient indicating whether he wants or does not want to use the suggested utterances.

The value of establishing the "personal voice" lies in both the patient's accepting and using the system and in the perception on the part of the conversational partners (staff and family) that they are communicating with the person and not with the preset AAC system. To that end, the more like the individual's natural speaking style the options are the better. Simply matching the speech output in terms of gender and pitch range does not accomplish making a good fit. On the other hand, we quickly discovered that we did not need to do wholesale revisions of our standard templates to achieve the personalization that would give patients a sense that it was their personal voice not merely a synthesized voice that was coming across. By customizing a mere handful of phrases, conversational partners readily acknowledge that they are communicating with a real person whose style and temperament comes through.

One interesting and extreme case involved a young adult female who requested that, if she could not use her own voice postoperatively, she wanted to sound like a "dirty old man." For her, the humor of having a lower, gravelly male voice functioned to mask the stereotypy of the utterances on her templates. There was no doubt that her choice lightened her interactions with staff and family members. She translated her penchant for joking from the novel content creation that was characteristic of communication style to a variation of speaker voices for different utterances. Thus, she was able to engage individuals and accomplish whatever communicative intention she had with a sense of personal ownership. She complemented this playing with voices with a few particular unique phrases she requested that we program for her. One that she suggested adding to parallel the standard request for medication for pain was "give my mom a valium." This utterance not only added to her arsenal of injecting humor but it also allowed her to communicate that her own condition was tolerable and that attention should be shifted to another individual; in this case her mother. The potency of that kind of an utterance set a tone for her postoperative care, by giving the staff and her family a focus beyond the physical issues associated with being intubated and having her head movements restrained with a cervical collar and then with a halo. That particular utterance entered into the AAC lore at our hospital and staff would mention it to new patients when describing the AAC protocol. It is remarkable how many patients landed up asking us to add that expression or a variant of it to their personal templates. Obviously, the example allowed patients to venture beyond thinking about how to communicate about pain and request particular care.

Many of the patients in intensive care settings receive their sustenance with a combination of IV and ENG feeding. Oral feeding is contraindicated in most cases because of either ventilatory support issues or a compromised swallowing mechanism. We have found it remarkable that patients who receive no oral feeding will nevertheless wish to talk about food. What is remarkable is not that they express the desire to eat, but that they will use the tube feeding as a vehicle for often humorous interchanges with the nursing staff. One young adolescent took to engaging the nurse in a regular exchange about the day's menu when the nurse prepared to set up the tube feeding. He would usually begin with a request to know what was on the day's menu, much the way patients who can eat ask what is on the tray that is being brought in. It was clear that he was not asking about either what was on food trays being delivered to the other patients or about the specific ingredients in the bag being hung on the IV pole by his bed. These discussions about food that we have observed in our patients are reminiscent of the thoughts about eating and food so eloquently put in Jean-Dominique Bauby's memoir: *The Diving Bell and the Butterfly.* One would think that such thoughts and talk would be painful in that they focus on what can not be enjoyed or savored. But it seems that as Bauby put it, one can savor the memory. In the case of our young adolescent, he would begin his interchange with the nurse with a series of questions inquiring whether she was bringing him a steak or a "Happy Meal." Some nurses would be comfortable enough to play along and make menu suggestions as if they were a waitress at a restaurant. It was clear that engaging in this lighthearted interchange put the patient at ease and made the issues surrounding tube feeding more tolerable. This engagement during a care procedure allowed the patient to assume an active role. As the nurse would be completing the setup and turning on the pump on the IV pole, the patient would say "You didn't forget the ketchup did you?" In this way of using humor, the patient was able to ask if everything with his tube feeding was set and ready to go. This behavior on the part of the patient not only amused the nursing staff, but created a context that led to considerably more natural conversational engagement. Nurses spent more time at his bedside talking about a wider variety of topics that were not necessarily related to the cares they were performing.

Very early on in our implementation of AAC systems in intensive care units, we began to get requests from our patients to add personal jokes. The patients wanted to be able to quickly tell a joke. In most cases, they wanted to be able to produce the joke as a family member came into the room. After several such requests we added a pop-up page to our standard templates to allow patients to access a set of jokes that they could customize. Individual patients varied in their use of this page and in the nature of the jokes they constructed. Pediatric patients were more likely to use the jokes pop-up option. Most often, the jokes were directed to family members and had a teasing nature to them. They often would focus on a particular behavior of the family member. These jokes were worked on with a member of the staff so that they could be sprung on the family member when they came to visit. The jokes functioned as ice-breakers that would set the tone for the ensuing interaction. This allows the patient to take control of the interaction and avoid the awkward moments engendered by the stereotypical question, "How are you feeling." The meaning of these jokes often is apparent only to the target of the joke. For example, one young boy asked that we program the phrase "Dad, did you smash the T-bird?" On the surface, it is not clear what the joke is, but the boy's father as well as the rest of his family found it a funny reference to the father's driving habits. Not only did it generate peals of laughter, but it allowed the boy to steer the conversation away from his medical condition which had been the focus of conversations on earlier visits and from the boy's perspective "upsetting, annoying, and boring."

Some patients utilized this use of humor to a far greater extent than others. One young patient with Duchene's muscular dystrophy had us revise his jokes on a daily basis and used them with family and staff. This ability to appear good natured and lighthearted, in spite of his medical condition, endeared him to everyone. It was evident that he came to understand the personalities of the nurses and that he constructed his jokes to fit those particular personalities. He tried to figure out ways to get a laugh out of everyone and, in that way, get them to engage with him on a more personal level. One day his mother brought him a stuffed animal toy. It was a 2-foot long snake. That evening when we made our rounds and asked what jokes he had planned for the next day, he asked that we program "lift the covers and see my snake." The following day he had his mom put the snake under his blanket and then when each nurse came in to see him he would greet them with the joke. He took great pleasure in the blushing he created. This display of humor in the context of a serious medical situation created a situation that enabled the patient to establish a strong personal relationship with the nurses that facilitated the manner in which his daily treatment/care was accomplished. This relationship transformed him from a patient who passively received treatments to one who was an active partner in his care plan.

C. DON'T ASSUME FULL UNDERSTANDING

The first AAC in acute care research protocol at Iowa involved assessing the efficacy of providing neurosurgery patients with an AAC device for the postsurgical intubation period. Dr. Menezes at UIHC has developed a surgical technique for repair of congenital cervical spinal defects. What is unique about this technique is that the surgeon uses an anterior transoral approach. As a consequence, there is considerable swelling of the tongue and oropharyngeal structures and so patients need to remain intubated until the swelling is reduced so that the airway is unobstructed. Depending on the length of the surgery and on the individual, the endotracheal tube remains in place for anywhere from a few days to at the longest a couple of weeks. Ideally, patients would be seen preoperatively to have a demonstration of the AAC system and to allow them to suggest customization of the content and to have some practice with the device. In some cases, the preoperative session was not possible and the team would introduce the system to the patient at the bedside when they were brought from the operating room to the intensive care unit.

One of our early pediatric cases involved a young boy who had not been set up for a preoperative visit. We were asked to come to the PICU and we demonstrated the system to him and his family. He was enthusiastic and immediately started using both the communication pages and the environmental control functions. His prior computer and gaming experience made access and navigation of the touch screen options very easy for him. About a half hour later we were summoned back to the PICU. The patient had become agitated and wanted the device removed. He appeared distressed and withdrew from all interactions with staff and his family. The device was removed from his bedside and we remained on the unit to be able to assist the staff in communicating with the patient. The staff and family made every effort to tell the patient that he was doing well; they indicated to him that he was likely to be extubated in the next few days. When he heard that, he instantaneously reverted to his earlier jovial and interactive mood. He gesticulated vigorously in the direction of the IV pole on which the AAC device was mounted indicating that he wanted the device back. One of the first messages he typed out with the on-screen keyboard was an explanation of why he had asked that it be taken away. It appeared that when we introduced the device he focused on the functionality being demonstrated and wanted to try it as quickly as possible. He reported not attending to our mentioning that the device was there to aid him during his "short" period of intubation. As a consequence, after the initial novelty of "playing" with the device wore off, he thought that the reason he was being given the device was that something had really gone wrong and that he would remain permanently intubated. The reassurance that the intubation was only to be short-term quickly disabused him of his misunderstanding and he was most eager to have the device back.

This case clearly illustrates the need to verify that patients clearly understand what they are being told about their condition and about the particular intervention they are consenting to. In this case, because the patient was so enthusiastic in his response to our introduction of the AAC system and because he immediately began to use it to engage in conversations with staff and his parents, everyone assumed that when he gave his assent to use the device that he had, in fact, attended to all of the information that he was presented. It was clear that he understood what we told him about the device and the instructions on how to use it. Our attention was focused on his willingness to use it and on whether he understood our instructions. Given that he embraced the use of the device and quickly mastered its use, we mistakenly assumed that he had equally understood everything else presented when his assent was obtained as part of the informed consent protocol. If he had not been so quick to take control of the conversations with his use of the device, the staff and his parents might have spent more time assuring him that he was doing exceptionally well postoperatively and that he would not remain intubated more than a few days. So, in a funny sense, because the AAC system empowered him to take control of his communicative interactions, he was not able to get the information that would have prevented his misunderstanding and the momentary distress that it engendered. The dynamics of the interactions observed in this case are not unusual in medical settings. A variety of factors influence selective listening. That is why it is commonly suggested to have a third party participate to write down what is being said and to also ask questions that the patient might not think of at the time. This can help to ensure that the critical information is noted and hopefully available for subsequent reflection and action. If one looks at adult-child interactions over a wide range of nonmedical situations, one can see similar misunderstandings occur. In some situations, the eagerness to get on with something generates responses like "yeah yeah I get it, let me do it."

The child may then demonstrate that he or she knows how to do step 1 of some instruction set but then may be incapable of producing the remainder of the sequence of steps. When what the child wants to do is potentially dangerous, like starting the lawnmower, parents will hold back and take greater care that the child understands the entire process. When there isn't an apparent danger with the use of some device, like an AAC device, adults may not be as cautious. As a consequence, the child either may fail to use the device appropriately or we get a situation of the sort we encountered in the PICU. Although there is no absolute metric of complete understanding, it is probably prudent to insist on continuing the instructional conversation to be able to probe understanding of the rationale as well as the utilization of the intervention being provided.

Even though the misunderstanding that occurred in this case was resolved quickly with no negative consequences, in retrospect it is clear that an additional

5 minutes when the system was introduced could have prevented the half hour or so of distress.

D. DON'T ASSUME TOO LITTLE UNDERSTANDING/ BE PREPARED FOR SURPRISES

Early on in our research development protocol we focused on working solely with the set of patients who were to undergo Dr. Menezes' transoral repair of cervical spine malformations. We chose to work with these patients in large part because we would be able to work with most of these patients prior to the surgery and the postsurgical intubation. It quickly became clear to the pediatric intensive care unit (PICU) nurses that giving their patients an effective means of communication enhanced their ability to care for their patients and also alleviated many of the psychological stresses associated with the intubation and other postsurgical procedures. On one occasion when one of our systems was being used in the PICU, a nurse caring for another child on the unit who was experiencing multiple organ failure inquired whether we could provide a unit for her patient. At that point, we had all ready obtained good success with both pediatric and adult patients and so we felt it was appropriate to request approval from our institutional review board (IRB) to extend the use of our protocol to the wider range of children and adults who might need AAC systems. We were able to quickly obtain permission from the IRB to extend the protocol. It is unclear whether in today's regulatory climate we would have been able to get approval in time to help this young girl.

The child was on the cardiac transplant waiting list and had suffered a stroke that limited her fine motor skills. Her cardiac and pulmonary status required her to be on ventilatory support. Over the course of a day, to accommodate her fairly labile state, we introduced her to our AAC system implemented on an IV pole mounted DynaMyte 3100. Although limited in fine motor control by hand contractures, with some effort she nevertheless was able to activate the touch screen and use a direct selection access mode to select phrases and environmental control options. By the end of the day, she was able to navigate from page to page and effectively communicate with the nurses and family members. Over the ensuing weeks, we worked with her to customize the message options to best meet her needs. This process involved bedside visits during which we would make programming changes on the spot. The patient had better and worse days as her medical status went back and forth from stable to crisis states. Various staff members expressed concern that her mental status might have been compromised by her condition and in particular by the stroke. There were many times when her attention appeared limited and she also would not always be able to track what was going on in her environment. On one occasion, when Hurtig was out of town, he received an urgent page from the PICU that something had gone wrong with the patient's device. When he called he was informed that somehow the device's voice output had changed from the young girl's voice we had programmed to a voice the nurse described as that of a breathy old man. We were all at a loss to explain how the voice could have "spontaneously" changed. Hurtig instructed the nurses how to reset the voice and upon his return to Iowa City stopped by to check on the device in order to better understand what happened. When he reached over to the side of the device to access the programming functions by depressing the on/off button, the patient's face lit up and she gave him what can only be described as a sly grin. As it turns out, she had been tracking what he was doing to program the device when he was doing all of the earlier bedside modifications. Although we thought that she was not cognitively intact, she turned out to have been able to watch and remember how we accessed the various programming functions. When she was alone, she explored the programming functions and discovered how to change the selected voice. She made the voice change in order to "surprise" the nurses.

Just as one needs to be sensitive to what is said at the bedside that the patient may be able to hear and process, one needs to take care of what we do when we program the device in front of the patient. Many devices have programming locks that require a password to enter programming mode and these can be used; but if a patient is carefully watching you program they can also watch you enter the password. But perhaps the most poignant lesson we learned from this case is that even a really sick child may want to be playful and have a laugh: at times at our expense!

E. VOICING ANGER CASE

Everyone working in a hospital setting wants compliant patients who treat staff respectfully. Yet we all realize that both the stress of the hospitalization as well as the patient's premorbid personality may lead patients to be less than cooperative and perhaps even abusive. Perhaps equally distressing to staff is the patient who withdraws and cannot actively participate in the care activities that need to be performed. A patient who does not have the means of reporting physical pain and psychological distress will be more difficult to treat. The failure to note a painful situation can lead to a failure to identify a potentially life-threatening condition. For patients who are bedridden and who have severely limited mobility, the need to monitor for potential tissue breakdown and pressure sores is critical. Often, the first indication may come from a report of pain or discomfort. Staff must attend to both unaided and aided communication that the patient has at his or her disposal. Because pain is generally seen as an aversive state, it can cause a wide range of responses that will shape the patients' communication.

The acute care setting, with the array of high technology and the large number of professionals who are involved in a single patient's care, is one in which the patient may be interacting with individuals who are strangers and with whom they have not been able to establish any relationship. It is not atypical for some member of the care team to come to the bedside and work on an IV pump, the ventilator, or some monitoring equipment and not engage the patient, let alone identify themselves. Although the lines of responsibility between physicians, nurses, respiratory therapists, physical therapists, occupational therapists, and speech-language pathologists are well known to the staff, patients and family members often have no way of distinguishing one from the other. Even if they read the ID badges, the alphabet soup after our names is not necessarily meaningful. The likely assumption, especially in the early stages of a hospitalization, is that anyone who enters the room could or should be able to address any of the patient's needs and should be in full control of all of the facts about the patient's state and every aspect of the treatment plan. So it is understandable that there might be confusion about why a staff member cannot directly respond to a patient request for some action or information. In a teaching hospital, this problem can be amplified as there also are students training in the varied allied health fields. Even if the individual at the bedside is keyed into being interactive and responsive, they may not know who the patient's nurse is and so may not be able to directly relay the request to the appropriate person so the request never "gets delivered" to the person who is in a position to address the patient's needs. This leads to situations where patients justifiably think they have made a request that has gone unattended to and that the staff "just doesn't care."

It is not uncommon in such situations for adults and children to utilize "coarse language" to express their reactions to pain and discomfort. For some individuals, the use of such language is limited to the most extreme situations and to communication with individuals with whom they have an established relationship. For others, the use of four-letter words is less restrictive and may not be seen as out of place even in conversations with doctors and nurses. Some individuals appear to code switch with ease as a function of communication setting, whereas others cannot. This is not unlike social dialect code switching (Labov, 1966).

Although medical personnel are trained to not let abusive language, or behavior, influence their treatment of patients, it is not unexpected that "nice people" get nicer treatment.

SS was scheduled for surgery to repair a congenital cervical spine defect. She and her family traveled from the east coast to Iowa for the surgery. SS was a spunky 10-year-old who was outspoken and had a certain tough kid demeanor. She had a medical history that also included cardiac problems that added risks to the transoral surgical procedure required to repair her spinal defect. SS was seen preoperatively to explain that she would be intubated postoperatively and that she could have access to an AAC device that would allow her to communicate while she was intubated. She was given the opportunity to become familiar with the device and to personalize the core messages of the Iowa Template pages that would allow her to make specific requests of the staff and of her parents. SS also requested having an on-screen keyboard so that she would have the option of creating a novel phrase if she needed to. In addition, she also requested to have ECU options that would allow her to summon the nurse, control her TV, and a fan in the room.

SS was admitted for preoperative cervical spine traction and the device was provide to her so that she would have an opportunity to practice using the device in advance of the surgery and the post-op intubation. It was not easy for this fairly active preteen to have to lie on her back with a halo and several pounds of traction. She made it clear that she was not a "happy camper." She developed some cardiac arrhythmias and needed to be put on ventilatory support. She was less than pleased about being intubated at this point. As soon as she was stabilized, she began using the AAC device again alternating between the preset templates and the on-screen keyboard. She was unrestrained in showing her displeasure and anger using language not often heard in the pediatric intensive care unit (PICU). Even though she was intubated and could not use her natural voice, it was evident that her personality was coming out in the tone of the messages she composed with the AAC device.

Over the next few days, as the staff was getting her stabilized and ready for the spinal surgery, she remained an engaged and at times demanding patient. On one occasion, as we were coming into the PICU, we crossed paths with the head of the Department of Pediatrics who thanked us for the work we had been doing with pediatric patients. He had, however, one request. Could we put a "four-letter filter" on the AAC device? Although in some settings such a request might lead to some form of limitations on novel utterance construction, we chose not to interfere with the child's choice of language. If she had not been intubated, she would certainly have used the same words.

After a few days, she had the surgery and remained intubated for about a week postoperatively. She continued to use the device for communication and for ECU functions during this period. One striking observation was that although she used the device for communicating her needs and wants, she also used it to engage the nurses and medical staff in conversations about a wide range of topics. Even though she was certainly still in some pain and not happy with having to lie supine; she used very little of the "angry voice" that we had seen in the first few days of her hospitalization. She continued to use the AAC device after she was extubated and moved to the step-down unit. As she regained her natural voice, she used the device less and less, although she continued to utilize the ECU functions until she was discharged. It is important to note that the little girl who started out as the hellion had turned into a favorite of the nurses. The salty language she used initially was not present in the utterances she was producing once she was over the worst. It was clear that the nurses acted professionally and probably understood where the child's anger was coming from. Had SS been withdrawn and non-communicative, the nurses would not have aware of and been able to address the critical needs of their patient. The better a patient can communicate his or her feelings, the easier it is for the staff to be responsive. If SS had been restricted to the template messages, she might very well have rejected the device because it could not accomplish the communicative acts she needed. It was clear that SS was a child who liked to be in control and her first experiences with traction and intubation were not only distressing but out of her control. Her choice of angry language perhaps reflected her distress with loss of control. The AAC device allowed her to effectively communicate and as such may very well have given her back a bit of control. Once sensing that she had some control, she found less need for the angry voice she had so effectively produced. SS like so many of our patients remarked at the discharge debriefing that what was good about the device was that "it allowed me to me when I couldn't speak." What she liked best was the ECU as she didn't need to ask for the TV to be turned on and she could get to her favorite channels quickly by herself.

F. CODEPENDENCY

The first in-patient case in the Iowa project involved a woman in her 60s who had been in a motor vehicle accident and sustained a severe cervical spinal injury which left her quadriplegic and ventilator dependent. At the time of the referral, she was medically stable and was a patient on the intermediate pulmonary care unit (IPCU). A member of the IPCU staff had heard of a presentation by one of the authors (RH) on some psycholinguistic research in which he used a voice actuated relay circuit to measure normal listeners' ability to process ambiguous sentences. In this experiment, the subject's vocal response tripped the circuit and allowed the measurement of the response latency from hearing the stimulus sentence to the beginning of subject's response. The IPCU staff member inquired whether we could adapt this circuit to serve as means by which this patient might access the nurse call system and perhaps do other things as well. The patient was totally dependent on others for all cares and, because she was on a ventilator, she was unable to speak. The only communicative behaviors she could consistently use were gaze shifts to indicate yes or no. The nurses indicated that she was able to make a weak clicking sound with her lips and that she would do that to try to get the nurses' attention. The problem was that the click was of fairly low amplitude and was not audible over all the sounds of the ventilator and the in-room TV unless someone was standing right by the bed. The use of a baby-intercom linked to the nurses' station was considered but given the poor signal-to-noise ratio, the clicking sound could not be heard.

Naively, we brought our head-mounted microphone and voice key circuit to the IPCU thinking that all that would be necessary to adapt it would be making a cable that would link the relay contacts on the voice key to the nurse call jack. We quickly discovered a range of problems. The first was that it was difficult to keep the head-mounted microphone in place in close proximity to the patient's mouth. Because of the need for continual shifting of the patient's position in the bed to avoid pressure sores, her head was not always oriented in the same direction and the pillows that would be used would cause the headband to shift and in some positions be uncomfortable for the patient. The much more serious problem was related to the sensitivity of the circuit microphone. Even with a reasonable placement in proximity to the patient's lips, we could not get the circuit to trip unless we had the input gain set to maximum. A consequence of that was that the much higher level of all the ambient noise would also trigger the voice key.

It became obvious that, if we wished to utilize the patient's clicking noise, we would have to develop something new for this unique application in an intensive care setting. We needed a solution that could differentiate the weak "intentional" signal from the much higher level background of noise. Our first step was to better understand the acoustic characteristics of the click so that we could design a circuit that might differentiate some component of the click from the other acoustic signals reaching the microphone. A spectral analysis revealed that the most distinguishing characteristic of the click was the transient, which was heavily weighted to the higher frequencies. After some experimentation, we designed a small circuit that had a 4-kHz high-pass filter on the front end and that utilized a small microprocessor that would sample the output of the filter and only close a solid-state relay if the output signal had a duration that was equivalent to the average durations of the patient's clicks. Thus, we eliminated most of the acoustic energy from the ambient noise. By filtering out everything below 4 kHz and only responding to acoustic signals that were shorter than 20 milliseconds, we had a circuit that was not triggered by the ventilator or even by others talking in the patient's vicinity. We resolved the problems of microphone positioning and sensitivity by using a hearing aid microphone mounted on a flexible piece of coated copper wire which, because of its size and weight, could be positioned at the corner of the patient's lips and held in place with tape on the patient's cheek or on the vent line coupling at the tracheostomy.

The design worked extremely well. It was easy for the nursing staff to keep it properly positioned and it was highly reliable. It detected the intentional clicks the patient made to attract the nurses and it rarely was triggered by some extraneous signal. The patient appeared to be pleased and less anxious about being left alone, as she now was able to get someone's attention whenever she needed. After a day or so, we thought we had really turned a corner and that we might be able to extend the use of the circuit so that the patient might also be able to use it to control the TV, a fan, and a light. We had developed a small microprocessor-based scanning circuit that would allow a patient who could only activate a single switch to control several electronic circuits. This small circuit had a series of LEDs mounted on the front and as the program switched from one LED to the next the patient's switch would toggle a relay set to a particular device. Our patient was enthusiastic that she might actually be able to control her own environment and began to use the scanning device with fairly high accuracy. Within a few days, she had mastered using her mouth clicks to call the nurse, turn a fan, and her TV on and off. To our dismay, as quickly as she accepted and mastered the switch, she abandoned using the switch and nonverbally indicated that she wanted it taken away. We along with the IPCU staff were baffled why our patient would give up given how successful she was. Our IRB-accepted protocol required us to withdraw our intervention if the patient indicated that she was not willing to continue.

Upon reflection and discussion with the psychiatric consult staff, we discovered what had occurred. This patient had a very devoted son who spent most of the day with her over the entire time she was in the hospital. Both she and her son realized that with the independence that the switch provided she was less dependent on her son to anticipate her every need. Her son could leave her bedside and be confident that she could on her own get the nurse to come to her bedside. She could turn the TV or fan on as she wanted rather than requiring someone to guess what she wanted or go through the laborious "20 questions" routine to figure out what she wanted. She and her son had developed a classical case of codependency that neither was prepared to abandon. As a result, the son didn't encourage her to use the switch and she declined to use it. For a variety of reasons, this patient remained in the hospital on one unit or another for almost 10 years and was never transferred to a long-term care facility. Depending on the status of her pulmonary function, there were times when the tracheal cuff did not need to be fully inflated and so on a very limited basis she was able to "talk around the trach." Over that long interval, we would periodically get requests from her and her son to see if we had some new technology that she might use. Over the years, we tried a variety of switches and even attempted a trial use of a high-tech AAC system for communication (Dynamyte). In each instance, we had an enthusiastic "first day" followed fairly quickly with a rejection of the assistive technology. The attention we provided the patient as we attempted to work on a new solution was always positively responded to by the patient and her family. However, in each case, when the codependency appeared to be threatened by the intervention, the patient rejected the solution.

We learned a great deal from working with this patient. The team's efforts to get something that would work led to a number of switch designs, mounting systems, as well as communicative content pages for AAC system. Perhaps the most important thing we learned was that we had begun to work with this patient too late. Had we established an effective switch and control system for this patient before the codependency had become entrenched, the patient might very well have continued to use the switch and learned to use a high-tech AAC system that would have provided enhanced communication as well as environmental control. Our experience working with subsequent trauma cases in the surgical intensive care unit (SICU) supported our realization that effective rehabilitation has to start as soon as possible.

G. FAILURE ALL AROUND

There are many reasons why, even with a well-trained staff and access to a range of AAC systems, enhancing communication for a particular patient may fail. These are cases where patient, family, and staff factors all conspire to lead to failure to achieve a favorable outcome. When an effective AAC services is in place, each of these individual factors can be addressed with technology, training, and counseling. However, in some cases, all the best efforts still fall short of achieving enhanced patient communication.

The codependency case we described above represents a situation where all the necessary adaptations were achievable. The patient, family, and staff showed an understanding of how to utilize the AAC system and were effective in using each system for a few days. In this case, gaining independence was not worth the loss of dependency that had unfortunately built up in the patient's early hospitalization. Such cases are frustrating because we appear to have found technology that would work and a system that the patient could learn to use and demonstrate that she could effectively use.

Although there are cases where we fail because we are unable to even get a reliable response from the patient that would enable the patient to utilize either a low-, mid-, or high-tech AAC system, advances in technology continually require less and less motor control on the patient's part. Likewise, in spite of an ongoing staff training program, there will be individual nurses who either have not had training on utilizing AAC or who would prefer not to communicate with their patients. Some choose to work in intensive care units because they prefer to care for unconscious and not responsive patients. For a patient who will need extra guidance and support to develop an effective alternative communication system, having such a nurse could be a prescription for failure. An institutional commitment to providing continual staff training and support in dealing with difficult patients is essential if we hope to provide patients with the support necessary to become active and interactive partners in their care. Patient factors such as diminished cognitive function and depression may also influence the likelihood of achieving success. The former factor can be addressed by keeping things simple and by providing ample training through repetitive modeling and support. The latter factor is often more intractable and requires a good interaction between nursing, psychiatry/psychology, and the AAC team in order to bring the patients out of their shells.

The case of ZZ is presented to highlight what happens when a conspiracy of factors keeps a patient from achieving an adequate level of communication. ZZ is a middle-aged woman with a complex medical history whose condition continued to deteriorate. She originally was admitted with a cardiac problem secondary to obesity and hypertension. Subsequently, she had a stroke which left her with a left hemiplegia and required ventilatory support. On top of that, clots in her right leg required amputation of the leg above the knee. This patient came to our facility from the federal prison system. Initially, she had around-the-lock guards at her beside and because she was not from the local area and had rare visits from family members. As her condition deteriorated, the federal prison system turned her over to the state as an indigent case and removed the guards. At a later point in her hospitalization when she was medically more stable, we were asked to see if we could provide the patient with some form of AAC to facilitate communication with the medical staff. At this point, the patient had limited mobility of her right arm and could on command activate a switch and reach up to the touch screen on the AAC device. Even when she was not sedated, it was difficult to get her attention and get her to direct her gaze at us or at the device. We began with a limited set of options that included summoning the nurse and turning the TV on or off. Both were ECU functions that her behavior pattern suggested she wanted. She would engage in a range of unwanted behaviors that patients resort to when they cannot use the standard nurse call system (see Chapter 5). It was clear to the nurses that these were intentional behaviors the patient used to get their attention. The problem was that once the nurse came to the bedside there was no way to determine what the patient wanted. The nurses basically made guesses based on the time of day and their "reading" of the patient's emotional state. Over several sessions, we attempted to determine whether the patient understood what we were offering, that the ECU options were ones the patient wanted to use and that the patient could produce a voluntary gesture. Our dilemma was that at one point it appeared that the patient had the cognitive requisites, attention, and physical ability to generate a response and yet at other times neither the nurses nor members of the AT team could elicit reliable responses from the patient. It appeared that the patient could learn to respond appropriately but she did not appear to use the response once the AT team left.

To further complicate developing even simple templates (1–3 buttons) for the patient, nothing in the patient's extensive history or in nursing notes provided us with information concerning the patient's literacy skills or visual acuity. Even when we resorted to large color-coded iconic symbols that we were certain the patient could recognize, we could not get much retention beyond our training sessions. We typically have nurses and family members practice with such patients to reinforce the training and get the patient to independently use the system. In this case, we could not get consistent practice across nursing shifts; some nurses took up the challenge and spent considerable time with the patient using both the high-tech system and a low-tech communication board; other nurses pushed the device aside and continued care as if the patient was unconscious. This was not a "bad nurse" behavior but rather a typical response of many nurses to patients who cannot communicate effectively. The nurses form the belief that the patient is physically and or mentally incapable of doing anything and so any effort to work on a communication system is wasted effort.

In this case, despite the best efforts of many nurses, the medical staff, and the speech pathologists, we failed. This failure is troublesome because we were able to identify some potential voluntary responses and could elicit patient behaviors that indicated both an understanding of the AAC system and apparent interest in using the system. This case taught us that ongoing support and practice with nurse and family members and the motivation associated with getting that support are essential to success. In many ways, this case is similar to our experience working with ALS patients, where success is often a function of family support and collaboration in getting an AAC system going. It is also clear that we were called in far too late and that the patient had by then developed significant depression that psychiatry consults could not alleviate. We can only speculate what might have happened if we had started sooner. We know from our work with trauma patients that we can be successful if we start within days, if not hours, of admission. The importance of some form of AT in-service training (see Chapter 12) for nurses and other medical staff might reduce the number of cases where referrals for AT services are made too late.

H. AGAINST-ALL-ODDS: SUCCESS

If we do our jobs well, there will be cases that have all the odds stacked against success, where nevertheless we are successful. FF is such a case. FF, a young adult male, was involved in a major motor vehicle accident and sustained a C3-C4 cervical spine injury that has left him a quadriplegic and ventilator dependent. Premorbidly, FF was a typical energetic fun-loving young adult whose lifestyle involved many risky activities that would predispose him to the accident he was involved in.

We were called in as soon as he was stabilized. When he was not sedated, he appeared to know where he was and what had happened to him and that he would most likely be a quadriplegic for the rest of his life. Within just a couple of days, he shut down and showed signs of depression. His initial interest in family members and friends disappeared and he became fairly passive with respect to the procedures and care the nurses and other medical staff carried out. At our first meeting, he was politely uninterested, but when we returned later in the day with a device and demonstrated how we could give him control of the TV and a fan at his bedside, he became more responsive. FF had his cervical spine stabilized with a halo brace and so we were able to use it as a platform to mount a charge transfer proximity switch by his cheek that he could activate by pushing his tongue into his cheek even though he was intubated. Within an hour, we had him reliably controlling a multiple button template that allowed him to call the nurse, control the fan at the bedside, turn the TV on and off, and ask for pain medication. He took to using the system the way many people take to a video game and became absorbed in figuring out how to get the desired function on the first scanning pass. He eagerly demonstrated his skill to the nurses, to his girlfriend, and to other family and friends. Because of his ability to quickly master control of the system, people treated him differently and provided encouragement and further opportunity to practice. By the end of the day, we were able to progress him to a multiple page system with a wide range of communication objects. By the end of the next day, he was adept at navigating through the system and working with us to make programming changes to suit his particular needs for communication and ECU. His TV page was laid out so that he could directly switch between his favorite channels. His relationship with his girlfriend grew and she spent long hours with him providing meaningful interactions in which he demonstrated to others as well as to himself that, even though he would be a quadriplegic, he could have autonomy and significant relationships. As his medical condition improved and he shed the halo and then the collar, we worked with him as a collaborator to develop a way of always keeping his switch accessible. He was one of our first patients to have a baseball cap mounted switch and also one of the first to use our auto suctioning system. Prior to his discharge from the ICU to a care facility, he married his girlfriend. His greatest concern at discharge was that he would be able to keep his switches and baseball cap so that his ability to control his environment would not be lost. Key to the success in this case was the early referral and the consistent support from the nurses and family and friends. That support is in part his "luck of the draw" in nurses and friends but also their natural response to an alert and motivated patient. FF, like Jean-Dominique Bauby, demonstrated that, when given a sense of autonomy and an ability to effectively communicate, being a quadriplegic is not the end of life.

12 Setting Up and Funding an AAC/Assistive Technology Service

CURRENT STATE OF AFFAIRS

Since the diagnosis and treatment of communication disorders, be they short or long term, are the primary responsibility of speech-language pathologists, SLPs typically have primary responsibility for addressing the communication needs of patients on inpatient units at most hospitals and care facilities. The organizational structure of hospitals and care facilities differs greatly across the United States. Speech-language pathologists may work as part of an independent service or as part of a rehabilitative services division. In smaller facilities, they may work for an external entity that is contracted to provide practicing registered nurse (PRN) services as needed. As such, the functioning of an Assistive Technology (AT) service may differ both in terms of the nature of the services provided and in terms of the organizational structure and funding scheme. It is unlikely that any single model will work equally well across all types of facilities. At this point in time, it is evident that provision of the full range of AAC and other AT is limited at most facilities. This can be attributed to many of the barriers to AAC discussed in earlier chapters. The limited training that many SLPs have received and the emphasis given to diagnosis and treatment of swallowing in most hospital practices has certainly had an impact on SLPs' overall scope of practice. This is evident in the names typically used for speech-language pathology services; among the most typical are "Speech and Swallowing" and "Speech Pathology." Over the past two decades, an ever greater portion of the SLP's day has been taken up with swallowing cases. There is no question that funding issues and the more straightforward nature of both assessment and treatment of patients with swallowing issues have contributed to this situation. Working on patients' language and communication issues involves a much larger set of skills and a greater amount of time. This time factor creates a financial problem in those settings in which the SLP service budgets and salaries are based on procedure-based billing codes. One consequence of this trend is that fewer language services are available and that nurses and medical staff may be unaware that SLPs can address the communication needs of their patients. Although neuropsychologists have in some institutions taken over the management of assessment and some treatment of aphasia cases, they are not trained or positioned to provide the range of AT for patients with non-neurogenic communication issues.

ORGANIZATION OF AN AT SERVICE

The following characterization of an ideal AT service structure is intended as a guide to clinicians who wish to expand the services they provide and/or establish a hospital-wide service. Although the clinicians and the hospital divide their world into discrete services and bill accordingly, patients and their families have only the holistic perspective of "I am sick and you all have a collective responsibility to take care of me." This justifiably egocentric perspective of the patient in need of AAC and AT services is captured in Figure 12-1. Any number of individuals, from a wide range of services, appear at the bedside to assess and treat the patient. The patients, regardless of their physical condition, have difficulty differentiating among these individuals and their particular responsibilities. At teaching hospitals, this may even be aggravated by the patients' inability to differentiate between staff and trainees. In any given 8- to 12-hour shift, a patient in intensive care may well come into contact with a dozen or more individuals who have some role to play in his or her care. Even their healthy family members have difficulty keeping track of "who does what and when do they do it." Perhaps with exception of the nurses, most of the rest of the staff members are involved in encounters that are fairly brief and tied to a particular care task or procedure. When one

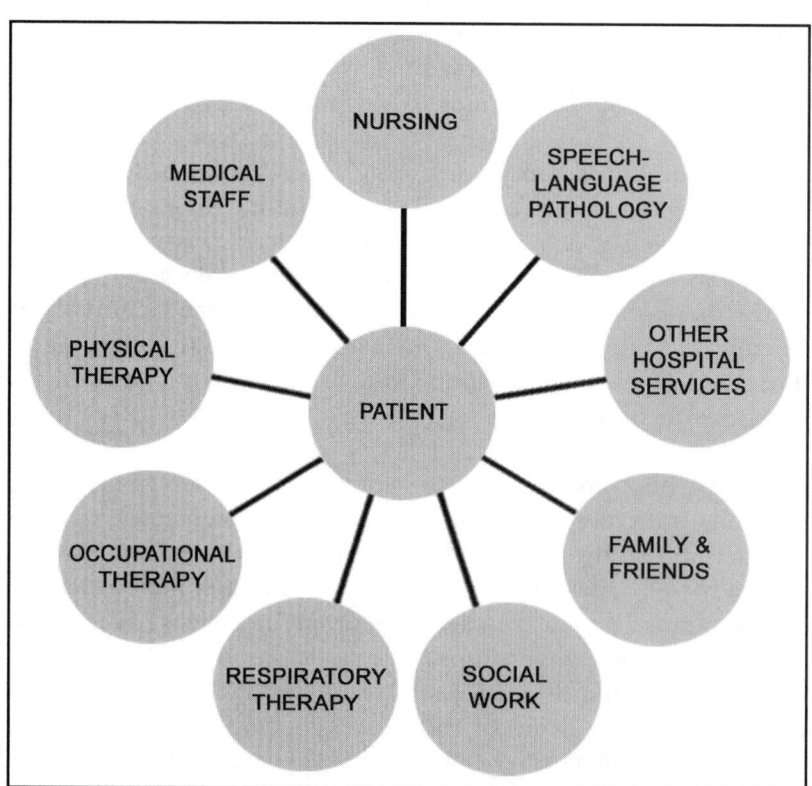

Figure 12–1. Patient's perspective on the care team.

adds to this situation a patient's inability to effectively communicate, the situation can be trying to say the least. Patients have unmet needs and what limited communication they are capable of may be directed to the wrong individual who may not be able to provide the particular assistance the patients may require (e.g., asking the SLP, OT or PT for medications, or asking the social worker to suction the airway).

In the model we are proposing, the SLP has primary responsibility for staffing an AT service. However, it should be evident that successful implementation of AAC systems and other AT require active collaboration across many disciplines (Figure 12-2). It is essential that, at some level, the hospital administration make a commitment to supporting an AT service. Our experience has shown that working with nurses and physicians staffing the ICUs to assist them in effectively communicating with their patients is a necessary first step in establishing an AT service. Physicians have the ultimate responsibility for the medical care of the patients. Much of their communication with critically ill patients and their families deals with decisions about treatment options and delicate end-of-life issues. When the patient is incapable of actively participating in that communication, the physician's role is more difficult. When the

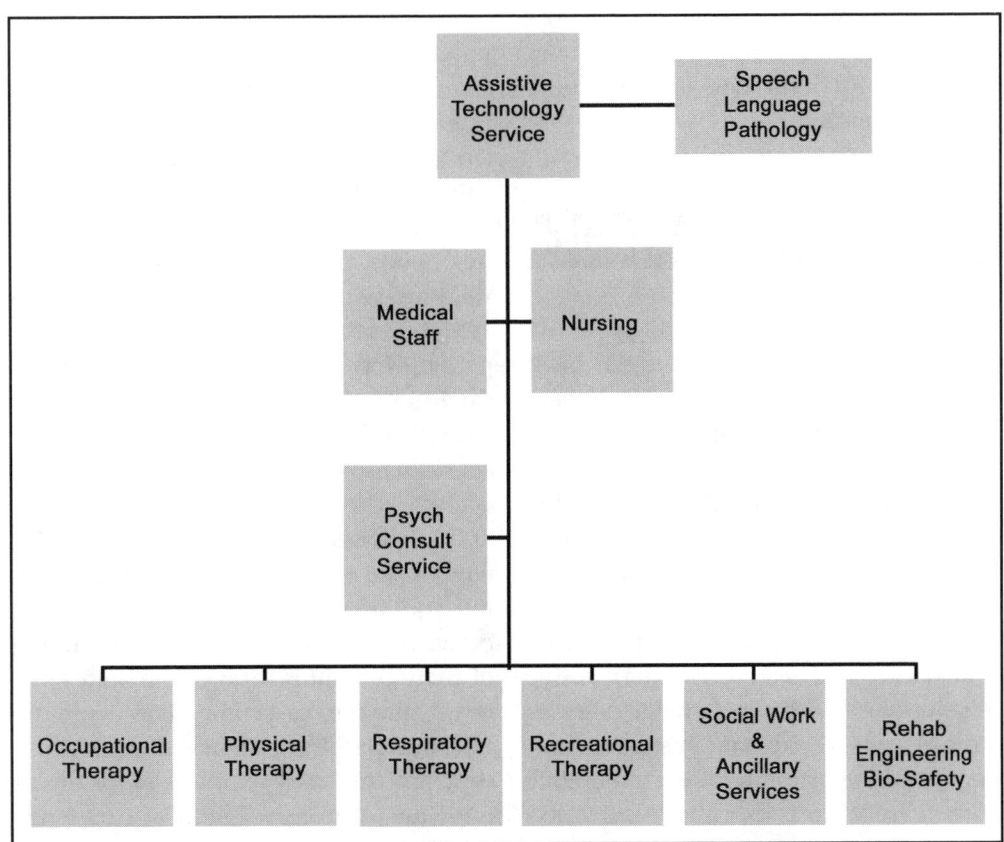

Figure 12–2. Multidisciplinary AAC/AT team.

physicians appreciate that the patient's communication can be enhanced, they are more likely to make the referrals for assessment and treatment of patient's communication problems. Hospital administrators, social workers, and pastoral services staff may also have critical issues that they need to deal with that require some communication with the patient. These may deal with the range of legal, ethical, and spiritual issues pertaining to patient care, possible discharge planning, and, if necessary, end-of-life planning. When either a language barrier or a disabling condition limits these individuals ability to effectively communicate with patients, they need to appreciate that the AT service and or language interpreters can be used. The resources needed to support an AT service fall into three major categories: staffing, training, and equipment. All of these resources require adequate funding.

STAFFING

The speech-language pathologist is by training and scope of practice the most likely leader of an AT service. That training should have exposed the SLP to a range of AAC strategies involving the full range of low- to high-tech AAC systems. Given the range of physical and cognitive limitations that patients on intensive care units face, a successful implementation will require a range of modifications or adaptations. These will require active collaborations with a wide range of other professionals on the patient's care team. Understanding the role of each member of the care team is essential to identifying how the skills of each can be brought to bear on the specific AT solution that will need to be put in place for a specific patient.

Nurses spend the most time with patients and often are the first to notice that a patient may need some form of AT to address communication and environmental control (e.g., adapted nurse call). Typically, they will be the ones to initiate the request for an AT service consult. Nurses are the functional interface between the health care system and the patients and their families. As such, they are an invaluable source of information when selecting the type of AAC system as well as the specific content for that system. Although a few critical care nurses prefer to work with unconscious patients, most see effective communication with their patients as critical to the range of cares they are responsible for. From the very beginning, when a patient is admitted to the unit, they are aware of the importance of the patient being able to summon assistance via the nurse call system and to be able to make his or her needs known to the nurse. Nurses working with the physicians are able to achieve optimal pain management when patients have the ability to indicate when they have pain as well as the locus and extent of the pain. Although each care/service provider should communicate directly with the patient about his or her condition and treatment plans, it often falls to the nurses to explain and elaborate on that communication with the patients and their families. When much of that communication can include "bad news," the nurses again end up being the interpreters of that information because they are the ones with the more direct ongoing relationship with the patients. But, even when we consider the standard elements of nursing care (e.g., taking vitals, administering medications, grooming), the nurses are best able to identify the elements of care and the type of nurse-patient communication associated with the care. Finally, because of their constant presence at or near the bedside, nurses are able to observe and assist patient-family interactions. Even though the physicians have the ultimate control of patient care, typically a member of the nursing staff functions as the case manager who coordinates all aspects of the patient's care. We have found that, because of this special status, the nurses are the ones best suited to provide the AT service with the critical information about types of communication that the patient needs and desires.

Physical therapists (PTs) are vital members of the hospital's ancillary services. It should be noted that their work environments also extend to outpatient settings, rehabilitation centers, nursing homes, private practice agencies, home health agencies, and schools. In general, the role of a PT is to evaluate and treat patients to allow them to achieve optimal function of gross and fine motor skills. The PT can also assist the patient in the management and relief of pain associated with large muscles, so that the patient is able to recover from physical aliments and/or regain his or her independence in the community or work place. A typical PT assessment includes evaluation of the patient's posture, body mechanics, joint and musculoskeletal system, neuromuscular system, and ambulation abilities. In addition, the PT can assist patients in obtaining any necessary durable medical equipment (i.e., modified foot orthotics, assistive ambulation devices) or prescribe needed therapeutic exercises. In the acute care setting, it is the PT who can assist the AT service in obtaining optimal device and switch positioning to decrease access barriers that might exist.

Occupational therapists (OTs), like the PTs, are, also, vital members of the hospital's ancillary services. Again, we note that OT services can also be found in outpatient settings, rehabilitation centers, nursing homes, private practice agencies, home health agencies, and schools. The OT assists patients in maintaining or improving their ability to perform activities of daily living. More specifically, the OT can assist the patient by identifying and/or adapting equipment that will allow the patient to be able to perform or participate in self-care, daily home tasks, work or school tasks, and leisure or play activities, The OT, too, can identify the necessary therapeutic exercises necessary to maintain function, reduce inflammation or prevent contractures, as well manage or reduce pain in the patient's extremities. OTs will also provide splints to facilitate writing, pointing and self-feeding as well as to prevent contracture of the joints. Finally, OTs also work with the nurses on positioning of the patient to minimize the impact of edema and the likelihood of tissue breakdown.

PTs and the OTs often work collaboratively to enhance patients' mobility and ability to perform activities of daily living as such they too engage in a fair amount of communication with patients. They can assist the AT service in two important ways. First, like the nurses, they can be involved providing important information about communication content to be included in an AAC system. The second involves providing technical expertise on positioning of devices and switches to maximize the patient's use of the

AAC system. In cases where an alternative pointing device needs to be attached directly to the patient, the splinting materials used by OTs can be adapted for that purpose. The PT and OT are in the best position to assess the safest positions and motions for the patient to use in accessing an AAC system.

Respiratory therapists (RT) are vital allied health professionals who work in a variety of settings with patients whose communication may be impaired. These settings include: hospital intensive care units, intermediate pulmonary care units, emergency rooms, operating rooms, delivery rooms, and medical flight teams. Unlike OTs, PTs, or SLPs, RTs are an essential member of hospital's life-saving response teams. Although it is more common to encounter RTs in a hospital setting, some now work outside of hospitals as patients can be maintained on ventilatory support outside of primary care facilities. In general, the role of the RT is to provide evaluation, treatment and care for individuals with respiratory problems. The RT is responsible for monitoring pulmonary function, for the operation and maintenance of the mechanical ventilation equipment, and maintaining the artificial airway. Typically, they assess all postsurgical patients' overall lung function and work on enhancing function with exercises. The RT also administers aerosol forms of medication to alleviate or reduce respiratory dysfunction or infection. RTs typically work under the supervision of either anesthesiologists or pulmonologists. They may play an important role in decisions about the feasibility of fitting the patient with a speaking valve (i.e., Passy-Muir, Figure 12–3) and/or reduction of the pressure on the inflatable cuff of the tracheostomy tube

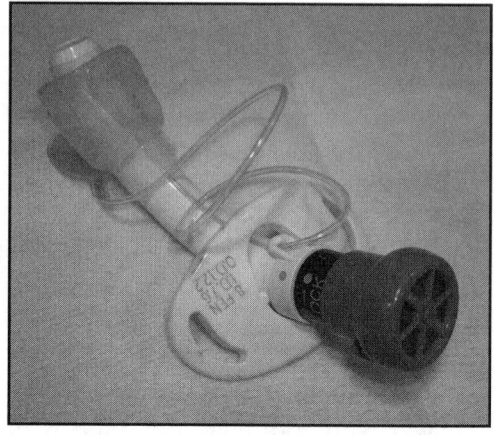

Figure 12–3. Passy-Muir speaking valve.

(Figure 12–4) to allow air up into the oral cavity for speech.

Rehab engineers play two important roles in any AT implementation. The first stems from their primary responsibility to ensure that all equipment used with patients meets bio-safety standards and is in proper working order. The second stems from their ability to design and fabricate adaptations to enhance patient access. This can involve anything from circuit design to bedside mounting systems.

Recreational therapists provide a range of activities for patients who may also require some level of effective communication, In addition, for the pediatric patients with long-term hospitalizations, there may also be an educational component to those services. As such they will need to provide input about the message content for the AAC systems so that the patients can actively participate in recreational and educational activities. As many of the activities are inherently pleasurable for the patients, working on AT solutions to allow patients to engage in those activities may serve to motivate patients to utilize the AAC systems in all interactions.

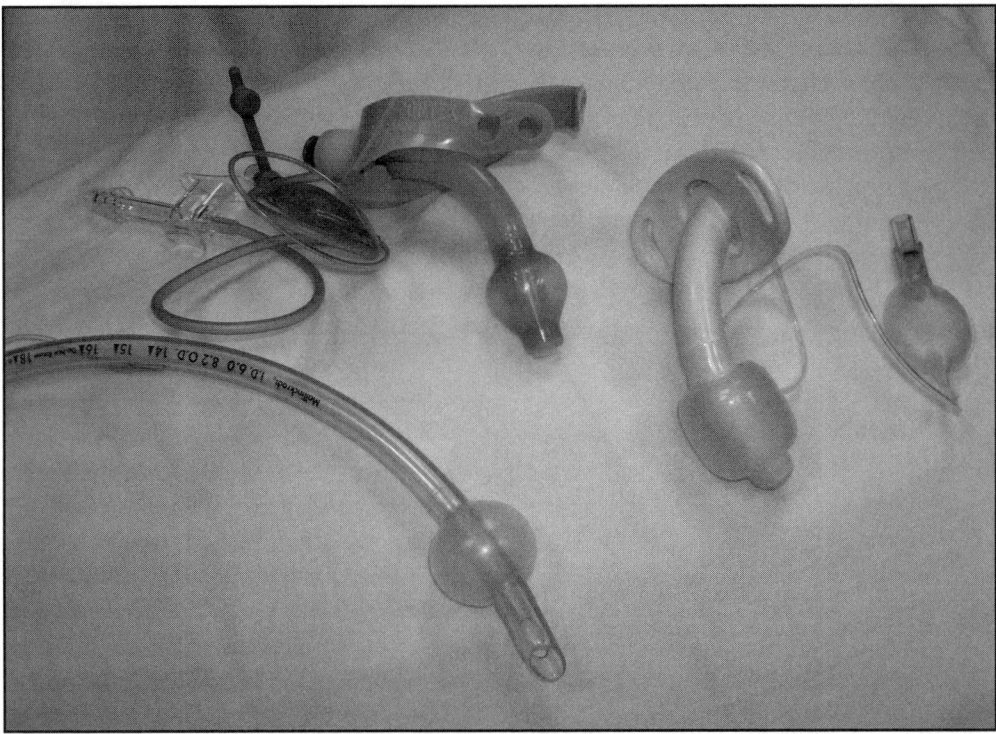

Figure 12–4. Inflatable cuff on endotracheal tubes and trachs.

EQUIPMENT

In an ideal setting, the services should have a sufficient number of communication systems to meet the needs of non-oral patients. Chapter 13 provides a list of the major AAC vendors from whom most of the equipment described in this text can be obtained. The inventory should include a range of low-tech communication boards that can be both generic as well as tailored to meet the needs of patients with particular etiologies (see Table 1-3A). In addition, the services should have a number of speech-generating devices. These can include mid-tech devices that will allow recording of patient specific messages (see Table 1-3B). In the case of patient's who are seen prior to intubation, such devices can be used to "bank" the patient's own renditions of the messages. Having a number of high-tech devices that are capable of providing both speech and environmental control will allow the AT service to meet the needs of the most critically ill patients (see Tables 1-3C and 1-3D). The advantage of such devices is that they can be used in both direct select and scanning access modes.

To ensure that the widest range of patients can take advantage of the assistive technology, services should also have a stock of access devices (e.g., pointers, switches, head/eye trackers). Chapter 5 provides details of the types of available switches. As we discussed in Chapter 7, the key to successful implementation is having devices and access switches mounted in such a way as to facilitate the patient's use of the technology. To that end, having dedicated IV poles as well as a range of flexible mounting systems is essential.

TRAINING

Assessing Staff Needs

Given that our work at the UIHC identified the nursing staff as key players in a successful implementation of high-end AAC systems in acute or critical care units, a needs assessment of the UIHC nursing staff's understanding of AAC was conducted in the summer of 2006. The needs assessment was aimed at obtaining information regarding:

1. The working knowledge of inpatient unit nurses' knowledge of AAC options for acute care patients.
2. The framework for future training needs of UIHC inpatient nurses as it pertains to AAC use with acute care patients.

The needs assessment solicited responses to an on-line anonymous nursing survey of 12 questions to obtain quantitative descriptive data concerning use of AAC at UIHC. A listing of the survey items is provided below.

1. Describe nursing role: (selection options: RN, APN).
2. Description of how long the surveyed had been a nurse: (selection options: 1 year or less, 2-5 years, 6-10 years, 11-15 years, 16-20 years, and >20 years).
3. Description of primary unit assignment (selection options: all intensive care and step down units at the UIHC).

Selection options for the following were yes/no unless otherwise indicated.

4. Have you ever had a patient with whom communication was difficult?
5. Have you ever had a patient who could not successfully use a conventional nurse call?
6. Have you ever used an alternative form of communication with a patient (i.e., paper/pencil, alphabet boards, sign language, electronic device, and/or lip reading)?
7. Are you aware of the term Augmentative/Alternative Communication (AAC)?
8. Do you know if there is an AAC service at UIHC?
9. Do you think that there are patients you serve who might benefit from AAC?
10. Do you think that a form of AAC might help your patients?
11. Would you like the opportunity to learn more about AAC for your patients?
12. If you answered "Yes" to Question 5 above, indicate the types of alternative communication you have tried with your patients: (Drop down box with the following options included: paper-pencil, alphabet board, picture or symbol board, sign language, electronic voice output device (computer), lip reading, and other—please specify).

An E-mail solicitation was sent to 822 registered nurses and/or advanced nurse practitioners at the UIHC. During the 2-week survey interval, 133 registered nurses and 2 advanced practitioner nurses responded to the survey. Although only 16% of UIHC nurses responded, those who did respond represented all levels of nursing experience (Table 12-1).

Only 35% of the nurses at UIHC indicated that they were aware of the term "augmentative/alternative communication." Thirty-four percent of the nurses surveyed indicated that that they were aware of an AAC Service at UIHC. Of the nurses surveyed, 95% indicated that they have had patients who would have benefited from the use of AAC; and 96% indicated that any form of AAC would most likely help their patients. Given these findings, it was not a surprise that 96% of the nurses desired an opportunity to learn more about AAC.

The percentage of nurses responding varied across the inpatient units at UIHC. It was clear that the units where Hurtig and Downey had been most active in implementing some form of AAC had higher response rates (Table 12-2). Clearly, the highest response rate came from the Surgical Intensive Care Units, which was 59%. This is not surprising as this unit is where the notion of AAC in acute care first began with Hurtig collaborating with neurosurgery in developing a communication system for temporarily ventilated patients. The mean response rate across the units was 16%. Other units with a response rate between 20 to 30% included: Medical Intensive Care Unit, Child Med Psych, Psych, Hematology/Oncology, Pediatric Intensive Care Unit, Pediatric Cardiology, Bone Marrow Unit, Oto/Eye/Oral surgery, GI Surgery/Transplant, Adult Psych, Intermediate Pulmonary Care Unit, and RCW-Medicine.

The most striking result was that 100% of the nurses surveyed indicated that they had had a patient for whom communication was difficult. Additionally, 98% of the UIHC nurses indicated that they have worked with patients who could not successfully access a conventional nurse call system. Ninety-nine percent of the nurses indicated that they have all used alternate forms of communication, the type of alternate communication most commonly used among those surveyed included:

- paper pencil 96%
- alphabet board 65%
- picture or symbol board 80%
- sign language 35%
- electronic voice output device 46%
- lip reading 70%
- other—please specify 18%
    - interpreter service
    - guessing
    - assistive technology
    - body gestures
    - the use of stethoscope—patient whispered into it

Table 12–1. UIHC Nursing AAC Survey-Nurse Experiences Level

Years of Nursing Experience	Experience Level
Less than 1 year	18
2–5 years	35
6–10 years	25
11–15 years	17
16–20 years	13
20+ years	27

Table 12–2. Multidisciplinary AAC/AT Team

UIHC Nursing Units	% of Response
1 JPE – CHILD PSYCH UNIT	27%
1 JPW – ADULT PSYC UNIT	0
2 JPE – GERIATRIC PSYCH UNIT	8%
2 JPW ADULT PSYCH UNIT	20%
4 SE – MED PSYCH	29%
PICU	24%
CWS SNU RN'S	0
2 JCP – PEDIATRICS CARDO	23%
3 JCP/7 RCE 2 PEDIATRIC HEMO	14%
CVICU	5%
IPCU	20%
MICU	29%
SICU/ALL BAYS	59%
2 RCE – NEUROLOGY	15%
4 RC – SURGERY/MED (MSCU)	13%
4 JCW – MED CARDO	6%
6 JCP – NEUROSURGERY/NEUROLOGY	4%
8 JCP – BURN CENTER	13%
3 RCW – ORTHO/UROLOGY	10%
3 JPW – OTO/EYE/ORAL SURGERY	22%
4 JPE – HEMATOLOGY/ONCOLOGY	25%
4 JPW – MED/SURG ONC	11%
6 RCE – MEDICINE	20%
6 RCW	19%
7 JCE/2 RCW – GI SURG/TRANSPLANT	21%
2 RCW	0%
7 RCW – BONE MARROW	23%
CRU RN'S	4%

A breakdown of the types of AAC interventions used on the critical care units at UICH is listed in Table 12–3. It is important to note that several forms of AAC options are being implemented on these units, thus confirming the nurses' recognition of the need for multiple AAC strategies.

Because the opportunity and need for nurses to interact and communicate with patients is high, it is important to address times during acute care when such interactions and "typical" communication patterns are altered. Atypical communication and altered interactions between nurses and patients occur at a high rate in critical care units (Etchels, 2003; Happ, 2000; Robillard, 1994). Clearly, there was compellingly evidence that all UIHC nurses encounter patients for whom communication and/or access to the nurse call is difficult. Additionally, the needs assessment highlights their strong desire to increase their ability to enhance communication opportunity for all patients. Although the units that were more vocal in this survey were those for whom AAC may have been more common (MICU, PICU, SICU, IPCU), these also are the units that are most likely to encounter more patients who cannot communicate in a typical fashion. Additionally, although the needs assessment indicated that several forms of AAC were implemented, it was clear that the higher end forms of AAC (i.e., voice output devices) were being implemented in the critical care units at UIHC only some of the time. The most common AAC interventions the nurses reported using were paper and pencil—96% and picture boards—80%. Both required the patients to have intact upper extremity function. In addition, both require that the patient have immediate and continual access to these aids; something that may not always occur. Thus, these highly implemented techniques may not always be accessible to the patient. And although 70% of the nurses reported that they used the technique of "lip reading," the needs assessment did not address how successful the nurses were at lip reading. Recalling that previous studies have documented that lip reading is often ineffective and may result in increased stress for the patient whose message is "unheard" (Etchels, et al., 2003; Robillard, 1994).

Table 12–3. Breakdown of Critical Care Units Use of Varying Forms of AAC

Forms of AAC	SICU	PICU	MICU	IPCU
Paper and Pencil	100%	92%	100%	100%
Alphabet Board	100%	75%	92%	100%
Picture Board	90%	92%	85%	100%
Sign Language	40%	41%	2%	0%
Electronic Device	50%	100%	50%	75%
Lip Reading	95%	83%	100%	25%

One last finding worthy of note was that 34% of the nurses surveyed indicated that they were aware that an AAC Service was available at UIHC, when in fact, no such formal service exists. Downey and Hurtig hypothesized that the nurses who responded positively to this question were confusing such a service with the research protocol based service currently being implemented by Hurtig and Downey. Perhaps the most important finding of this needs assessment was the nurses' willingness to learn more about AAC with 96% of the respondents indicated a desire for additional training. It is important to note that this needs assessment was based on the perspective of the nursing staff who deal with patients with communication problems.

These findings echo the recurring theme noted in literature review highlighting the importance of nursing in the implementation of AAC in acute care settings and the need for nurse training as it relates to AAC implementation. The need to assist the nurse in understanding how to communicate with a nonoral patient is paramount to the implementation of any AAC system, particularly when we consider that nursing is the discipline on the frontline and the profession with the most opportunity and/or need for the greatest amount of direct patient communication. To proceed in the implementation of any form of AAC within the acute care setting without the active participation of the "nurse" would be less than optimal.

Nursing training should provide a framework to allow for successful implementation of all forms of AAC system (i.e., low- to high-end options). Furthermore, the literature supports that the education of nursing staff regarding patients' perceived frustration and increased stress levels when low-end AAC options fail. The development of any nursing in-service(s) or training session(s) must include:

1. Screening protocols placing specific prominence on a hierarchy of assessment tasks permitting rapid decision making and minimal efforts by the acutely ill patient (Dowden, Honsinger, & Beukelman, 1986).
2. A thorough assessment of communication needs related to communication, partners, environment, and desired messages, as these patients are unable to participate in lengthy evaluations/trials (Dowden et al., 1986).
3. A set of strategies to allow the nursing staff to learn new communication techniques to allow for immediate enhancement of the patient's ability to communicate.

In-Service Training

Our nursing tutorial was developed in response to overcoming the practice barriers and attitude barriers noted to be in place in acute care hospitals. Several researchers (Garrett et al., 2007)) have identified the need for nurses, the healthcare professionals manning the frontlines, to be trained to enhance communication options for with nonoral patients. As stated earlier, nurses tend to minimize their interactions with patients they view as being less responsive and instead provide opportunities for communication which are limited to task-related events (Ashworth, 1980; Sayler, & Stuart, 1985).

In developing the tutorial, it became clear that nurses need to be educated about commonly identified communication strategies used with nonoral patients and its perceived effectiveness by the patient (Downey & Hurtig, 2004; Happ et al. 2004; Leathart, 1994). Often patients report that the method of communication used by family members or nursing staff was not effective and the inability to communicate increased their level of frustration and stress. It is imperative that nurses be aware of what works for patients and what does not. If the nurse is unaware that the strategy he or she is using is not helpful, then the nurse's perception may be that it is helpful or at least not harmful. The need to correct this is compounded by the fact that any frustration or anxiety experienced by the patient can have lasting effects on the patient beyond the hospital stay (Jones et al. 2001).

The use of simple communication strategies can greatly improve the patient's ability to communicate and can be accomplished easily at the bedside without the benefit of any high-end electronic devices. Consequently, we thought that any tutorial should include pertinent information regarding the establishment and implementation of a simple "yes/no" response. The use of the yes/no response allows family members and nursing staff to communicate about most, if not all, necessary items. Additionally, it does not require the use of any equipment. But, it does require the element of consistency. Yes/no responses tend to be most effective when the same motor responses (i.e., looking up for "yes" and blinking for "no") is used by all potential communication partners.

Although the use of a yes/no response is helpful in an acute care setting, it does not allow the patient to initiate communication independently. Therefore, the use of a low- to high-end AAC device may be necessary to further augment the patient's ability to communicate. Currently, educational preparation for nurses does not provide the nursing student with much information on "how to communicate with nonoral patients" let alone on the use of AAC systems. It is imperative that nurses be exposed to the range of AAC systems, preferable in a tutorial, prior to encountering the system(s) at the bedside. Lessening the burden and work demands for the nurse must be central to any tutorial regarding AAC implementation in an acute care setting. We must be cognizant of the fact the nurse, at any given time, may be providing life-saving medical care to the patient that must take priority over all other tasks the nurse must manage for the patient. Accordingly, the objectives of our tutorial were fourfold.

1. To provide nurses with an understanding of the basic communication parameters associated with nonoral communicators;
2. To help nurses develop a working knowledge of issues related to communication between nurses and nonoral communicators;
3. To educate nurses about the importance of establishing and using a functional yes/no response;
4. To increase nurses' ability to identify a range (low to high tech) of communication options for nonoral patients.

Online Tutorials

One can develop tutorials using presentation software like PowerPoint and Adobe Premier that can be deployed on individual workstations or on a hospital server that is used for staff training. Some rules of thumb for constructing tutorials include:

1. Remember to keep the tutorials fairly short. Most existing skills tutorials

take no more than 10 to 15 minutes to go through.
2. Keep the text on each slide as short as possible.
3. When selecting the content, one should assume little technical background on the part of the end users.
4. Use graphic organizers to guide the user from topic to topic.
5. Use embedded pictures and video vignettes to illustrate key points.
6. Provide detail annotation notes that the user can either hear or read along with viewing the slide presentation.
7. We provide a longer version of the tutorial we have developed on the CD/DVD accompanying this text.

Competency Assessment

With hospitals and care facilities facing increasing regulatory requirements, the need to regularly assess the competency of care providers over a range of skills has become standard. Simple assessment tools can be constructed to tap basic knowledge of core AAC concepts (Table 12–4). Instruments like this can also be deployed as part of a hospital's on-line mandatory competency testing system. In order to test the ability of the care provider to utilize knowledge to enhance communication with nonoral patients, one can also construct an assessment tool in which the nurses are presented with a scenario and then asked to identify the actions they would take to address the problems posed in the scenarios. These scenarios can be presented in either written form or as short video vignettes (see Appendix A for examples). Finally, if a simulator facility is available, the scenarios can be set up so that the assessment involves observations of the caregiver's actual responses to the problems presented in the simulations. The latter approach not only requires a simulator facility but considerably more time on the part of both the care provider and the assessment team. Many of the vignettes used for this text were produced at the UIHC Nursing Clinical Education Center (http://www.nursing.uiowa.edu/students/resources/NCEC.htm) simulator facility.

Table 12–4. Assessing Caregiver's Knowledge of AAC

1. The prevalence for patients who experience some form of temporary or permanent forms of ventilation is
    A. Less than 100,000 per year
    B. Less than 1,000,000 per year
    C. More than 1,000,000 per year
    D. More than 2,000,000 per year

2. The Joint Commission's standard implemented in January of 2006 focusing on patient's communication stipulates
    A. The identification of all patient's communication status
    B. The use AAC techniques with all nonoral patients
    C. That all bilingual patients be provided with an interpreter
    D. All of the above

Table 12–4. *continued*

3. Nurses tend to have more positive communication encounters with patients they perceive as being
   A. Uncomfortable
   B. More responsive
   C. Having difficulties communicating
   D. Younger

4. The amount and quality of nurse-patient communication may be constrained by the nurse's level of experience.
   True
   False

5. The use of AAC may improve the patient's communication abilities with his/her family and reduce their level of frustration.
   True
   False

6. Which of the following behaviors have been reported to be ineffective in critical care settings?
   A. Mouthing words
   B. Gestures
   C. Head nods
   D. All of the above

7. The use of lip reading as a communication strategy causes a great amount of frustration on the part of the nonoral patient.
   True
   False

8. Criteria for use of AAC with nonoral patients do not include:
   A. A functional yes/no response
   B. A significant amount of hand or head movement
   C. The most minimal amount of movement
   D. None of the above

9. Examples of acceptable yes/no responses include:
   A. Shift in eye gaze
   B. Squeezing of a hand
   C. Thumbs up/down
   D. All of the above

10. Strategies for promoting the use of yes/no responses include
    A. The use of open-ended questions
    B. Having different yes/no response for nursing, family members and physicians
    C. Changing the yes/no response daily
    D. None of the above

11. The use of a yes/no response empowers the patient and allows them to communicate with family members, loved ones and health professionals.
    True
    False

continues

Table 12–4. *continued*

12. Implementation of a yes/no response requires the use of equipment available at the beside?
    True
    False

13. Communication boards used by patients should be
    A. Printed in black and white
    B. Printed in color
    C. Customized
    D. Okayed by a speech pathologist prior to implementation

14. If an ACC device, mounted on an IV pole, is not functioning which of the following trouble shooting techniques would you employ?
    A. Check that the device is on.
    B. Check to see that the AC power pack is plugged in at the power strip, wall outlet, and device itself.
    C. Hit the reset button
    D. All of the above

15. Common items that might be available on a nursing unit to assist in adapting an AAC System include:
    A. Custom switch purchased for each unit
    B. A yankaur
    C. Stethoscope placed on the lamina of the thyroid
    D. None of the above

16. The use of the picture boards, electronic voice output devices and alphabet boards are not considered forms of AAC.
    True
    False

17. The nurse's ability to communicate with his or her patient is an issue that is vital to the patient's recovery period.
    True
    False

18. Speech-language pathology, as an ancillary service in the hospital, can affect significant change in the nurse's ability to communicate with his/her nonoral patients.
    True
    False

19. The use of computer generated voice output devices are considered to be forms of AAC which are appropriate for individuals in critical care settings (i.e., PICU, IPCU, MICU, SICU)
    True
    False

20. The term AAC refers to Assessing All Communication?
    True
    False

Answers: 1. C, 2. A, 3. B, 4. True, 5. True, 6. D, 7. True, 8. B, 9. D, 10. D, 11. True, 12. False, 13. C, 14. D, 15. B, 16. False, 17. True, 18. True, 19. True, 20. False.

FUNDING ISSUES

As with traditional AAC implementations funding creates a barrier that must be overcome. Funding issues can be broken down into two major components; equipment and personnel. Existing billing codes for Speech-Language Pathology as well as Physical/Occupational Therapy can be used to cover assessment, device programming as well as therapy/training services (Table 12–5). Unlike the traditional AAC implementations with individuals who have either developmental disabilities or conditions that result in permanent need for AAC, the AAC systems for individuals with shorter term needs must be acquired by the hospital. This equipment (low, mid, and high tech) should be viewed in the same manner that we view hospital beds, wheelchairs, IV pumps, ventilators, and other standard hospital equipment. After having demonstrated the efficacy of providing AAC services to patients with communication needs, the UIHC Nursing Department began including AAC equipment in its capital budget. This represents an understanding of the role that AAC can play to ensure that the hospital is meeting the JAHCO standard of insuring that the communication needs of patients are addressed.

There is no question that, at this time, there is no single funding model that can

Table 12–5. AAC/AT Billing Codes

CPT/HCPC Codes	Description	Provider
92506	Speech, Language, Auditory Process Evaluation	SLP/AuD
92507	Speech, Language, Auditory Process Treatment	SLP/AuD
92597	Voice Prosthetic Evaluation	SLP
92605	Evaluation for nonspeech generating device. (Bundled)	SLP
92606	Nonspeech generating device services. (Bundled)	SLP
92607	Evaluation for speech generating device; First hour	SLP
92608	Evaluation for speech generating device; additional ½ hour	SLP
92609	Speech generating device services	SLP
96105	Assessment of Aphasia	SLP
97001	Physical Therapy Evaluation	PT
97003	Occupational Therapy Evaluation	OT
97755	Assistive Technology Assessment (Prior Authorization)	PT
95851	Range of motion testing 1	PT
95852	Range of motion testing 2	PT

Source: Based on Health and Recovery Services Administration (HRSA) Reimbursement Tables: Effective January 1, 2008)

be applied across hospitals. There is no question that it is a challenge to staff and to fund an AT service with a combination of professional service fees and capital expenditures that need be charged to different departmental budget lines. In an ideal situation, an AT service's budget would be supported in part by a fraction of the hospital's per diem charge. In such a model, individual patients would receive the level of professional services commensurate with their needs and the clinicians would not be under the same pressures they face when their salaries can only be justified based on CMS billable services. To get to this ideal model will require both a commitment on the part of hospital administrations as well as a change of mind set on the part of clinicians with regard for how their services are reimbursed. To some extent, it may also require some cooperation from third party payers in terms of what they are willing to incorporate in the allowable per diem charges.

13 Useful Products and Links

THE MACGYVER KIT: ESSENTIAL TOOLS AND MATERIALS

Given the need to make adaptations to switches and mounting to meet the individual needs of patients, we have found it useful to put together a portable kit that can be brought to the bedside (Figure 13-1). This makes it possible to make the necessary modifications and cut down on extra back and forth trips from the lab to the bedside. We have found that the basic kit should include:

Tools
1. Small screwdriver set
2. Allen wrench set
3. Small vise grip pliers
4. Needle nose pliers
5. Wire cutters
6. Razor blades/ scalpels
7. Loc-Line wrench
8. Small hot air hair dryer
9. Small hot glue gun

Fasteners
1. Short cable ties
2. Medium cable ties
3. Long cable ties
4. Assorted twist ties
5. Assorted self adhesive Velcro fasteners (standard and heavy duty)
6. Ball clamps
7. Loc-Line tubing (http://www.loc-line.com/)
8. Vent line adapter rings
9. Bogen Magic Arm/Super Clamp (http://www.manfrotto.com/)

Other supplies
1. Tongue depressors
2. Assorted bandage and plastic tape
3. Safety pins
4. Tubing and straws (for sip and puff switches)
5. Adapter cables (to convert from standard to mini phone plugs)
6. Roll of Dycem (http://www.dycem-ns.com/)
7. Pieces of Thermoplast
8. Elastic bands/straps
9. Angled Plexiglas brackets
10. Weighted bean bags (small and large)
11. Small tape measure
12. X-10 Modules (appliance and relay modules) (http://www.x10.com)

182 AUGMENTATIVE AND ALTERNATIVE COMMUNICATION

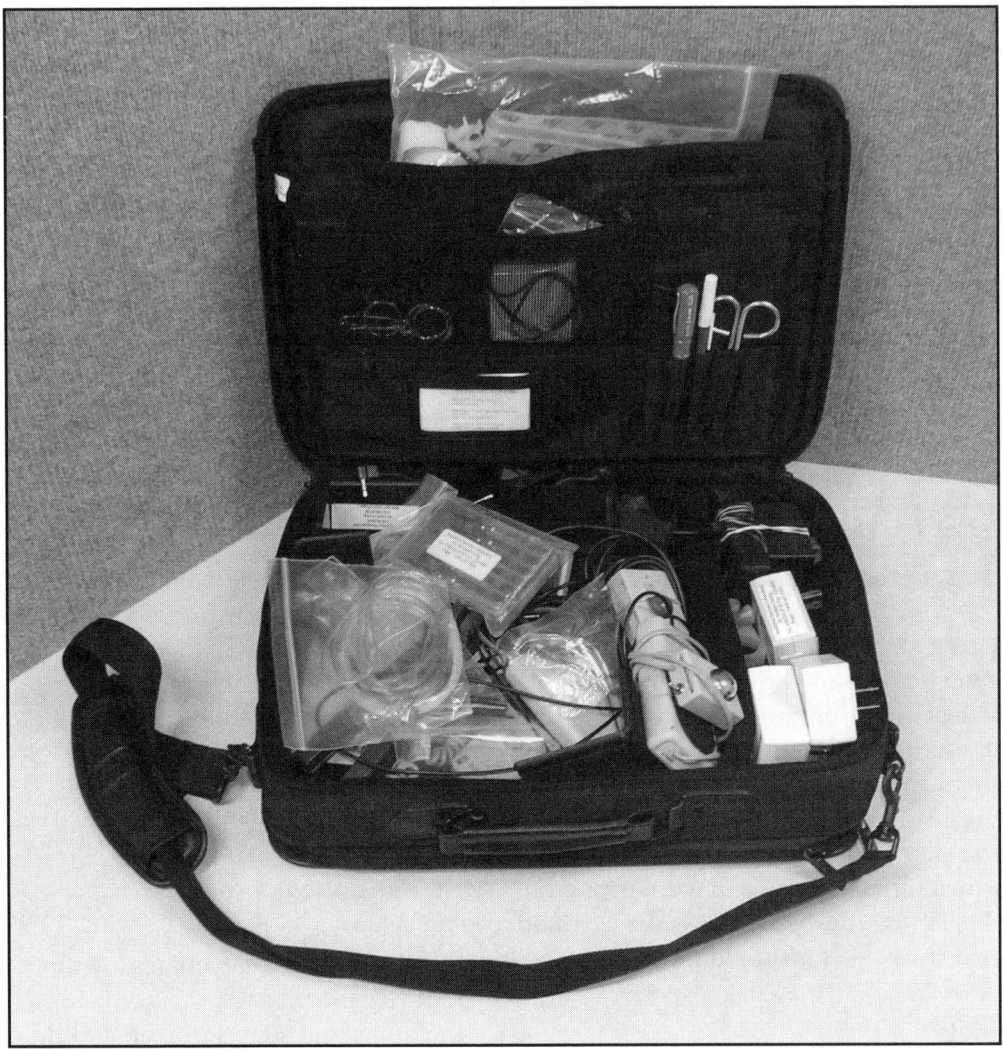

Figure 13–1. MacGyver Kit: Supply kit for bedside adaptation of devices and switches.

AAC MANUFACTURER LINKS

Appendix B provides a partial listing of the major manufacturers of AAC devices and switches of the sort that can be utilized in acute care settings.

AAC RESOURCE LINKS

Appendix C provides a listing of AAC/AT resources that represent the major government, university, industry, and professional organizations involved in AAC/AT.

Appendix A
Assessment Scenarios

SCENARIO 1: HALO PATIENT WITH AAC SYSTEM IN PLACE

You have a patient in a halo who has a tracheostomy; the patient has suffered a fall and is not able to move his hands, arms, or shoulders. From a cognitive standpoint, he is intact. The AAC service has already been called to see this patient and has set up a voice output device for the patient. The patient is using the device in scan mode. He accesses the device by using a switch that is mounted from the ring of his trach hub. At shift change, his nurse tells you that the device works well and that he has been using it to communicate. The nurse lets you know that the patient sticks his tongue into the side of his mouth to access the switch. She tells you that the switch can be easily moved if the patient requires any kind of mouth care. She instructs you to simply move the switch out of the way and then pull it back when you are finished with the care. She adds that the switch should not touch the patient's cheek but should be close enough to allow him to make contact when he sticks his tongue into the right side of his cheek. She lets you know that the patient is also using the device to access the nurse call button. The nurse also lets you know that the patient can communicate by looking up for "yes" and blinking his eyes twice for "no."

Question/Problem

You enter the patient's room and find the device off to the side of the bed and notice that the patient has a switch mounted on his trach hub but note that it is placed off to the side of his face and pulled away from the patient's cheek. What do you do to help this patient communicate?

Scoring Criteria

1. Using the patient's yes/no response the nurse asks if the patient would like the system back in place. (2 points)
2. The nurse repositions the device where she thinks that the patient can see the device. (2 points)
3. The nurse uses the patient's yes/no response to verify that the patient can see the device. (2 points)
4. The nurse repositions the switch so that the patient can access the switch. (2 points)
5. The nurse verifies that the patient can access the switch and that it is

comfortable for the patient, again, by using the yes/no response. (2 points)
6. The nurse uses the system to communicate with the patient. (2 points)
7. The nurse checks to verify that nurse call is functional for the patient. (2 points)

SCENARIO 2: LOW-TECH PATIENT WITH AAC SYSTEM IN PLACE

You have an 80-year-old female patient on a ventilator; the patient had transoral surgery and cannot talk. The patient does not have any type of motor or cognitive dysfunction. The AAC service has already been called to see this patient and left communication boards for the patient to use. The patient has been using two types of boards: one regarding basic needs and an alphabet board with four boxes along the bottom of the page allowing the patient to request: "suctioning," "glasses," "Mary" (her daughter), and "pain medicine" (all items frequently requested by the patient). At shift change, her nurse tells you that the communication boards work okay for the patient but that the patient continues to try to mouth words. The nurse adds the patient is using a Yaunkaur to access/point to the communication board and reports that they are on the over-the-bed table. According to the nurse, family members continue to try to have the patient write on a piece of paper but the patient is too weak. The nurse instructs you to use the boards with the patient and to encourage the family to do the same. The nurse lets you know the patient is using a gray flat pad nurse call system. She adds that if the pad is off to the side the patient will be too weak to reach or look for the call pad. The nurse also lets you know the patient can communicate by shaking her head up and down for "yes" and side to side for "no."

Question/Problem

You enter the patient's room and find the communication boards on the over-the-bed table along with a Yankaur and several of the patient's personal belongs, pictures of her family, cards, and glasses. You notice that the gray flat-pad nurse call button appears to be within the patient's reach. You observe family members asking the patient to write how she is feeling but sense the patient is ignoring the family, what should you do to help this patient communicate better?

Scoring Criteria

1. The nurse uses the patient's yes/no response to ask if the patient if she feels okay. (2 points)
2. The nurse tells the patient why mouthing words is difficult for the family and medical personnel to understand and encourages the use of the communication board. (2 points)
3. The nurse checks to make sure the patient is wearing her glasses. (2 points)
4. The nurse uses the patient's yes/no response to verify that the patient can see the board. (2 points)
5. The nurse offers the Yankaur to the patient so that she can make a selection using the board. (2 points)

6. The nurse attempts to use the communication boards left at the bedside. (2 points)
7. The nurse verifies that the patient can access the flat-pad nurse call system and that it is comfortable for the patient, again, by using the patient's yes/no response. (2 points)
8. The nurse checks to verify that the nurse call is functional for the patient. (2 points)
9. The nurse encourages the family to use the yes/no response and/or the communication board to communicate with the patient. (2 points)

SCENARIO 3: MVA PATIENT WITHOUT AN AAC SYSTEM IN PLACE

You have a 27-year-old motor vechicle accident (MVA) patient who has just arrived on your unit and is on a ventilator. The patient has a C-4 spinal fracture. From a cognitive standpoint, he is intact. The AAC service has not been called to see this patient. The patient arrived on the unit 30 minutes prior to shift change. At shift change, his nurse tells you that he is unable to communicate and appears to be depressed. The nurse lets you know that the patient is unable to access a conventional nurse call button. The nurse also lets you know that the patient's brother is here and upset that he cannot communicate with the patient.

Question/Problem

You enter the patient's room and find the brothers crying. Using what you learned from the AAC tutorial outline, what you would do to help establish a communication system for this patient.

Scoring Criteria

1. The nurse attempts to identify volitional responses that the patient can use? (3 points)
    a. Identify one area of the body the patient can volitionally control
        i. Eye blink
        ii. Squeeze hand
        iii. Shoulder shrug
        iv. Move tongue
        v. Eye gaze
        vi. Pointing
2. The nurse defines a usable yes/no response (2 points)
    a. Look up for yes/ blink eyes once for yes/squeeze hand once for yes
    b. Look down for no/blink eyes twice for no/squeeze hand twice for no
    c. Stick tongue into check for yes/ stick tongue out for no
3. The nurse uses the identified volitional response in an attempt to assess the alertness level of the patient with answers to yes/no questions (*the patient is considered alert if 3 correct responses are elicited*). (3 points)
    a. Is your name _____?
    b. Are your eyes blue?
    c. Is _____ the current President?
    d. Is your spouse/child/parent's name _____?
    e. Do you live in the State of Iowa?
4. The nurse uses yes/no questions with the identified motor response to communicate with the patient. (2 points)

5. The nurse uses the volitional response to have the patient indicate selected choices on preprinted communication cards. (2 points)
6. The nurse generates a consult to the AT service to obtain a modified nurse call and a communication system. (2 points)

SCENARIO 4: MVA PATIENT WITH AN AAC SYSTEM IN PLACE

You have a 42-year-old MVA patient who is on a ventilator. The patient has a C-6 spinal fracture. From a cognitive standpoint, he is intact. The AAC service has seen this patient and left a high-tech voice output system for the patient to use. The patient has had the device for less than a day. He is using the device to access nurse call and control the TV. He is not using it yet for any other function. The AAC service has indicated that they will return to advance the patient's communication options within the next hour. Staff fears the patient is spiraling into a deep depression. At shift change, his nurse tells you that he is able to communicate by looking up for "yes" and down for "no." The nurse lets you know that the patient has used the device to turn "on" and "off" the television and has consistently used the device to trigger the nurse call system. The nurse adds the patient is accessing the device by shrugging his right shoulder to hit a switch that is pinned to his pillow. The nurse also lets you know that the patient's wife continues to suggest the patient is in pain and thinks his leg, which was broken during the accident, is bothering him.

Question/Problem

As you pass the patient's room, you see the call light button illuminated. You enter the patient's room and notice the device at the bedside and see the switched pinned to the pillow. You note that the patient is watching a Cub's baseball game but appears uncomfortable. His wife enters the room and approaches you demanding pain medication for his broken leg. You agree that the patient appears to be uncomfortable. Assume something is bothering this patient. What can you do immediately to verify what is bothering the patient in a way that lets his wife believe you are managing his care appropriately?

Scoring Criteria

1. The nurse attempts to use the patient's yes/no response to ask if the patient is in pain. (2 points)
2. The nurse asks yes/no questions to determine what is bothering the patient; for example:

    Is your _____ hurting? (Eye, mouth, head, etc.)

    or

    The nurse divides the body into two sections and proceeds with yes/no questioning to locate the area of discomfort. (e.g., Is what's bothering you above your waistline/below your waistline, located on your head, chest, etc.)? (2 points)

3. The nurse uses yes/no questions with the identified motor response to communicate with the patient. (2 points)

4. The nurse educates the wife on how to communicate with the patient by using his yes/no response. (2 points)
5. The nurse checks to make sure that the patient can access his switch. (2 points)
6. The nurse encourages patient to use the high-tech system. (2 points)
7. The nurse verifies that the nurse call is accessible and functional. (2 points)

SCENARIO 5: PEDIATRIC PATIENT WITH AN AAC SYSTEM IN PLACE

You have a 12-year-old boy who is temporarily trached following surgery. He has been uncooperative and is now in restraints. Although the patient can move his hands, the restraints limit his movement and he no longer can write on a clip board. We believe his cognitive status to be unremarkable. He is able to demonstrate a yes/no response by nodding his head up and down for "yes" and shaking his head from side to side for "no." The AAC service has seen this patient and left a high-tech voice output system for him to use. He is accessing the device via a hand held mouse without difficulty. The device has been left at his bedside. He has been using the device successfully to communicate almost everything. He uses the device to access the television, play computer games, and access the nurse call system. The patient has been using the device functionally for the past 2 days. At shift change, his nurse tells you the day has been difficult. He has been using the device to type out inappropriate comments laced with vulgarity. She has removed the device and placed it in the corner of his room as she was tired of his inappropriate comments. Since this has occurred the patient has been less responsive. The nurse lets you know the patient's parents are not here today.

Question/Problem

You enter the patient's room and notice the device is in the corner of the room. The television is on CNN and the patient does appear to want to communicate with you. You notice him rolling his eyes toward the device. You think the patient wants his device back, what should you do and how can you be sure you are doing the right thing?

Scoring Criteria

1. The nurse attempts to use the patient's yes/no response to ask patient if he wants his communication system back. (2 points)
2. The nurse places the communication device bedside. (2 points)
3. The nurse uses a yes/no question to make sure that the patient can see the device. (2 points)
4. The nurse gives the patient the handheld mouse to access the device and verifies that it is functional for the patient. (2 points)
5. The nurse uses the device to communicate with the patient. (2 points)
6. The nurse educates other staff that, regardless of the content of the patient's comments, the device should be accessible to the patient if the patient so desires. (2 points)
7. The nurse encourages patient to use the high-tech system. (2 points)
8. The nurse verifies that the nurse call is accessible and functional. (2 points)

SCENARIO 6: CEREBRAL PALSY PATIENT WITH AN AAC SYSTEM IN PLACE

You have a 54-year-old male with cerebral palsy, quadriplegia, and severe dysarthria. The patient has used a voice output system for the majority of his life. From a cognitive standpoint, he is intact. The AAC service has seen this patient and made his high-tech voice output system functional for his hospital stay. He is using the device to access the nurse call system, control the TV, and access communication pages related to medical needs. The patient is also able to communicate via spelling novel messages with his voice output device. At shift change, his nurse tells you that he is able to communicate by looking up for "yes" and down for "no." The nurse lets you know that the patient has used the device to turn the television "on" and "off," trigger the nurse call system, and communicate his daily needs. She adds the patient is accessing the device by shrugging his right shoulder to hit a switch that is pinned to his pillow.

Question/Problem

As you pass the patient's room, you see the call light button illuminated. You enter the patient's room and notice the device at the bedside and see the switch pinned to the pillow. You note that the patient is watching a Cubs baseball game but appears uncomfortable. Assume something is bothering this patient. You try to have him use the communication device but notice that the screen is frozen. You follow the instructions hanging from the device to reset it, but to no avail. What can you do immediately to identify what is bothering the patient in way that lets you believe you are managing his care appropriately?

Scoring Criteria

1. The nurse attempts to use the patient's yes/no response to ask if the patient is in pain. (2 points)
2. The nurse asks yes/no questions to determine what is bothering the patient; for example:

   Is your _____ hurting? (Eye, mouth, head, etc.)

   or

   The nurse divides the body into 2 sections and proceeds with yes/no questioning to locate the area of discomfort. (e.g., is what's bothering you above your waistline/below your waistline, located on your head, chest, etc.)? (2 points)
3. The nurse use yes/no questions with the identified motor response to communicate with the patient beyond just talking about nursing cares? (2 points)
4. The nurse contacts the AAC service to report a problem with the communication device. (2 points)

SCENARIO 7: LOW-TECH PATIENT WITH AAC SYSTEM IN PLACE

You have a 65-year-old male patient on a ventilator; the patient had transoral surgery and cannot talk. The patient does not have any type of motor or cognitive dysfunction. The AAC service has already been called to see this patient and left communication boards for the patient to use. The patient has been using two types of boards: one regarding basic needs allowing the patient to request: "suctioning," "glasses," "blanket," "hearing aids," dentures," and "wipe my lips" (all items frequently requested by the patient), and a pain scale board. At shift change, his nurse tells you that the communication boards work okay for the patient but the patient continues to try to mouth words. The nurse adds the patient is using his right index finger to access/point to the communication boards, which are on the patient's bed tray along with his personal belongs. According to the nurse, family members continue to try to have the patient write on a piece of paper but the patient is too weak. The nurse instructs you to use the boards with the patient and to encourage the family to do the same. The nurse lets you know the patient is using a pneumatic bulb nurse call system. She adds that, if the bulb is off to the side, the patient will not be able to reach the bulb. The nurse also lets you know the patient can communicate by shaking his head up and down for "yes" and side to side for "no."

Question/Problem

You enter the patient's room and find the communication boards on the bed tray along with the patient's personal belongings. You notice that the nurse call appears to be within the patient's reach. You observe family members asking the patient to write how he is feeling but sense the patient continues to try to mouth words; what should you do to help this patient communicate better?

Scoring Criteria

1. The nurse checks to make sure the patient is wearing his hearing aids. (2 points)
2. The nurse uses the patient's yes/no response to verify that the patient can see the board. (2 points)
3. The nurse uses patient's yes/no response and the pain scale board to ask the patient if he feels okay or has any pain. (2 points)
4. The nurse attempts to use the communication boards left at the bedside. (2 points)
5. The nurse reminds the patient to use his right index finger to make his selections on the board. (2 points)
6. The nurse tells the patient why mouthing words is difficulty for the family and medical personnel to understand and encourages the use of the communication board. (2 points)
7. The nurse verifies that the patient can access the nurse call system and that it is comfortable for the patient, again, by using the patient's yes/no response. (2 points)
8. The nurse checks to verify that nurse call is functional for this patient. (2 points)
9. The nurse encourages the family to use the yes/no response and/or the communication board to communicate with the patient. (2 points)

SCENARIO 8: PEDIATRIC HALO PATIENT WITH AAC SYSTEM IN PLACE

You have a 13-year-old female patient in a halo who is on a ventilator; the patient has suffered a fall and is not able to move her hands, arms, or shoulders. From a cognitive standpoint, she is intact. The AAC service has already been called to see this patient and has set up a voice output device for the patient. The patient uses the device in scan mode. She accesses the device by using a switch that is mounted onto a bar of the halo. At shift change, her nurse tells you that the device works well and that she has been using it to communicate. The nurse lets you know that the patient sticks her tongue into the side of her mouth to access the switch. She tells you that the switch can be easily moved if the patient requires any kind of mouth care. She instructs you to simply move the switch out of the way and then pull it back when you are finished with the care. She adds that the switch should not touch the patient's cheek but should be close enough to allow her to make contact when she sticks her tongue into the right side of her cheek. She lets you know that the patient is using the device to access the nurse call system. The nurse also lets you know that the patient can communicate by looking up for "yes" and blinking her eyes twice for "no."

Question/Problem

You enter the patient's room and find the device off to the side of the bed and notice that the patient has a switch mounted on her halo but note that it is placed off to the side and pulled away from the patient's cheek. What do you do to help this patient communicate?

Scoring Criteria

1. The nurse uses the patient's yes/no response to ask if the patient would like the system back in place. (2 points)
2. The nurse repositions the device so that the patient can see the device. (2 points)
3. The nurse uses the yes/no response to verify that the patient can see the device. (2 points)
4. The nurse repositions the switch so that the patient can access the switch. (2 points)
5. The nurse verifies that the patient can access the switch and that it is comfortable for the patient, again, by using the patient's yes/no response. (2 points)
6. The nurse uses the system to communicate with the patient. (2 points)
7. The nurse checks to verify that the nurse call is functional for this patient. (2 points)

SCENARIO 9: C-4 FRACTURE PATIENT WITHOUT AN AAC SYSTEM IN PLACE

You have a 17-year-old football player who sustained an injury during the game. He has just arrived on your unit and is on a ventilator. The patient has a C-4 spinal fracture. From a cognitive standpoint, he is intact. The AAC service has not been called to see this patient. The patient arrived on the unit 30 minutes prior to shift change. At shift change, his nurse tells you that he is unable to communicate and appears to be depressed. The nurse lets you know that the patient is unable to access a conventional nurse call button. The nurse also lets you know that the patient's parents are here and upset that they cannot communicate with the patient.

Question/Problem

You enter the patient's room and find the family distressed that they cannot communicate with their son. Using what you learned from the AAC tutorial what you would do to help establish a communication system for this patient.

Scoring Criteria

1. The nurse attempts to identify volitional responses that the patient can use? (3 points)
   a. Identify one area of the body the patient can volitionally control
      i. Eye blink
      ii. Squeeze hand
      iii. Shoulder shrug
      iv. Move tongue
      v. Eye gaze
      vi. Pointing
2. The nurse defines a usable yes/no response. (2 points)
   a. Look up for yes/ blink eyes once for yes/squeeze hand once for yes
   b. Look down for no/blink eyes twice for no/ squeeze hand twice for no
   c. Stick tongue into check for yes/ stick tongue out for no
3. The nurse uses the identified volitional response in an attempt to assess the alertness level of the patient with answers to yes/no questions (*the patient is considered alert if 3 correct responses are elicited*). (3 points)
   a. Is your name _____?
   b. Are your eyes blue?
   c. Is _____ the current President?
   d. Is your spouse/child/parent's name _____?
   e. Do you live in the State of Iowa?
4. The nurse uses the volitional response to have the patient indicate selected choices on preprinted communication cards. (2 points)
5. The nurse uses yes/no questions with the identified motor response to communicate with the patient. (2 points)
6. The nurse generates a consult to the AAC service to obtain a modified nurse call and a communication system. (2 points)

Appendix B
Major AAC Manufacturers

ABLENET
http://www.ablenetinc.com/

ADAPTIVATION, INC.
http://www.adaptivation.com/

ADVANCED MULTIMEDIA DEVICES, INC.
http://www.amdi.net/

DEDALUS TECHNOLOGIES, INC. (DAESSY)
http://www.daessy.com/

DYNAVOX-MAYER JOHNSON
http://www.dynavoxtech.com/

PRENTKE ROMICH COMPANY
http://www.prentrom.com/

TASH (ABLENET)
http://www.tashinc.com/

TOBii-ATI. (Assistive Technology Inc.)
http://www.assistivetech.com/

WORDS+
http://www.words-plus.com/

ZYGO Industries Inc
http://www.zygo-usa.com/

Appendix C
AAC/AT Resources

ABLEDATA, NIDRR
8630 Fenton Street, Suite 930
Silver Spring, MD 20910
http://www.abledata.com/

AMERICAN ASSOCIATION OF CRITICAL-CARE NURSES
101 Columbia
Aliso Viejo, CA 92656-4109
http://www.aacn.org/

AMERICAN ASSOCIATION OF SPINAL CORD INJURY NURSES
75-20 Astoria Blvd
Jackson Heights, NY 11370
http://www.aascin.org/

AMERICAN OCCUPATIONAL THERAPY ASSOCIATION
4720 Montgomery Lane
P.O. Box 31220
Bethesda, Maryland 20824-1220
http://www.aota.org/

AMERICAN PHYSICAL THERAPY ASSOCIATION
1111 North Fairfax Street
Alexandria, VA 22314-1488
http://www.apta.org/

AMERICAN SPEECH-LANGUAGE-HEARING ASSOCIATION
2200 Research Boulevard
Rockville, MD 20850-3289
http://www.asha.org/

ASSISTIVE TECHNOLOGY INDUSTRY ASSOCIATION
401 North Michigan Avenue,
Chicago, IL 60611-4267, USA
http://www.atia.org/

AUGMENTATIVE COMMUNICATION COMMUNITY PARTNERSHIPS CANADA (ACCPC)
131 Barber Greene Rd.,
Toronto ON M3C 3Y5
http://www.accpc.ca/

INTERNATIONAL SOCIETY FOR AUGMENTATIVE AND ALTERNATIVE COMMUNICATION
http://www.isaac-online.org/

IOWA COMPASS
Center for Disabilities and
    Development
University of Iowa
Iowa City, IA 52242
http://www.iowacompass.org/

NATIONAL INSTITUTE ON DISABILTY AND REHABILITATION RESEARCH
U.S. Department of Education
400 Maryland Avenue, SW
Washington, D.C. 20202
http://www.ed.gov/about/offices/list/
    osers/nidrr/index.html

REHABILITATION ENGINEERING AND ASSISTIVE TECHNOLOGY SOCIETY OF NORTH AMERICA
1700 NORTH Moore Street
Suite 1540
Arlington, VA 22209-1903
http:///www.resna.org/

REHABILITATION ENGINEERING RESEARCH CENTER ON COMMUNICATION ENHANCEMENT
http://aac-rerc.com/

TRACE RESEARCH AND DEVELOPMENT CENTER
University of Wisconsin-Madison
2107 Engineering Centers Bldg.
1550 Engineering Drive
Madison, WI 53706
http://trace.wisc.edu/

UNITED STATES SOCIETY FOR AUGMENTATIVE AND ALTERNATIVE COMMUNICATION (USSAC)
P.O. Box 1195
Burlingame, CA 94011
http://www.ussaac.org/

UNIVERSITY OF NEBRASKA, LINCOLN: AAC
University of Nebraska-Lincoln
Department of Special Education and
    Communication Disorders
318 Barkley Memorial Center
P.O. Box 830738
Lincoln, NE 68583-0738
http://aac.unl.edu/

References

American Speech and Hearing Association. (1981). Position statement on nonspeech communication. *ASHA, 23,* 577-581.

American Speech and Hearing Association. (2004). *Roles and responsibilities of speech language pathologist with respect to augmentative and alternative communication* [Technical report]. Rockville, MD: Author.

American Speech and Hearing Association. (2005). *Roles and responsibilities of speech language pathologist with respect to augmentative and alternative communication* [Position statement]. Rockville, MD: Author.

Angus, D. (2004). Use of intensive care at the end of life in the United States: An epidemiological study. *Critical Care Medicine, 32,* 638-643.

Ashworth, P. (1980). *Care to communicate—An investigation into problems of communication between patients and nurses in intensive therapy unit.* London: Royal College.

Baker, C., & Melby, V. (1996). An investigation into the attitudes and practices of intensive care nurses towards verbal communication with unconscious patients. *Journal of Clinical Nursing, 5,* 185-192.

Ball, L. J., Beukelman, D. R., & Bardach, L. (2007). Amyotrophic lateral sclerosis. In D. R. Beukelman, K. L. Garrett, & K. M. Yorkston (Eds.), *Augmentative communication strategies for adults with acute or chronic medical conditions* (pp. 287-316). Baltimore: Paul H. Brookes.

Bauby, Jean Dominique. (1997). *The diving bell and the butterfly.* New York: Alfred A Knopf.

Benner, P. (1984). *From novice to expert excellence and power in clinical nursing practice.* Menlo Park, CA: Addison-Wesley.

Bergbom-Enberg, I., & Halijamae H. (1993). The communication process with ventilator patients in the ICU as perceived by the nursing staff. *Intensive and Critical Care Nursing, 9,* 40-47.

Beukelman, D. R., Fager, S., Ball, L., & Dietz, A. (2007). AAC for adults with acquired neurological conditions: A review. *Augmentative and Alternative Communication, 23*(3), 230-242.

Beukelman, D. R., & Garrett, K. (1988). Augmentative and alternative communication for adults with acquired severe communication disorders. *Augmentaive and Alternative Communication, 4,* 104-121.

Beukelman, D., & Mirenda, P. (1988). Communication options for persons who cannot speak. In C. A. Coston (Ed.), *Proceedings of the National Planners Conference on Assistive Device Service Delivery* (pp. 151-165). Washington, DC: Association for the Advancement of Rehabilitation Technology.

Beukelman, D., & Mirenda, P. (1998). *Augmentative and alternative communication* (2nd ed.). Baltimore: Paul H. Brookes.

Beukelman, D., & Mirenda, P. (2005). *Augmentative and alternative communication: Management of severe communication, supporting children and adults with complex communication needs* (3rd ed.) Baltimore: Paul H. Brookes.

Blackstone, S. (1989). Augmentative communication services in the schools. *ASHA, 33,* 61-64.

Bourgeois, M. S., & Hickey, E. M. (2007). Dementia. In D. R. Beukelman, K. L. Garrett, & K. M. Yorkston (Eds.), *Augmentative communication strategies for adults with acute or chronic medical conditions* (pp. 243-286). Baltimore: Paul H. Brookes.

Britton, D., & Baarslag-Benson, R., (2007). Spinal cord injury. In D. R. Beukelman, K. L. Garrett, & K. M. Yorkston (Eds.), *Augmentative communication strategies for adults with acute or chronic medical conditions* (pp. 91-130). Baltimore: Paul H. Brookes.

Brown, C. (1954). *My left foot.* London: Secker and Warbug.

Byock, I. (1997). *Dying well.* New York: Riverhead Books, G. P. Putnam & Sons.

Carlson, D., & Ehrlich, N. (2005). *Assistive technology and information technology use and need by persons with disabilities in the United States.* Washington, DC: U.S. Department of Education, National Institute on Disability and Rehabilitation Research.

Coleman, C. L., Cook, A. M., & Meyers, L. S. (1980). Assessing non-oral clients for assistive communication devices. *Journal of Speech and Hearing Disorders, 45,* 185-191.

Costello, J. (2000). AAC intervention in the intensive care unit: The Children's Hospital Boston model. *AAC Augmentative and Alternative Communication, 16,* 137-153.

Culp, D., Beukelman, D.D., & Fager, S.K. (2007). Brainstem impairment. In D. R. Beukelman, K. L. Garrett, & K. M. Yorkston (Eds.), *Augmentative communication strategies for adults with acute or chronic medical conditions* (pp. 59-90). Baltimore: Paul H. Brookes.

Curtis, J. R. (2000). Communicating with patients and their families about advanced care planning and end-of-life care. *Respiratory Care, 45*(11), 1385-1394.

Curtis, J. R. (2004) Communicating about end-of-life care with patients and families in the intensive care unit. *Critical Care Clinics, 20*(3), 363-380.

Curtis, J. R., Engelberg, R. A , Wenrich, M. D., Nielsen, E. L., Shannon, S. E., Treece, P. D., et al. (2002). Studying the communication about end-of-life care during the ICU family conference: development of a framework. *Journal of Critical Care. 17*(3), 147-160.

Curtis, J. R., Patrick, D. L., Shannon, S. E., Treece, P. D., Engelberg, R. A. & Rubenfeld, G. D. (2001) The family conference as a focus to improve communication about end-of-life care in the intensive care unit: opportunities for improvement. *Critical Care Medicine, 29*(2 Suppl.), N26-N33.

Devitt, J., Kurrek, M., Cohen, M., & Cleave-Hogg, D. (2001). The validity of performance assessments using simulation. *Anesthesiology, 95,* 36-42.

Dowden, P., Honsinger, M., & Beukelman, D. (1986). Serving nonspeaking patients in acute care settings: An intervention approach. *Augmentative and Alternative Communication, 2,* 25-32.

Downey, D., & Hurtig, R. (2006). Rethinking the use of AAC in acute care settings. *Perspectives on AAC, 15*(4), 3-8.

Etchels, M., MacAulay, F., Judson, A., Ashraf, S., Ricketts, I., Walter, A., et al. (2003). ICU-Talk: The development of computerized communication aid for patients in ICU. *Care of the Critically Ill, 19,* 4-9.

Fadiman, A. (1997). *The spirit catches you and you fall down.* New York: Noonday Press, Farrar, Straus and Giroux.

Fager, S. K., Doyle, M., & Karantounis, R. (2007). Traumatic Brain Injury. In D. R. Beukelman, K. L. Garrett, & K. M. Yorkston (Eds.), *Augmentative communication strategies for adults with acute or chronic medical conditions* (pp. 131-162). Baltimore: Paul H. Brookes.

Fitch, M. (1987). Patient perceptions: Being unable to speak on a ventilator. RRT: *Canadian Journal of Respiratory Therapy, 23*(3), 21-23.

Fitch, M. (1994). How much do I say to whom? *Journal of Palliative Care*, *10*(3) 90-100.

Foreman, P., & Crews G. (1998). Using augmentative communication with infants and young children with Down syndrome. *Down Syndrome Research and Practice*, *5*, 16-25.

Fowler, E. (2004). An ethical dilemma. Is it ever acceptable to lie to a patient? *British Journal of Perioperative Nursing*, *14*(10), 448-451.

Fowler, S. B (1997). Impaired verbal communication during short term oral intubation. *International Journal of Nursing Terminologies and Classifications*, *8*(3), 93-98.

Fried-Oken, M., Howard, J., & Stewart, S. (1991). Feedback on AAC intervention from adults who are temporarily unable to speak. *Augmentative and Alternative Communication*, *7*, 43-50.

Garrett K. L., Happ M. B., Costello, J. M., & Fried-Oken, M. B. (2007). AAC in the Intensive Care Unit. In D. R. Beukelman, K. L. Garrett, & K. M. Yorkston (Eds.), *Augmentative communication strategies for adults with acute or chronic medical conditions*. Baltimore: Paul H. Brookes.

Glennen, S., & Decoste, D. (Eds.) (1997). *Handbook of augmentative and alternative communication*. San Diego, CA: Singular.

Gries, M. L. (1988). Patient perceptions of the mechanical ventilation experience. *Focus on Critical Care*, *15(2)*, 52.

Hafsteindóttir, T. B. (1996). Patient's experiences of communication during the respirator treatment period. *Intensive and Critical Care Nursing*, *12*(5), 261-271.

Happ, M. (2000). Using a best practice approach to prevent treatment interference in critical care. *Progress in Cardiovascular Nursing*, *15*, 58-62.

Happ, M. (2001). Communicating with mechanically ventilated patients: State of the science. *AACN Clinical Issues*, *2*, 247-258.

Happ, M., Roesch, T., & Kagan, S. (2005). Patient communication following head and neck cancer surgery: A pilot study using electronic speech-generating devices. *Oncology Nursing Forum*, *32*, 1179-1187.

Happ, M., Tuite, P., DiVirgilio-Thomas, D., & Kitutu, J (2004). Communication ability, method, and content among nonspeaking nonsurviving patients treated with mechanical ventilation in the intensive care unit. *American Journal of Critical Care*, *13*, 210-220.

Higdon, C., & Higdon, L. (2004). A missing link: People, practice and some precarious research. *Topics in Language Disorders*, *24*, 5-13.

Honsinger, M. (1989). Midcourse intervention in multiple sclerosis: An inpatient model. *Augmentative and Alternative Communication*, *5*, 71-73.

Hudelson, E. L. (1977). Mechanical ventilation from the patient's point of view. *Respiratory Care*, *22*(6), 654-656.

Hurtig, R., & Downey, D. (2005, November). *Implementing AAC in acute care settings.* A short course. Presented at the American Speech and Hearing Association Convention, San Diego, CA.

Hurtig, R., & Downey, D. (2006, November). *Implementing AAC in acute care settings.* Presented at the Assertive Technology Industry Association Conference, Orlando, FL.

Jablonski, R. S. (1994). The experience of being mechanically ventilated. *Qualitative Health Research*, *4*(2), 186-207.

Jacobs, B. Drew, R., Ogletree, B., & Pierce, K. (2004). Augmentative and alternative communication (AAC) for adults with severe aphasia: Where we stand and how we can go further. *Disability and Rehabilitation*, *26*, 1231-1240.

Joint Commission on Accreditation of Healthcare Organizations. (2005). *Comprehensive accreditation manual for hospitals: The official handbook*. Oakbrook Terrace, IL: Author.

Jones, C., Griffiths, R. D., Humphris, G., & Skirrow, P. M. (2001). Memory, delusions, and the development of acute posttraumatic stress disorder-related symptoms after intensive care. *Critical Care Medicine, 29*(3), 573.

Kangas, K., & Lloyd, L. (1988). Early cognitive skills as prerequisites to AAC use: What are we waiting for? *Augmentative and Alternative Communication, 3,* 211-221.

Kladde, A. G. (1974). Nonoral communication techniques: Project summary #1, August 1967. In Beverly Vicker (Ed.), *Nonoral Communication System Project 1964/1973* (pp. 57-104). Iowa City: Campus Stores.

King, J. M., Alarcon, N., & Rogers, M. A. (2007) Primary Progressive Aphasia. In D. R. Beukelman, K. L. Garrett, & K. M. Yorkston (Eds.). *Augmentative communication strategies for adults with acute or chronic medical conditions* (pp. 207-242). Baltimore: Paul H. Brookes.

Labov, W. (1966). *The social stratification of English in New York City.* Washington DC: Center for Applied Linguistics

Lasker, J. P., Garrett, K. & Fox, L. E. (2007). Severe aphasia. In D. R. Beukelman, K. L. Garrett, & K. M. Yorkston (Eds.), *Augmentative communication strategies for adults with acute or chronic medical conditions* (pp. 163-206). Baltimore: Paul H. Brookes.

Leathart, A. (1994). Communication and socialization (1): an exploratory study and explanation for nurse-patient communication in an ITU. *Intensive and Critical Care Nursing, 10*(2), 93-104.

Light, J. (1988). Interaction involving individuals using augmentative and alternative communication systems: State of the art and future directions. *Augmentative and Alternative Communication, 4*(2), 66.

Lloyd, L. L. (1985). Comments on terminology. *Augmentative and Alternative Communication, 1,* 95-97.

Matas, J., Mathy-Laikko, P., Beukelman, D., & Legreseley, K. (1985). Identifying the nonspeaking population: A demographic study. *Augmentative and Alternative Communication, 1,* 17-31.

Maxwell, C. (2000). The future of work—understanding the role of technology. *BT Technology Journal, 18,* 55-56.

Menzel, L. (1994). Need for communication-related research in mechanically ventilated patients. *American Journal of Critical Care Nursing, 3,* 165-167.

Miller, D, Light, J., & Schlosser, R. (2006). The impact of augmentative and alternative communication intervention on the speech production of individuals with developmental disabilities: A research review. *Journal of Speech, Language, and Hearing Research, 49,* 248-264.

Miller, J., & Carpenter, C. (1964). Electronics for communication: Approaches to the problem of communication in children with severe cerebral palsy. *American Journal of Occupational Therapy, 18,* 20-23.

Miller, J., Sedey, A., Miolo, G., Rosin, M., & Murray-Branch, D. (1991, November). *Spoken and sign vocabulary acquisition in children with Down syndrome.* Poster session presented at the annual meeting of the American Speech-Language-Hearing Association, Atlanta, GA.

Mirenda, P. (2003). Toward functional augmentative and alternative communication for students with autism: Manual signs, graphic symbols, and voice output communication aids. *Language Speech and Hearing Services in Schools, 7,* 203-216.

Mitsuda, P., Baarslag-Benson, R., Hazel, K., & Therriault, T. (1992). Augmentative communication in intensive and acute care unit settings. In K. M. Yorkston (Ed.), *Augmentative communication in the medical setting* (pp. 5-57). Austin, TX: Pro-Ed.

Munson, J. Nordquist, C., & Thuma-Rew, S. (1987). *Communication systems for persons with severe neuromotor impairment: An Iowa interdisciplinary approach.* Iowa City: The University of Iowa.

Musselwhite, C. R., & St. Louis, K. W. (1982). *Communication programming for the severely handicapped: Vocal and nonvocal strategies.* Houston, TX: College-Hill Press.

National Joint Committee for the Communication Needs of Persons with Severe Disabilities. (1992). Guidelines for meeting the communication needs of persons with severe disabilities *ASHA, 34*(Suppl. 71). 1-8.

Nelson, J. E., Meier, D. E., Litke, A., Natale, D. A.,Siegel, R. E., & Morrison, R. S. (2004). The symptom burden of chronic critical illness. *Critical Care Medicine, 32*, 1527-1534.

Owens, R. E., & House, L. I. (1984). Decision-making processes in augmentative communication. *Journal of Speech and Hearing Disorders, 49*, 18-25.

Ratcliff, A., & Beukelman, D. (1995). Preprofessional preparation in augmentative and alternative communication: State-of-the-art report. *Augmentative and Alternative Communication, 11*, 61-73.

Reichle, J., & Karlan, G. (1985) The selection of an augmentative system in communication intervention: A critique of decision rules. *Journal of the Association for Persons with Severe Handicaps, 10*(3), 146-156.

Reichle,J., & Karlan, G. (1987). Decision rules for the adoption of augmentative techniques. In R. L. Schiefelbusch & L. L. Lloyd (Eds.), *Language perspectives II* (pp. 321-339). Austin, TX: Pro-Ed.

Reichle,J., & Karlan, G. (1988). Selecting augmentative communication interventions: A critique of candidacy criteria and a proposed alternative. In R. L. Schiefelbusch & L. L. Lloyd (Eds.), *Language Perspectives: Acquisition, retardation and intervention* (2nd ed., pp. 321-329). Austin, TX: Pro-Ed.

Reichle, J., York, J., & Sigafoos, J. (1991). *Implementing augmentative and alternative communication: Strategies for learners with severe disabilities.* Baltimore: Paul H. Brookes.

Robillard, A. (1994). Communication problems in the intensive care unit. *Qualitative Sociology, 17*, 383-395.

Romski, M., & Sevcik, R. (1988). Augmentative and alternative communication systems: Considerations for individuals with severe intellectual disabilities. *Augmentative and Alternative Communication, 2*, 83-93.

Romski, M., & Sevcik, R. (1996). *Breaking the speech barrier: Language development through augmentative means.* Baltimore: Paul H. Brookes.

Romski, M., & Sevcik, R. (2005). Augmentative communication and early intervention: myths and realities. *Infant and Young Child Journal, 18*, 174-190.

Saylor, J., & Stuart, B. J. (1985). Nurse-patient interactions in the intensive care unit. *Heart and Lung, 14*, 20-24.

Shane, H., & Bashir, A. S. (1980). Election criteria for the adoption of an augmentative communication system: Preliminary considerations. *Journal of Speech and Hearing Disorders, 45*, 408-414.

Silverman, F. (1980). *Communication for the speechless.* Englewood Cliffs, NJ: Prentice-Hall.

Stovsky, B. Rudy, E., & Dragonette, P. (1988). Caring for mechanically ventilated patients; comparison of two types of communication methods used after cardiac surgery with patients with endotracheal tubes. *Heart and Lung, 17*(3), 281-289.

Sullivan, M. D., Gaebler, C. & Ball, L. J. (2007). AAC for people with head and neck cancer. In D. R. Beukelman, K. L. Garrett, & K. M. Yorkston (Eds.), *Augmentative communication strategies for adults with acute or chronic medical conditions* (pp. 347-368). Baltimore: Paul H. Brookes

Tavalaro, J. (1997). *Look up for yes.* New York: Kodansha International

Treece, J., & Treece, E. (1977). *Elements of research in nursing* (2nd ed.). St. Louis, MO: Mosby.

Villaire, M. (1995, February). ICU from the patient's point of view. *Critical Nurse*, pp. 81-87.

Waters, C. M. (1999). Professional nursing support for culturally diverse family members of critically ill adults. *Research in Nursing and Health, 22*(2), 107-117.

Weissman, D. (2003). Measuring the quality of pain management. *Journal of Palliative Medicine, 6*, 185-187.

Wilkinson, K., & Hennig, S. (2007). The state of research and practice in augmentative for children with developmental/intellectual disabilities. *Mental Retardation and Developmental Disabilities Research Reviews, 13*, 58-69.

Yorkston, K. M., & Beukelman, D. R. (2007). AAC intervention for progressive conditions: Multiple sclerosis, Parkinson's diseases, and Huntington's disease. In D. R. Beukelman, K. L. Garrett, & K. M. Yorkston (Eds.), *Augmentative communication strategies for adults with acute or chronic medical conditions* (pp. 317-346). Baltimore: Paul H. Brookes.

Zangari, C., Lloyd, L. L., & Vicker, B. (1994). Augmentative and alternative communication: An historic perspective. *Augmentative and Alternative Communication, 10*, 27-59.

Index

A

AAC/assistive technology service provision
   competency assessment, 176-178
   current state of affairs, 163
   equipment, 169-170
   funding, 179-180
   in-service training, 174-175
   multidisciplinary team, 164-165
   nurses, 166-167
   online tutorials, 174-175
   organization of, 164-166
   OTs (occupational therapists), 167-168
   and patient view of care team, 164
   PTs (physical therapists), 167-168
   rehab engineers, 168
   RTs (respiratory therapists), 168
   SLP leadership, 166
   staffing, 166-168
   staff needs assessment, 170-174
   training, 170-178
   tutorials, online, 175-176
Abledata, 195
Ablenet, 193
Access
   angle brackets, 108, 109, 110, 111
   baseball cap as platform, 122-123
   bean bag stabilization, 109, 112
   bed rail implementations, 96, 98
   bed tray implementations, 91, 94-96
   Bogen Magic Arm, 98, 99, 112
   call pendant mounting, 103-105
   and cervical collar brace, 117, 119
   challenges, 16-17
   ETRAN position, 93
   eyeglasses as platform, 121-122
   foot movement, 116
   gooseneck mounting arms, 96, 97, 112, 113
   and halo brace, 117, 118, 122
   hand elastic strap, 115
   hand-held implementations, 91, 92, 93
   hand movement, 116
   hand splint, 115
   intubation special case, 123-124
   issue overview, 89-90
   IV pole implementations, 98-102
   Loc-Line tubing, 96, 97, 112, 114, 117, 118, 119, 120, 123, 124, 181
   medical device as platform, 117-121
   mounting solutions, 90-102, 103-124
   patient body as platform, 114-117
   Silastic pressure bulb, 121
   soft cloth/bedding mount problems, 105
   switch pinned to gown/sheet, 106
   switch pinned to pillow/towel roll, 107
   switch strapped to bed rail, 108
   and thermoplast mounting, 108, 109
   visor (head) as platform, 122-123
Acute care setting overview
   caregiver relationship, 23
   communications boards, 22, 24
   DynaMyte, 25
   DynaVox, 25, 26
   ECU (environmental control unit) options, 25, 27
   electrolarynx use, 23-24
   equipment barriers as practice barriers, 24
   and family concerns, 23
   high-tech AAC implementation, 23-24

Acute care setting overview *(continued)*
    ICU-Talk software, 26
    IV poles as AAC mounting platforms, 24
    low-tech supplemental communication options, 22–23
    Message Mate, 25
    nurses
        and needs determination, 21–23
        nonverbal communication training lack, 22–23
    patients
        assistance needs communication, 23
        gesture misinterpretation, 22–23
        self-control sense, 27
    pen and pencil communication options, 22, 24
    Step-by-Step, 25
Adaptivation, Inc., 193
Advanced Multimedia Devices, Inc., 193
ALS (amyotrophic lateral sclerosis), 12, 161
    communication rate enhancement, 18–19
    message generation, 32
    on ventilatory support: PC/microswitches, text-to-speech, 18–19
American Association of Critical-Care Nurses, 195
American Association of Spinal Cord Injury Nurses, 195
American Occupational Therapy Association, 195
American Physical Therapy Association, 195
American Speech-Language-Hearing Association, 195
    Ad Hoc Committee on the Communication Processes of Non-speaking Persons, 4
    postions on AAC, 12–14
Aphasia, 12
Assessment
    alertness level determination, 33
    array comfort level determination, 33–34
    family input, 29, 30
    and hearing aids, 29–30
    instruction compliance determination, 33–34
    motor skill nursing summary, 30
    nurse input, 29, 30
    overview, 29
    and patient arousal status, 30
    patient awareness of condition, 33
    patient orientation to examiner, 30
    patient reliability considerations, 31, 34
    and prescription glasses, 29–30
    questions to be addresses, 29
    question types, 30
    responsiveness of patient, 30
    scanning technique introduction, 34
    scenarios
        cerebral palsy patient/AAC in place, 188
        C-4 spinal fracture, 185–186
        C-4 spinal fracture/no AAC in place, 190–191
        C-6 spinal fracture, 186–187
        halo patient/AAC in place, 183–184
        halo pediatric patient/AAC in place, 189–190
        low-tech/AAC in place, 184–185, 188–189
        motor vehicle accident (MVA) patient/AAC in place, 186–187
        motor vehicle accident (MVA) patient/no AAC in place, 185–186
        pediatric halo patient/AAC in place, 189–190
        pediatric patient/AAC in place, 187
        tracheostomy, 183–184
        transoral surgery, 188–189
    sensory status preliminary review, 29–30
    staff competency, 176–178
    staff needs, 170–174
    and switch access issues, 31
    volitional control identification, 31–32
Assistive Technology Inc., 193
Assistive Technology Industry Association, 195
Assistive technology, 3
Augmentative Communication Community Partnerships Canada, 195
Autism, 12

B

Bad news delivery. *See* Communication
Bauby, Jean-Dominique
    empowerment lack, 75, 135-136
    letter frequency of occurrence, 83
    and memories, 149-150
    oral scanning needs, 91
    overview, 32
    yes/no question technique, 83
BIGMack, 9
Bill of Rights for Communication, 5
Bogen Magic Arm, 98, 99, 112
Brainstem stroke, 12
Burn victims, 12

C

Cases
    anger voicing, 154-156
    cardiac problems/obesity/hypertension/stroke, 160-161
    C3-C4 cervical spine injury, 161-162
    Chiari malformation Type I, 142-147
    codependency, 157-159
    DynaMyte, 153-154
    humor/joking, 149-151, 154
    intervention communication, 151-153
    language barrier
        AAC familiarization, 142-143
        admission interview, 142
        bilingual device setup, 144
        and crown halo traction, 144
        cultural understanding, 144
        and family, 143, 144
        feedback, patient, 146
        graphic symbol selection, 143
        lessons learned, 146-147
        overview, 141-142
        postoperative, 144, 146
        and Tech/Speak, 143, 144
    pediatric multiple-system failure, 153-154
    personal voice maintenance
        and AAC acceptance, 147-148
        anger voicing, 154-156
        and dignity, 148
        humor/joking, 149-151
        phrase customization, 148-149
        and tube feeding, 149-150
        programming passwords, 154
    quadriplegia, 157-159, 161-162
    success against odds, 161-162
    ventilatory dependency, 157-159, 161-162
Cerebral palsy, 11, 12, 32, 188
Challenges
    of access, 16-17
    of bedside examination, 16-17
    and computers, 17-18
    end-of-life decision making, 18
    and equipment supplies, 17-18
    of opportunity, 17-19
    overview, 15-16
Chiari malformation Type I case study, 142-147
Chipper, 9
Communication
    about dying, 133-134, 136
    bad news delivery, 133-140
    competency issues, 135
    cultural miscues, 134-135, 140
    customization of options' presentations, 139-140
    and family, 134-135, 138
    giver of information, 134-135
    with infants/toddlers, 135
    interaction example, 137
    on life-support withdrawal, 137-138
    negative reaction fear, 133
    options presentation, 138-139
    patient autonomy, 136, 138
    patient expressions of comprehension, 136-137
    and teens, 135
    timing of bad news, 135-136
    yes/no as only patient options, 139
Communication Bill of Rights, 5
Communication boards, 3, 22, 24, 138-139, 148
Convertible, 11

D

Daessy, 193
Dedalus Technologies, Inc., 193
Defining AAC, 2-3
Dementia, 12

The Diving Bell and the Butterfly
  (Bauby), 32, 149–150. *See also*
  Bauby, Jean-Dominique
DynaMyte, 25, 153–154
DynaVox, 25, 26
Dynavox-Mayer Johnson, 193
Dynawrite, 11

E

ECUs (environmental control units), 25, 27
  overview, 127
  remotes
    home automation, 128–130
    universal models, 127, 128
    voice-activated, 127–128 (*See also main heading* X-10 modules)
    room-control ECU pop-up page, 72, 73, 74
Electrolarynx use, 23–24
Engineers, rehab, 168
ERICA, 10
Etiologies benefiting from AAC, 11–12
ETRAN boards, 54–57
ETRAN position, 93

F

Fadiman, Anne, 134

G

Go-Talk, 9
Guillain-Barré syndrome, 12, 27

H

History
  Ad Hoc Committee on the Communication Processes of Non-speaking Persons, ASHA, 4
  Communication Bill of Rights, 5
  communication boards, 3
  Communication Disorders graduate programs, 6
  Journal of Augmentative/Alternative Communication, 4
  Kladde: 9 criteria for AAC clients, 3–4
  laryngectomy patients, 11
  and mainstreaming, 4
  Non-Oral Communication Systems Project, 3–4
  nonoral term, 3
  Public Law 94-142, 4
  Rehabilitation Act of 1973, 4
Hmong family communication, 134–135, 140
Huntington's disease, 12

I

ICU (intensive care unit) overview, 2
ICU-Talk software, 26
IM (instant messaging), 85–86
Instant messaging (IM), 85–86
International Society for Augmentative and Alternative Communication, 195
Iowa AAC templates
  abbreviation expansion, 85–86
  alphabetic keyboard, 83
  alphabetic keyboard with bailout buttons, 83
  alternative keyboard layouts, 83–85
  bed control pop-up, 74
  body parts pop-up, 77
  chat page, 71
  clinician auditory scanning, 83
  entertainment pop-up page, 69, 71 (*See also* chat page *in this section;* jokes pop-up page *in this section*)
  eye/head tracking layout, 87
  feelings pop-up page, 68–69
  frequency keyboard, 84
  get me pop-up, 76
  grid-pattern button, 62
  help pop-up, 75, 76, 77
  and instant messaging (IM), 85–86
  jokes pop-up page, 72, 73, 151 (*See also* entertainment pop-up page *in this section*)
  and keyboard experience, 81
  keyboard experience lacking, 81, 82, 83
  medical questions pop-up page, 71–72
  mouth care pop-up, 78
  novel message generation, 79–81

number pop-up, 80
one-button, 60–61, 63
overview, 59–60
pain pop-up page, 69, 70
personal pop-up, 77, 79
punctuation pop-up, 80
QWERTY keyboard, 80, 81, 83
rate enhancement strategies, 81, 83, 85–87
room-control ECU pop-up page, 72, 73, 74 (*See also main heading* ECUs (environmental control units))
simple buttons with links, 62, 65, 66
Spanish version, 88
top-level menu page, 66–67
TV control pop-up, 74–75
two-to-three-button, 61, 63, 64
wipe my pop-up, 78
word prediction buttons, 83, 85
Iowa COMPASS, 195
Iowa smart switch, 57–58

J

Joint Commission on the Accreditation of Healthcare Organizations (JC), 19, 125
Journal of Augmentative/Alternative Communication, 4

L

Laryngectomy, 11
L*E*O, 9
LightWRITERS
 in acute care setting, 25–26
 overview, 11
Link, 11
Loc-Line tubing. *See under* Access

M

M3, 9
MacGyver tools/materials kit, 181–182
Materials. *See* Tools/materials
Menezes, Arnold, 141–142, 151
Mercury II/MiniMerc, 10
Message Mate, 9, 25
Mounting overview, 89–90

MS (multiple sclerosis), 12
Multidisciplinary teams, 164–165
Myths/realities of AAC, 7

N

National Institute on Disability and Rehabilitation Research (NIDRR), 19, 195
Nurse call systems, 89. *See also* Switches
 alternatives to, 42–47
 bed rail button, 40
 call pendant, 39, 40, 89–90, 103–105
 door illuminator, 38
 and family concerns, 40
 and nursing protocols, 89–90
 overview, 37–38
 patient alternative choices, 41
 patient maneuver dangers, 40–41
 patient room call panel, 39
 placement of/access to, 40, 41
 pneumatic bulb switches, 43, 44, 105
 pressure place switch, 43, 44, 45, 46
 pull cord, 42
 push-button switches, 42–43
 versus shouting for assistance, 41
 station call enunciator, 38
 ventilator patients, 41
Nurses, 166–167

O

One Step, 9
OTs (occupational therapists), 167–168

P

Pain management, 90, 125–126
Parkinson's disease, 12
Partner One/Partner Two/Partner Four, 9
Pathfinder, 32
Patients
 arousal status assessment, 30
 assistance needs communication, 23
 awareness of condition assessment, 33
 body as access platform, 114–117
 cerebral palsy patient/AAC in place, 188
 gesture misinterpretation, 22–23

Patients *(continued)*
   halo patient/AAC in place, 183–184
   halo pediatric patient/AAC in place,
      189–190
   and humor/joking, 149–151, 154
   with language barrier, 141–147
   motor vehicle accident (MVA)
      patient/AAC in place, 186–187
   motor vehicle accident (MVA)
      patient/no AAC in place, 185–186
   orientation to examiner assessment, 30
   pediatric halo patient/AAC in place,
      189–190
   pediatric multiple-system failure,
      153–154
   pediatric patient/AAC in place, 187
   personal voice maintenance, 147–150
   reliability of, 31, 34
   responsiveness assessment, 30
   self-control sense, 27, 125, 136, 138
   view of care team, 164
PCA (patient-controlled analgesia) pumps,
      90, 125–126
   X-10 modules, 129–131
PICU (pediatric intensive care unit), 2
Prentke Romich Company, 193
PTs (physical therapists), 167–168

R

Rehabilitation Engineering and Assistive
   Technology Society of North
   America, 196
Rehabilitation Engineering Research
   Center on Communication
   Enhancement, 196
Resources, 195–196
Respiratory insufficiency, 12
Retardation, 12
RTs (respiratory therapists), 168

S

Say-it Sam, 10
Shakespeare, 133
Sophocles (442 BC), 133
Spinal cord injury, 12
*The Spirit Catches You and You Fall
   Down* (Fadiman), 134

SpringBoard Plus/SpringBoard Lite, 9
Step-by-Step, 25
Stroke, brainstem, 12
Switches. *See also main heading* Access
   adaptation, 102–103, 102–105
   advanced technology, 49–57
   charge transfer/proximity, 49, 50
   computer-based systems, 52–53
   and ETRAN, 54–57
   eye movement/gaze, 54–57
   head position, 53–54
   Iowa smart switch, 57–58
   IR-blink, 49–50, 51
   jelly bean/spec, 47
   nurse call systems, 37–47 (*See also
      main heading* Nurse call systems)
   and nursing protocols, 89–90
   overview, 37, 40
   and PCA (patient-controlled analgesia)
      pumps, 90, 126
   P-switch, 49, 50
   rocker, 47, 48
   sip and puff, 47, 49
   speech recognition circuitry, 52
   standard, 47–49
   tongue, 47, 48
   voice-activated, 50–51, 52, 53

T

TANGO, 10
Tash, Inc., 193
Tavalaro, Julia, 31, 32, 135–136
Technology overview
   and computers, personal, 6–8
   devices, 9–11
   high-tech devices, 10
   low-tech devices, 9
   mid-tech devices, 9
   overview, 6
   portability, 8
   speech synthesis, 6
   text-to-speech devices, 11
Tech/Speak, 143, 144
Tech 8/Tech 32, 9
Tech Touch, 10
Templates. *See* Iowa AAC templates
Tobii-ATI, 193
Tools/materials MacGyver kit, 181–182

Trace Research and Development Center, 196
Traumatic brain injury, 12

U

United States Society for Augmentative and Alternative Communication (USSAC), 196
University of Nebraska, Lincoln: AAC, 196

V

Vanguard Plus/Vantage Plus, 10
V/Vmax, 10

W

Web sites
  AAC: University of Nebraska, Lincoln, 196
  Abledata, 195
  Ablenet, 193
  Adaptivation, Inc., 193
  Advanced Multimedia Devices, Inc., 193
  American Association of Critical-Care Nurses, 195
  American Association of Spinal Cord Injury Nurses, 195
  American Occupational Therapy Association, 195
  American Physical Therapy Association, 195
  American Speech-Language-Hearing Association, 195
  Assistive Technology Inc., 193
  Assistive Technology Industry Association, 195
  Augmentative Communication Community Partnerships Canada, 195
  Bogen Magic Arm, 181
  Daessy, 193
  Dedalus Technologies, Inc., 193
  Dynavox-Mayer Johnson, 193
  International Society for Augmentative and Alternative Communication, 195
  Iowa COMPASS, 195
  Loc-Line tubing, 181
  National Institute on Disability and Rehabilitation Research (NIDRR), 195
  Prentke Romich Company, 193
  Rehabilitation Engineering and Assistive Technology Society of North America, 196
  Rehabilitation Engineering Research Center on Communication Enhancement, 196
  Tash, Inc., 193
  Tobii-ATI, 193
  Trace Research and Development Center, 196
  United States Society for Augmentative and Alternative Communication (USSAC), 196
  Words+, 193
  X-10 modules, 181
  ZYGO Industries Inc., 193

X

X-10 modules
  and AC circuit, 100
  bed control, 74
  custom wall switch, 130
  ECU, 72, 126
  and free-standing remotes, 52, 53
  IR (infrared) receiver, 129
  nurse relay, 68
  relays requiring switch closure, 131
  RF (radio frequency) receiver, 129
  and top-level menu page, 66–67
  Web site, 181

Z

ZYGO Industries Inc., 193